Anatomy and Physiology Workbook for Paramedics

PAUL D. ANDERSON, PhD

Middlesex Community College

UK Editor:

JOHN KNIGHT, PhD

Swansea University, UK

JONES & BARTLETT
LEARNING

World Headquarters
Jones & Bartlett Learning
5 Wall Street
Burlington, MA 01803
978-443-5000
info@jblearning.com
www.psglearning.com

To order this product, use ISBN: 978-1-284-18300-9

6048

23 22 21 20 10 9 8 7 6 5 4 3

Contents

Introduction

Anatomy and physiology are both key underpinning areas of science on a variety of professional and non-professional undergraduate degree programmes. Paramedics, nurses, midwives, and doctors all require a solid grasp of these subjects to inform their practice and provide the best quality of care for their patients. Paramedic Science degree programmes in the UK expect students to demonstrate an awareness of anatomy and physiology in order to systematically assess, analyse, and evaluate the ill or injured patient and make effective clinical judgments in their practice. This knowledge is vital for paramedics' understanding of disease, illness, and dysfunction in a patient and the impact that this may have on the human body.

In order for students to successfully graduate and enter clinical practice, most current programmes in the healthcare sciences assess anatomy and physiology extensively through a combination of formal written exam papers, practical laboratory sessions and objective structured practical exams (OSPEs), and objective structured clinical exams (OSCEs). Learning and understanding anatomy and physiology often poses a considerable challenge to many students due to the vast amount of information that is embedded in many syllabuses and the complex and often abstract concepts students are required to learn and apply.

There are a multitude of excellent textbooks available that thoroughly explore all aspects of human anatomy and physiology, and this textbook forms an ideal companion to help the student develop their knowledge base and assess their current level of understanding. Anatomy and physiology, by their very nature, are both very visual subjects and the colouring exercises and structured self-assessment tests within this study guide provide the student with an excellent opportunity to consolidate their understanding of key areas that are frequently assessed in examinations.

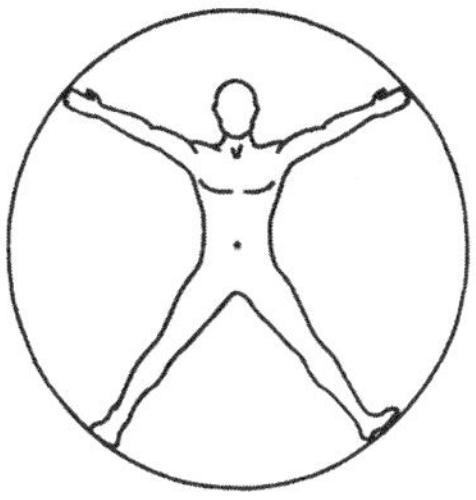 1

Basic Anatomy

I. CHAPTER SYNOPSIS

This chapter introduces the student to the organisational pattern of the entire body. Among the topics considered are the location and contents of the principal body cavities, the characteristics of the anatomical terms (with common names of body regions), the use of directional terms, planes and sections of the body, and the linear units of measurement in the metric system and how one unit converts to another.

II. OBJECTIVES

After reading this chapter, the student should be able to:

- Describe the pH scale and relate its significance.
- Name the planes of the body using proper anatomical terms.
- Name the important regions of the body and the body cavities.
- Name the nine abdominal regions.
- Differentiate between the Imperial and metric systems of measurement by comparing the different units of length.

III. IMPORTANT TERMS

Using your textbook, define the following terms:

abdominal (ab-do′min-al) ______________________________

____

abdominopelvic (ab-do′min-o-pel′vik) ______________________________

____

acid (as′id) ______________________________

____

acidosis (as-i-do′sis) ______________________________

____

alkaline (base) (al′kah-line) ______________________________

____

alkalosis (al-kah-lo′sis) ______________________________

____

anterior (ant-ter′eor) ______________________________

____

bilateral (bye-lat′ur-ul) ______________________________

____

cranial (superior) (kra′ne-al) ______________________________

____

deep (dee′p) ______________________________

____

distal (dis′tal) ______________________________

____

dorsal (posterior) (dor′sal) ______________________________

____

epigastric (epi-gas′trik) ______________________________

____

frontal (frun′tal) ______________________________

____

hypochondriac (hi-po-kon′dre-ak) ______________________________

____

hypogastric (hi-po-gas′trik) ______________________________

____

iliac (il′e-ak) ____________________

inferior (in-fer′eor) ____________________

inguinal (ing′gwi-nal) ____________________

lateral (lat′er-al) ____________________

lumbar (lum′bar) ____________________

medial (me′de-al) ____________________

pelvic (pel′vik) ____________________

posterior (po-ster′eor) ____________________

proximal (prok′si-mal) ____________________

spinal (spi′nal) ____________________

sagittal (saj′i-tal) ____________________

superficial (soo′pa-fish′al) ____________________

superior (soo-per′eor) ____________________

thoracic (tho-ras′ik) ____________________

transverse (trans-vers′) ____________________

umbilical (um-bil′i-kal) ____________________

ventral (anterior) (ven′tral) ____________________

vertebral (vur′te-brul) ____________________

IV. EXERCISES

Complete the following exercises in the order given. A precise set of terms and planes has evolved to describe positions, relationships, and directions within the human body.

Exercise 1.1

Fill in the Blanks. Place the terms from the Key list into the correct blank spaces in the text on the right.

Key:
Acid
Alkaline
H^+
OH^-
neutral

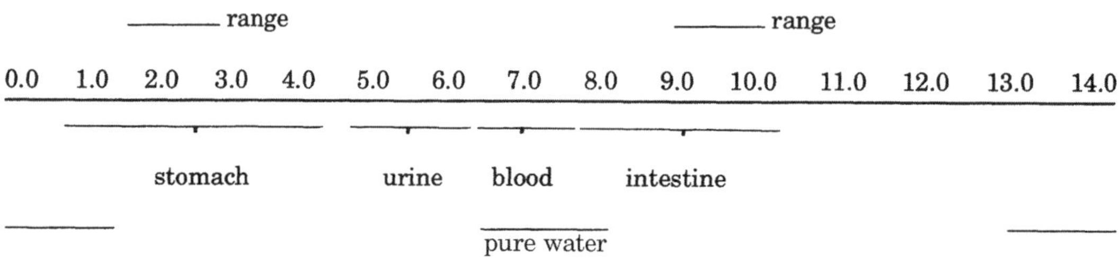

Figure 1.1 The pH scale.

Key:
acid
acid-base
acidity
acidosis
alkaline
alkalosis
higher
lower
H^+
OH^-
neutral
pH

It is essential to understand that a number on the ______ scale is actually the result of dividing the numeral 1 by a mathematical value called *logarithm*. The result is that the ______ the concentration of ______ and consequently the greater the ______, the ______ the pH value. Thus pH 4.0 indicates a ______ concentration of H^+, and a higher ______, than does pH of 5.0.

Most cells are extremely sensitive to changes in the pH of their environment. The pH of human blood plasma is usually maintained at a value between 7.35 and 7.45 – that is, blood plasma is slightly ______. The normal metabolism of food by the cells releases carbon dioxide (CO_2), which forms carbonic acid when combined with water. The foods we commonly eat contain sodium, potassium, magnesium, and calcium, and these substances form ______ compounds within the body. When the normal limits of the blood plasma pH are greatly exceeded in either direction along the scale, ______ (pH below 6.8) or ______ (pH above 7.8) can lead to illness and even death, unless a proper ______ balance is restored.

Exercise 1.2

Labelling. Write the name of each numbered body plane and the direction on the corresponding lines. Select different colours for the separate planes – do not colour the body.

Key:
dorsal, posterior
frontal (coronal) plane
inferior
sagittal plane
superior
transverse plane
ventral, anterior

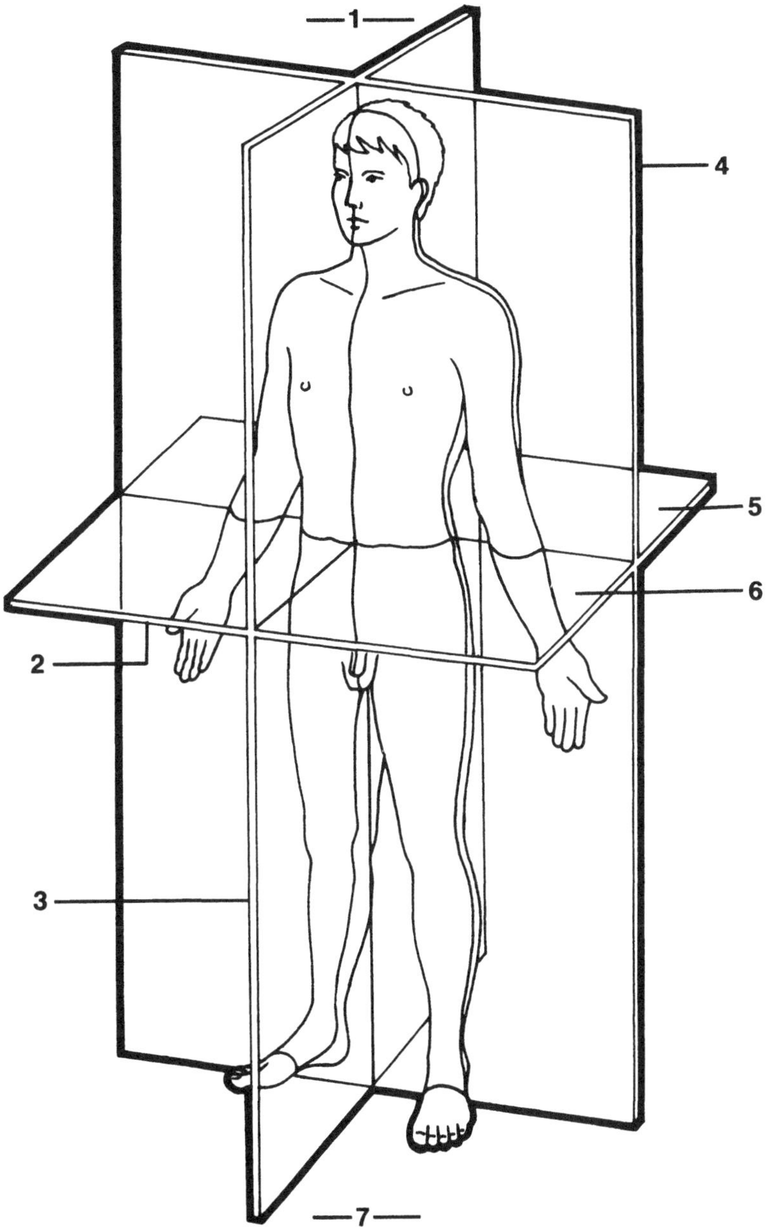

Figure 1.2 Body planes and directions.

1. ______________________
2. ______________________
3. ______________________
4. ______________________
5. ______________________
6. ______________________
7. ______________________

Exercise 1.3

Labelling. Write the name of each numbered body cavity or cavities on the corresponding lines below. Colour the dorsal and ventral cavities a different colour.

Key:
abdominal cavity
abdominopelvic cavity
cranial cavity
diaphragm
dorsal body cavities
pelvic cavity
pericardial cavity
pleural cavity
spinal cavity
thoracic cavity
ventral body cavities
vertebral column

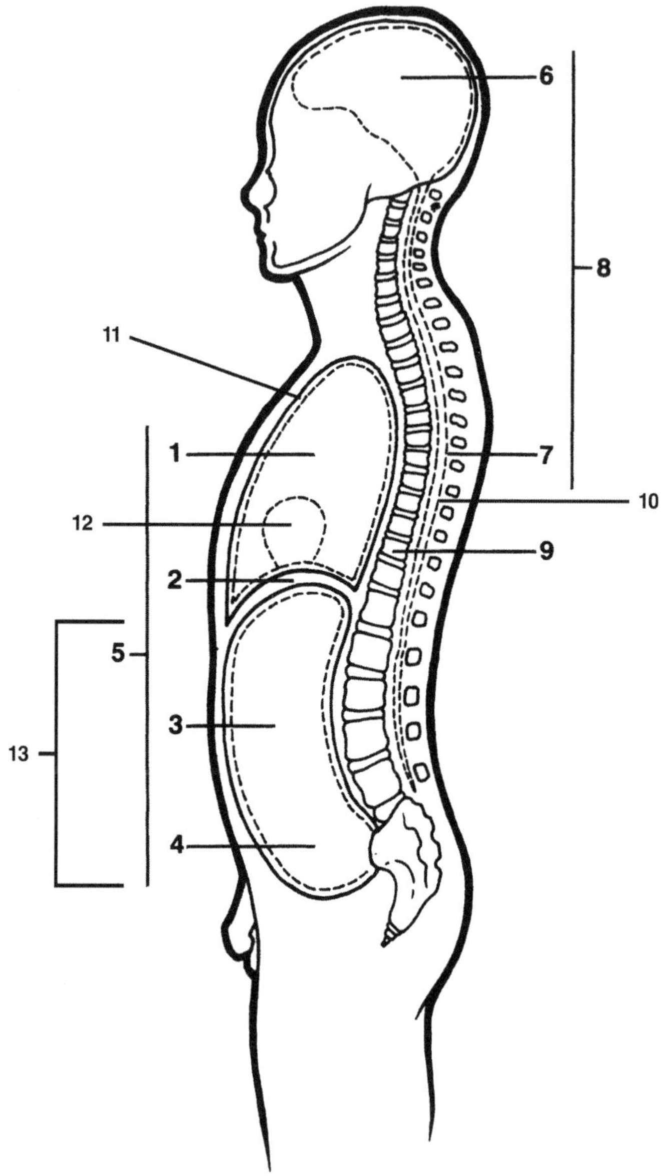

Figure 1.3 Sagittal section of the body, showing the dorsal and ventral body cavities.

1. ____________________
2. ____________________
3. ____________________
4. ____________________
5. ____________________
6. ____________________
7. ____________________
8. ____________________
9. ____________________
10. ____________________
11. ____________________
12. ____________________
13. ____________________

Exercise 1.4

Labelling. Write the name of each numbered region of the abdomen on the corresponding lines. Select a different colour for each of the nine regions.

Key:
epigastric
hypogastric
left hypochondriac
left inguinal
left lumbar
right hypochondriac
right inguinal
right lumbar
umbilical

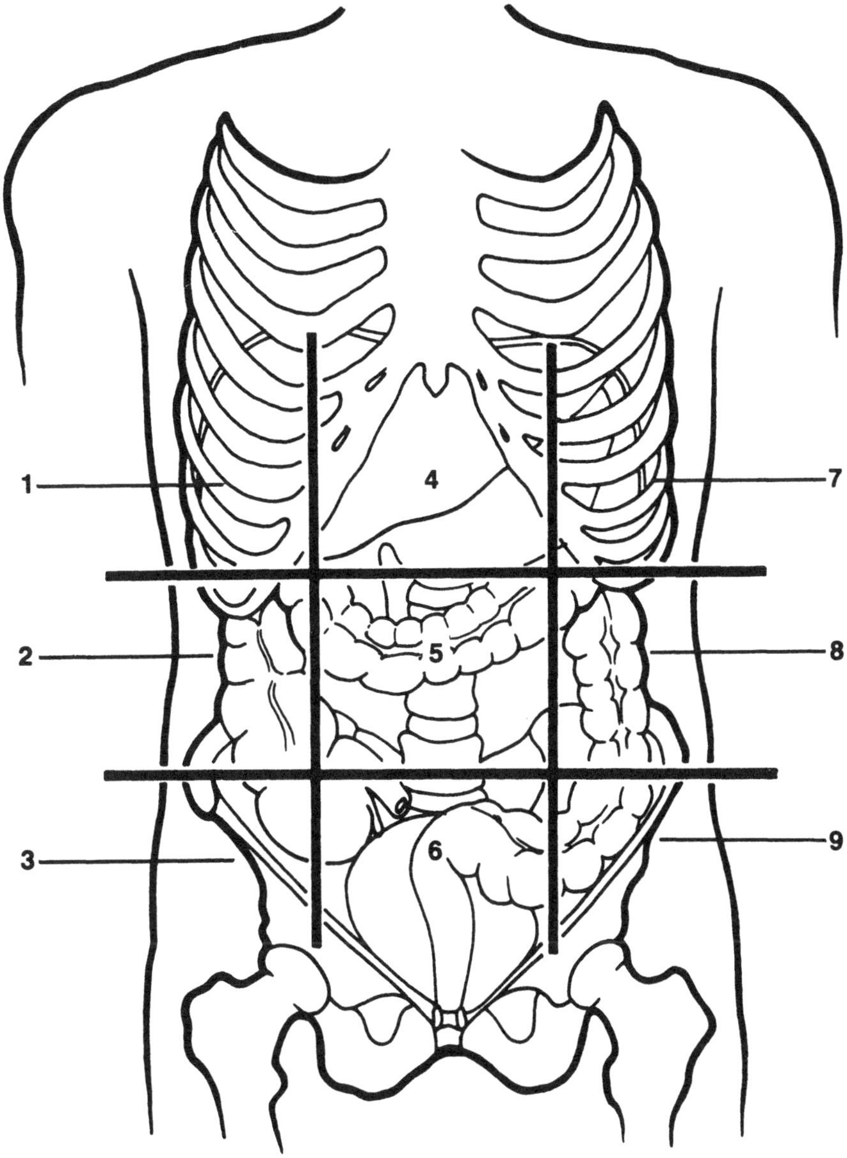

Figure 1.4 Abdominal regions.

1. ______________________
2. ______________________
3. ______________________
4. ______________________
5. ______________________
6. ______________________
7. ______________________
8. ______________________
9. ______________________

Exercise 1.5

The Metric System

Table 1.1 *Units of Measurement*

Unit	Symbol = Equivalent
Centimetre	cm = 0.4 inch
Millimetre	mm = 0.1 cm
Micron (Micrometre)*	μ = 0.001 mm (μm)
Millimicron (Nanometre)*	mμ = 0.001 μ (nm)
Angstrom	Å = 0.1 mμ

*The terms in parentheses have been adopted by the new international system of units of measurement to replace the ones given. However, the more familiar terms have not gone out of use as yet.

To demonstrate that you understand the relationship of one metric unit to another, fill in the blanks that follow.

1 mm = ______ μ   1 μ = ______ mm

1.5 mm = ______ μ   1,500 μ = ______ mm

0.25 mm = ______ μ   250 μ = ______ mm

1.5 cm = ______ mm = ______ μ

5,000 μ = ______ mm = ______ cm

V. TEST ITEMS

A. *Multiple Choice.* There is only one answer that is either correct or most appropriate. Circle the best answer for each question.

1. Which of the following is the preferred primary source of energy for human cells?
   a. fats
   b. carbohydrates
   c. proteins
   d. nucleic acids

2. The building blocks of DNA are
   a. fatty acids
   b. amino acids
   c. nucleotides
   d. cholesterol

3. The chest is known as what region?
   a. lumbar
   b. spinal
   c. thoracic
   d. abdominal

4. A frontal (coronal) section will cut the body into
   a. right and left halves
   b. superior and inferior halves
   c. dorsal and ventral halves
   d. lateral and medial portions

5. Which term describes the location of the foot in reference to the knee?
   a. anterior
   b. proximal
   c. inferior
   d. posterior

6. Which term best describes the relative constancy of the interval environment of the body?
   a. stress
   b. pathology
   c. homeostasis
   d. metastasis

7. The pH of blood is slightly basic. Which of the following numbers would be appropriate?
   a. 6.4
   b. 4.6
   c. 4.7
   d. 7.4
   e. 13.8

8. The term used to describe the acid or base content of fluids is
   a. endocytosis
   b. pH
   c. exocytosis
   d. filtration

9. If you were to assume the anatomical position you would
   a. lie face down
   b. lie face up
   c. stand erect with palms facing forward
   d. stand erect with thumbs backward

10. Which term describes the location of the hand in reference to the arm?
    a. anterior
    b. proximal
    c. distal
    d. posterior

11. The study of how the body functions is called
    a. physiology
    b. anatomy
    c. homeostasis
    d. dissection

12. Of the nine abdominal regions which of the following groups are medial?
    a. hypochondriac, lumbar, and iliac or inguinal
    b. epigastric, umbilical, and hypogastric
    c. epigastric, umbilical, and iliac
    d. hypochondriac, umbilical, and hypogastric

13. If you wanted to separate the abdominal from the thoracic cavity, which plane would you use?
    a. sagittal
    b. transverse
    c. frontal
    d. coronal

14. A graze injury on the arm would be described as
    a. dorsal
    b. lateral
    c. superficial
    d. deep

15. The peritoneum (peritoneal membrane) lines which cavity?
a. abdominopelvic
b. thoracic
c. cardiac
d. cranial

16. The diaphragm separates which cavities from each other?
a. abdominal and pelvic
b. cranial and vertebral
c. thoracic and abdominal
d. dorsal and ventral

17. A pulled muscle in the femoral region might affect your ability to
a. turn your head
b. bend your arm
c. walk
d. move your fingers

18. Which of the following is a monosaccharide?
a. lactose
b. glucose
c. sucrose
d. maltose

19. Liver and muscle cells are able to store chains of glucose as
a. cellulose
b. protein
c. cholesterol
d. glycogen

20. Which term best describes the relationship of the elbow to the wrist?
a. medial
b. lateral
c. proximal
d. external

B. *Matching.* Each of the phrases in Column B refers to a word in Column A. Insert the letter of the phrase from Column B that best describes each word in Column A. Some words or phrases may be used more than once or not at all.

Column A		*Column B*
1.	___ proximal	**a.** toward the feet
2.	___ inferior	**b.** further from the point of origin
3.	___ parietal	**c.** toward the back
4.	___ distal	**d.** toward one side of the body
5.	___ visceral	**e.** in close proximity to body walls
6.	___ ventral	**f.** nearer to the point of origin
7.	___ dorsal	**g.** toward the front of the abdomen
8.	___ medial	**h.** toward the head
9.	___ superior	**i.** next to the internal organs
10.	___ lateral	**j.** toward the midline of the body

C. *True or False.* Place a *T* or an *F* in the space provided to indicate true or false.

___ **1.** Neurology is the branch of anatomy that deals with the structure of tissues.

___ **2.** In the standard anatomical position, the body is erect with the feet together, the arms hanging at the sides, and the palms facing forward.

___ **3.** Most feedback mechanisms are negative in nature.

___ **4.** Sagittal and coronal planes divide the body into upper and lower parts.

___ **5.** Cranial and vertebral portions are subdivisions of the dorsal body cavity.

___ **6.** The hands are the proximal portion of the upper extremities.

___ **7.** Water is essential to biological processes.

___ **8.** The numerical value of pH increases with increasing hydrogen ion concentration.

___ **9.** Because K^+, Na^+, Cl^-, and HCO_3^- all have charges, they are classified as ions.

___ **10.** The degree of acidity or alkalinity of a given solution is referred to as its pH.

Answer Sheet—Chapter 1

Exercise 1.1

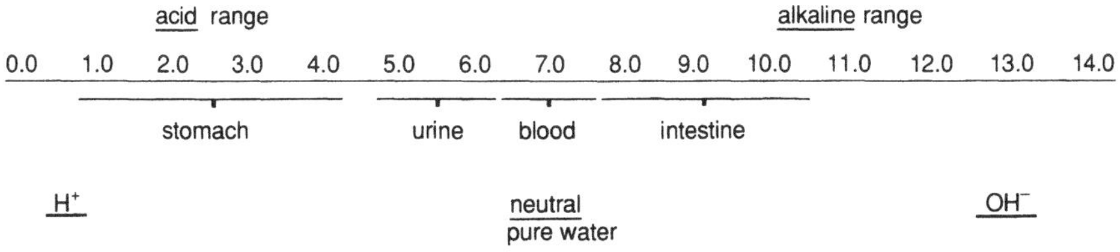

Figure 1.1 The pH scale.

It is essential to understand that a number on the pH scale is actually the result of dividing the number 1 by a mathematical value called a *logarithm*. The result is that the higher the concentration of H^+, and consequently the greater the acidity, the lower the pH value. Thus pH 4.0 indicates a higher concentration of H^+, and a higher acidity, than does pH 5.0.

Most cells are extremely sensitive to changes in the pH of their environment. The pH of human blood plasma is usually maintained at a value between 7.35 and 7.45—that is, blood plasma is slightly alkaline. The normal metabolism of food by the cells releases carbon dioxide (CO_2), which forms carbonic acid when combined with water. The foods we commonly eat contain sodium, potassium, magnesium, and calcium, and these substances form alkaline compounds within the body. When the normal limits of the blood plasma pH are greatly exceeded in either direction along the scale, acidosis (pH below 6.8) or alkalosis (pH above 7.8) can lead to serious illness and even death, unless a proper acid-base balance is restored.

Exercise 1.2

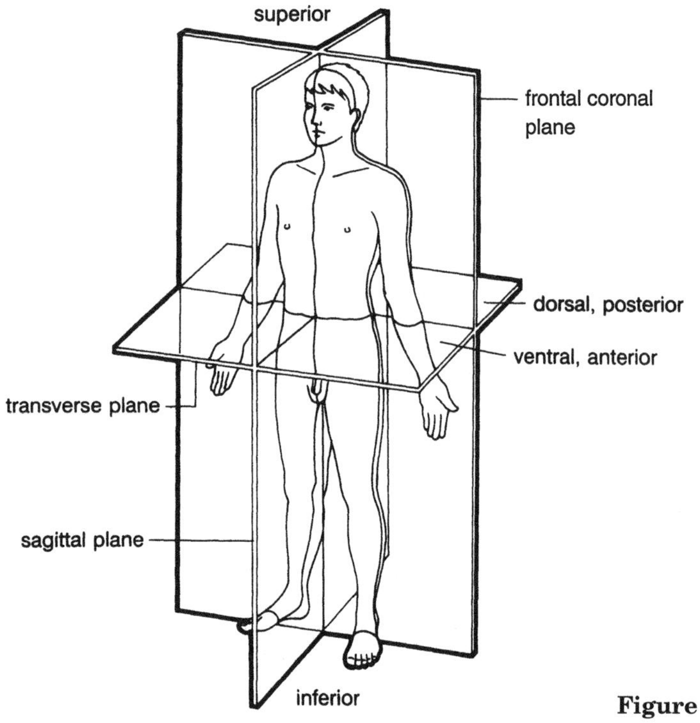

Figure 1.2 Body planes and directions.

Exercise 1.3

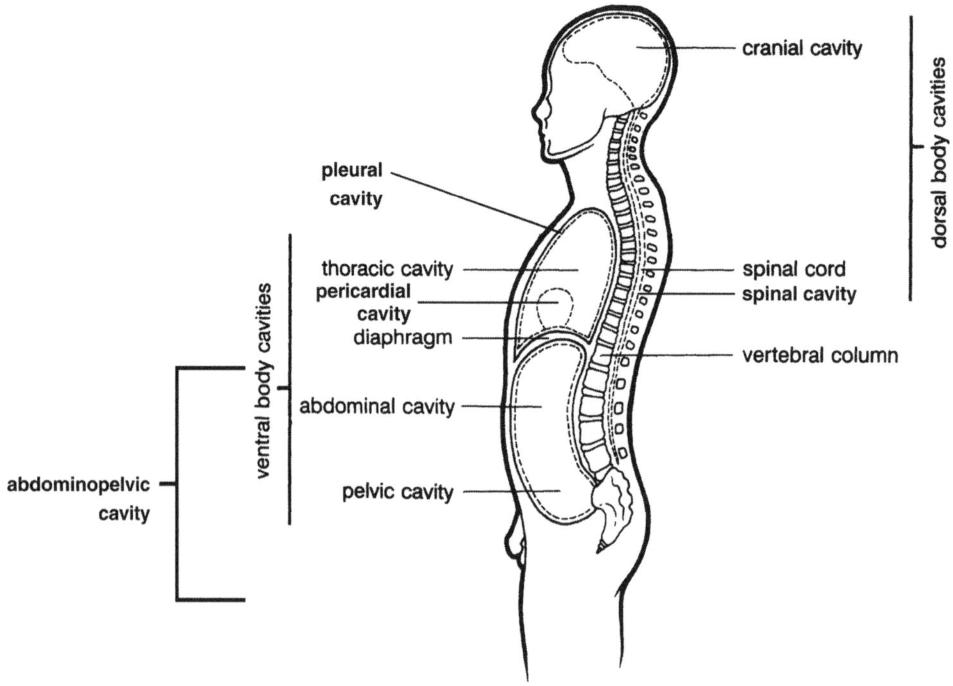

Figure 1.3 Sagittal section of the body, showing the dorsal and ventral body cavities.

Exercise 1.4

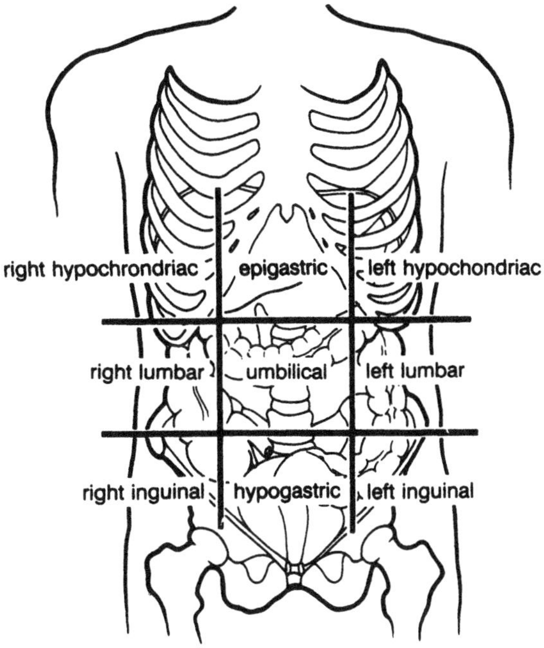

Figure 1.4 Abdominal regions.

Exercise 1.5

1 mm	=	1,000	μ			
1.5 mm	=	1,500	μ			
0.25 mm	=	250	μ			
1.5 cm	=	15	mm	=	15,000	μ
5,000 μ	=	5	mm	=	0.5	cm

1 μ	=	0.001	mm
1,500 μ	=	1.5	mm
250 μ	=	0.25	mm

Test Items

A. 1. b, 2. c, 3. c, 4. c, 5. c, 6. c, 7. d, 8. b, 9. c, 10. c, 11. a, 12. b, 13. b, 14. c, 15. a, 16. c, 17. c, 18. b, 19. d, 20. c.

B. 1. f, 2. a, 3. e, 4. b, 5. i, 6. g, 7. c, 8. j, 9. h, 10. d.

C. 1. F, 2. T, 3. T, 4. F, 5. T, 6. F, 7. T, 8. F, 9. T, 10. T.

2

The Living Cell

I. CHAPTER SYNOPSIS

Living things or organisms display a remarkable fundamental similarity in both structure and function. All living forms are essentially made up of one or more basic units or structural compartments called cells.

The living substance of the cell is called protoplasm. It refers to the living matter within the cell or plasma membrane. Within the protoplasm are structures called organelles, each playing a major role in the total physiology of the cell.

II. OBJECTIVES

After reading the chapter, the student should be able to:

- Describe the basic cellular organisation.
- Give one or more important functions for each of the major organelles.
- Describe mitochondria, ribosomes, and lysosomes and show their relation to cellular metabolism.
- Explain the possible roles of microtubules and microfilaments in the shape of a cell.
- Describe the structure and chemical nature of DNA.
- Explain the complementary pairing of nucleic acids in the structure of DNA.
- Cite the main function of DNA contained in the nucleus of a cell.

- Distinguish between DNA and RNA.
- Describe the chemical and mechanical phases of mitosis.

III. IMPORTANT TERMS

Using your textbook, define the following terms:

adenosine triphosphate (ATP) (uh-de′n-uh-seen try-fo′ss-fate; ATP) ____________________

____

anaphase (an′ah-faze) ____

____

autolysis (aw-tol′i-sis) ____

____

autosome (aw′to-some) ____

____

centriole (sen′tre-ol) ____

____

chromatin (kro′mah-tin) ____

____

chromosome (kro′mo-some) ____

____

cisternae (sis-ter′ne) ____

____

codon (kod′on) ____

____

cristae (Kris′ta) ____

____

cytoskelleton (si′to-skel-i-tn) ____

____

cytosol (si-to-sawl) ____

____

cytoplasm (si′to-plazm) ____

____

deoxyribonucleic acid (DNA) (dee-ah′k-see rye′-boh-noo-klay-ikk acid; DNA) ____________

____

endoplasmic reticulum (en-do-plaz′mic re-tik′u-lum) ____________________

____

enzyme (en′zime) ______

Golgi apparatus (gol′je apah-ra′tus) ______

interphase (in′ter-faze) ______

lysosome (li′so-some) ______

meiosis (mi-o′sis) ______

metaphase (met′ah-faze) ______

microfilament (mi-kro-fil′ah-ment) ______

microtubule (mi-kro-tu′bule) ______

mitochondria (mi-to-kon′dria) ______

mitosis (mi-to′sis) ______

nucleolus (nu-klee′o-lus) ______

nucleoplasm (nu′-klee-o-plaz-em) ______

nucleotides (nu′-klee-o-tahyd) ______

organelle (or-gah-nel′) ______

prophase (pro′-faze) ______

protoplasm (prot′-ah-plaz-em) ______

ribonucleic acid (RNA) (ry′e-boh-noo-klay-ikk acid; RNA) ______

ribosome (ri′-bo-some) ______

telophase (tel′-o-faze) ______________________________

____

transcription (trans-krip′-shun) ______________________________

____

translation (tranz-lay′-shun) ______________________________

____

IV. EXERCISES

Complete the following exercises in the order given. A precise set of terms and structures has evolved to describe the cell and DNA/RNA.

Exercise 2.1

Labelling. Write the name of each numbered part of the cell on the corresponding blank space. Use a different colour to depict a common function.

Key:

centriole
rough endoplasmic reticulum (rough ER)
smooth endoplasmic reticulum (smooth ER)
globular heads
Golgi apparatus
lipid droplets
lysosome
mitochondrion
nuclear envelope
nucleolus
secretory granules

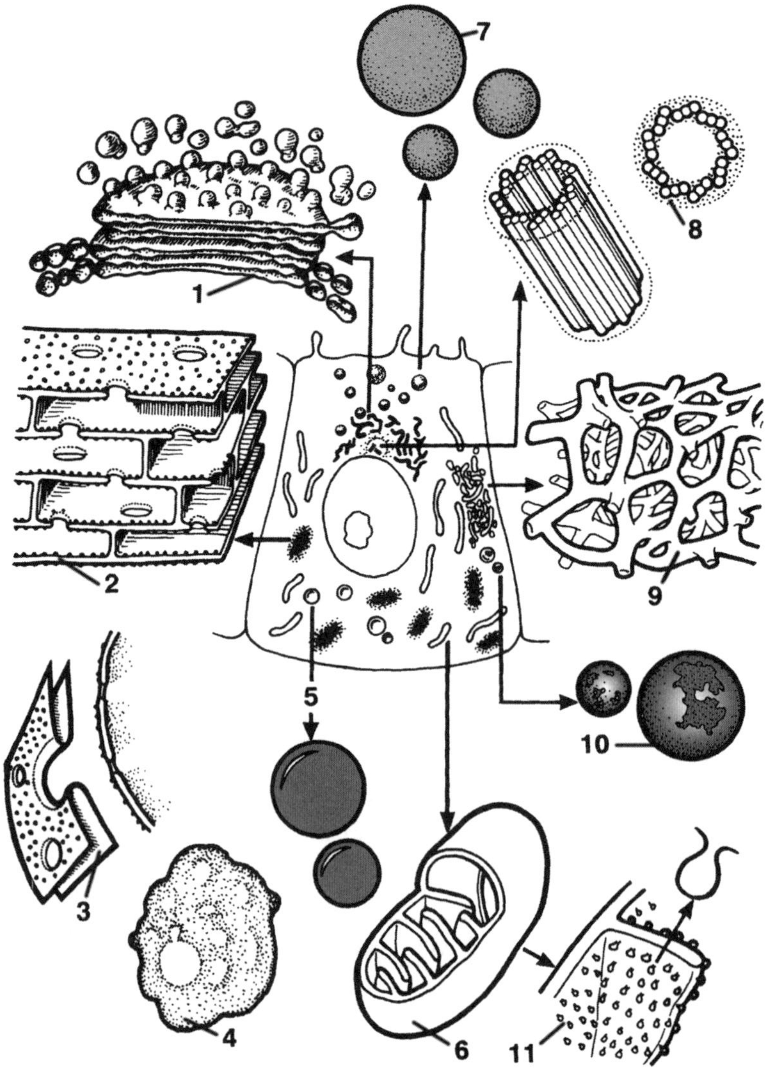

Figure 2.1 Cell (centre).

1. ______________________
2. ______________________
3. ______________________
4. ______________________
5. ______________________
6. ______________________
7. ______________________
8. ______________________
9. ______________________
10. ______________________
11. ______________________

Exercise 2.2

Labelling. Write the name of each numbered part of the nucleus on the corresponding line of the answer sheet.

Key:
chromosomes
nucleotides
nucleolus
nucleus

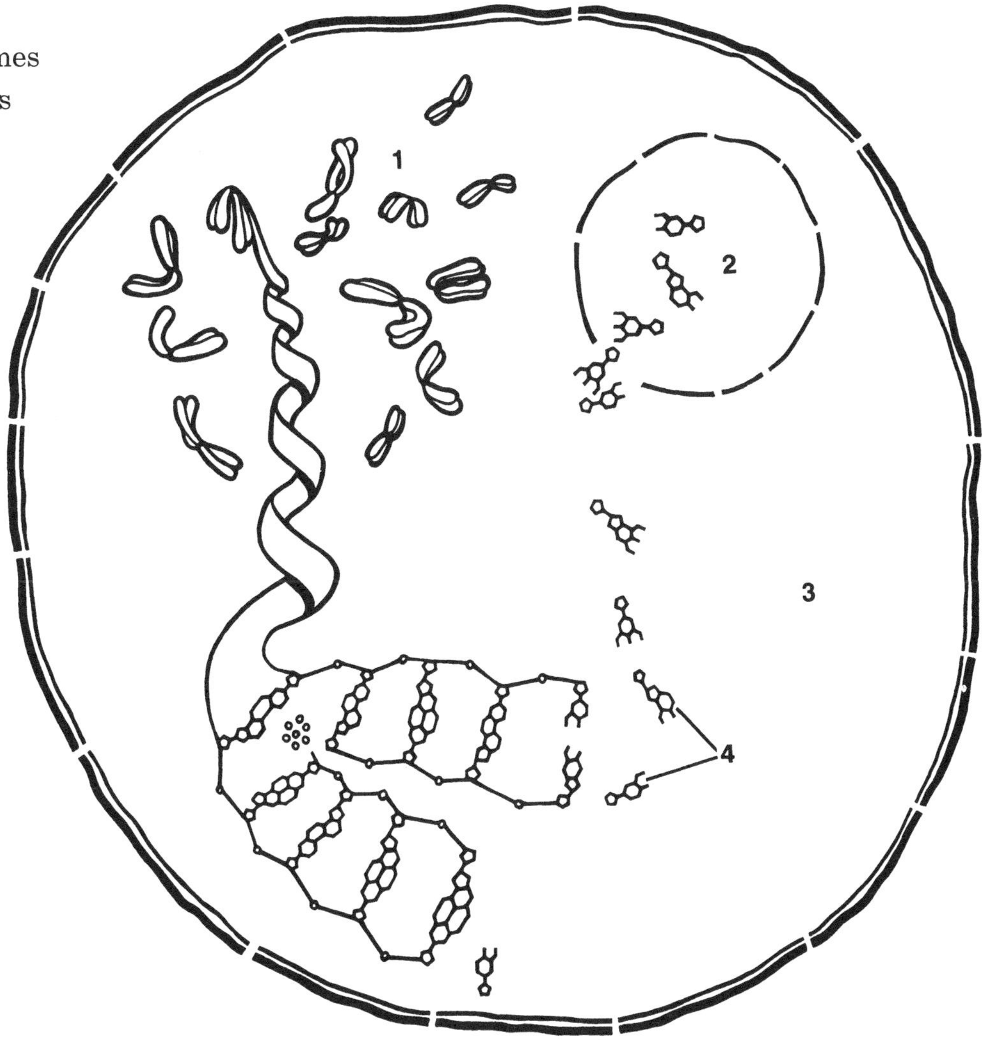

Figure 2.2 DNA molecule, showing replication in the nucleus.

1. ______________________
2. ______________________
3. ______________________
4. ______________________

Exercise 2.3

Labelling. Write the name (symbol) of each numbered part on the corresponding blank space. Colour the reciprocal base pairings to match their codons.

Key:
A
C
G
protein
T
transcription
translation
U

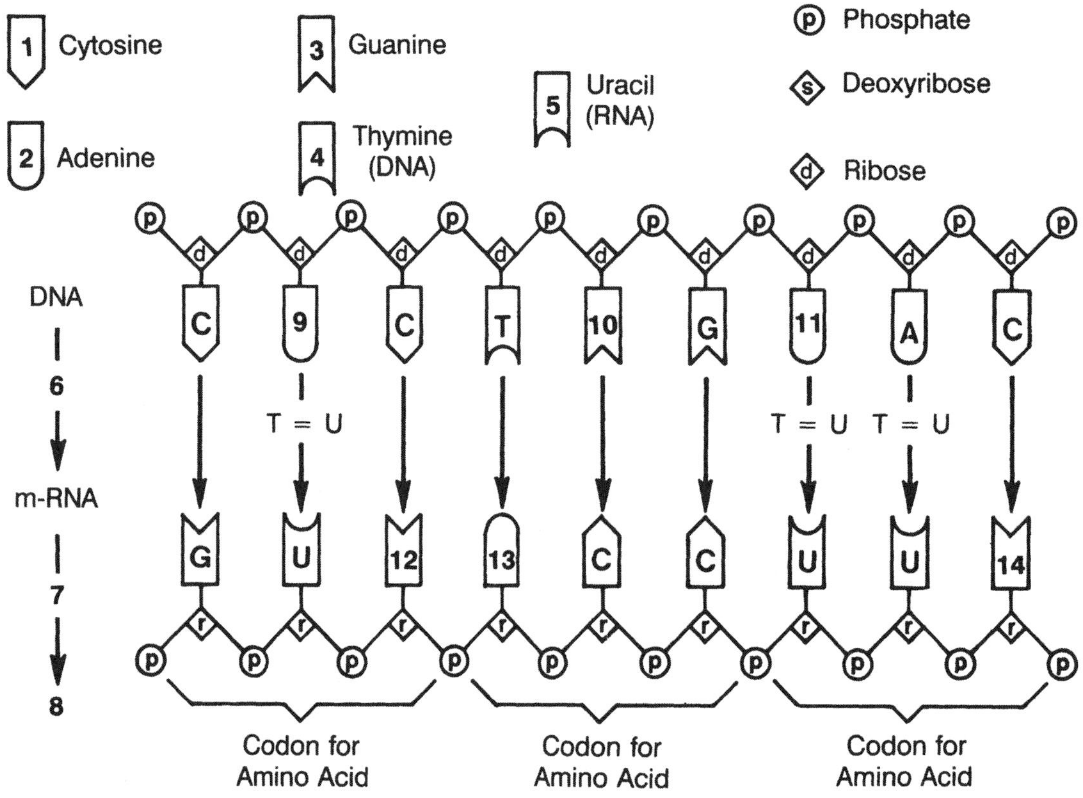

Figure 2.3 Transcription from one DNA strand to m-RNA showing codons that specify amino acids. Phosphates connect deoxyribose molecules in DNA and ribose molecules in RNA. Abbreviations: A, adenine; d, deoxyribose sugar; T, thymine; C, cytosine; r, ribose sugar; U, uracil; p, phosphate molecules.

1. ______________________
2. ______________________
3. ______________________
4. ______________________
5. ______________________
6. ______________________
7. ______________________
8. ______________________
9. ______________________
10. ______________________
11. ______________________
12. ______________________
13. ______________________
14. ______________________

Exercise 2.4

Labelling. Write the name of the part or phase of mitosis of a living cell. Colour the nuclear components a different colour than the cytoplasm.

Key:
anaphase
cell membrane
centrioles
chromosomes
early prophase
early telophase
interphase
interphase
late prophase
late telophase
metaphase
nuclear membrane

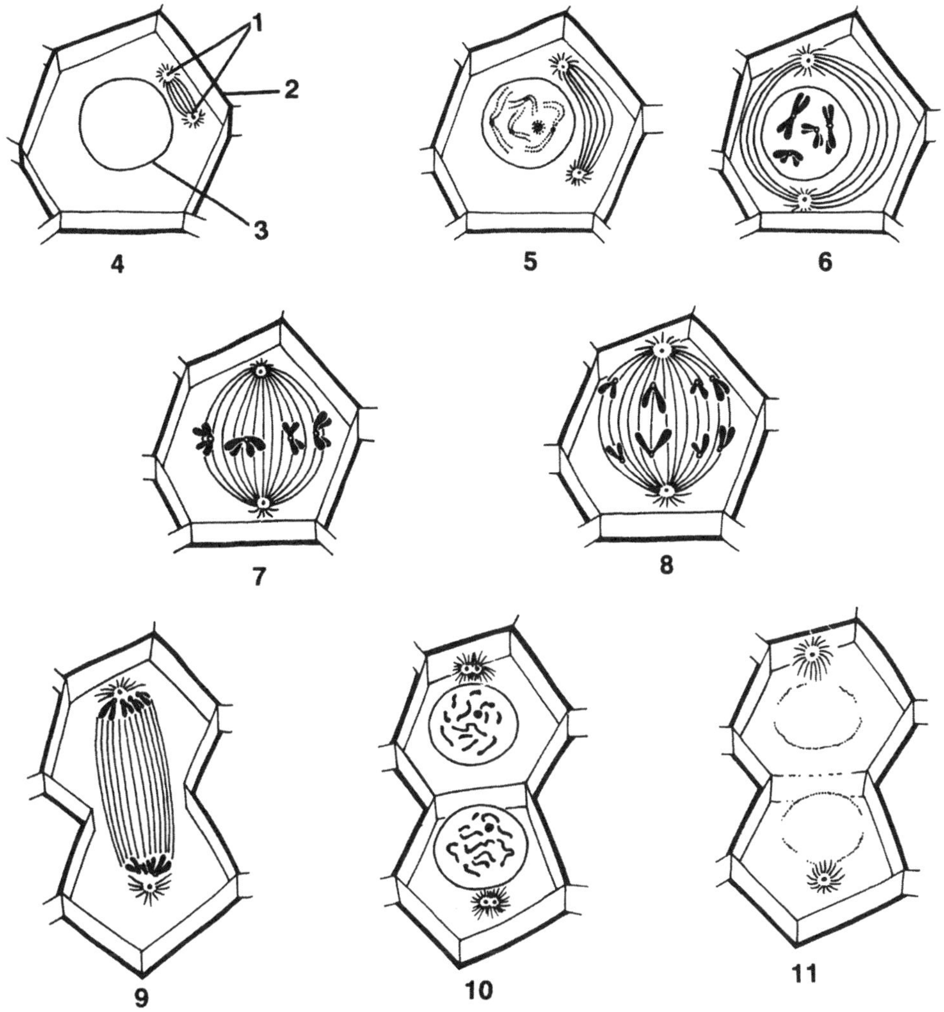

Figure 2.4 Schematic representation of mitosis of a cell. See text for an account of what happens during each of the various stages.

1. ______________________
2. ______________________
3. ______________________
4. ______________________
5. ______________________
6. ______________________
7. ______________________
8. ______________________
9. ______________________
10. ______________________
11. ______________________
12. ______________________

V. TEST ITEMS

A. *Multiple Choice.* There is only one answer that is either correct or most appropriate. Circle the best answer for each question.

1. Most of the cell's ATP is manufactured in organelles called
   a. mitochondria
   b. Golgi apparatus
   c. ribosomes
   d. lysosomes

2. The major role of smooth endoplasmic reticulum (ER) is
   a. protein synthesis
   b. energy release
   c. intracellular digestion
   d. lipid synthesis

3. Which of the following organelles packages substances synthesised by the cell?
   a. Golgi apparatus
   b. mitochondria
   c. lysosomes
   d. ribosomes

4. Which of the following molecules forms the genetic blueprint in the nucleus of the cell?
   a. DNA
   b. RNA
   c. proteins
   d. none of the foregoing

5. During which stage of mitosis does DNA replication occur?
   a. interphase
   b. metaphase
   c. prophase
   d. telophase

6. The site of protein synthesis is
   a. ribosomes
   b. smooth endoplasmic reticulum
   c. lysosomes
   d. none of the above

7. Which of the following nucleotide base pairings is inaccurate?
   a. G-T
   b. T-A
   c. C-G
   d. G-C

8. The endoplasmic reticulum (ER)
   a. functions as an extracellular network
   b. attaches to chromosomes during division
   c. forms the cleavage furrow during division
   d. serves as an internal framework and an intracellular passageway

9. As a result of mitotic cell division, each daughter cell has
   a. half as many chromosomes as its parent cell
   b. twice as many chromosomes as its parent cell
   c. the same number of chromosomes as its parent cell
   d. one quarter as many chromosomes as its parent cell

10. With the exception of sex cells (sperm and ova) nucleated human cells have
   a. 23 chromosomes
   b. 46 chromosomes
   c. 26 chromosomes
   d. 43 chromosomes

11. 65% of the mass of the human body is composed of
a. water
b. fats
c. carbohydrates
d. proteins

12. The linkage of bases in DNA follows a pattern in which a purine base is always linked with a pyrimidine base. Possible linkages are
a. A-G
b. A-T
c. C-U
d. T-C

13. The unit of structure and function of living things is
a. protoplasm
b. the cell
c. an organ
d. a nucleus

14. The smallest unit of structure is considered to be at the
a. organ level
b. chemical level
c. cellular level
d. system level

15. Select the base that is not found in both DNA and RNA.
a. adenine
b. uracil
c. guanine
d. cytosine

16. Rough endoplasmic reticulum is mostly associated with
a. ribosome and protein formation
b. mitochondria and respiration
c. centrosome and mitosis
d. ribosome and respiration

17. Which of the following structures transmits genetic traits?
a. lysosome
b. chromosome
c. ribosome
d. centriole

18. Phagocytosis and pinocytosis occur at the
a. cell (plasma) membrane
b. endoplasmic reticulum (ER)
c. nucleus
d. nucleolus

19. The prominent folds on the inner membrane of a mitochondrion are termed
a. cristae
b. rugae
c. villi
d. microvilli

20. An acid
a. has a pH greater than 7
b. has a pH less than 7
c. has more OH^- ions
d. has a pH of 7

B. *Matching.* Each of the words or phrases in Column B refers to a word or phrase in Column A. Insert the letter of the word or phrase from Column B that best describes each word or phrase in Column A. Some words or phrases may be used more than once or not at all.

	Column A		*Column B*
1. ___	synthesis of ATP	**a.**	Golgi apparatus
2. ___	package and storage of cellular secretions	**b.**	nucleolus
3. ___	digestion of material within the cell	**c.**	mitochondria
4. ___	synthesis of protein	**d.**	ribosomes
5. ___	synthesis of mitotic spindle	**e.**	microtubules
6. ___	storage of solid or fluid substance	**f.**	centrioles
7. ___	shape of the cell	**g.**	lysosomes
8. ___	channels for passage of substance within the cell	**h.**	chromosomes
9. ___	transmission of genetic information	**i.**	vacuoles
10. ___	synthesis of ribosomal RNA	**j.**	endoplasmic reticulum (ER)
		k.	plasma membrane

	Column A		*Column B*
1. ___	chromosomes move to opposite poles of cell	**a.**	prophase
2. ___	centrioles reach poles; line up on equator	**b.**	interphase
3. ___	genetic information replicated	**c.**	telophase
4. ___	nuclear membrane disappears	**d.**	anaphase
5. ___	two daughter cells are produced	**e.**	metaphase
6. ___	chromatin condenses into chromosomes		

C. *True or False.* Place a *T* or an *F* in the space provided to indicate true or false.

___ **1.** The science that deals with the study of cells is cytology.

___ **2.** In DNA and RNA, the backbone of the nucleic acid chain consists of alternating units of phosphate and a five-carbon sugar.

___ **3.** The nuclear envelope disintegrates in the metaphase.

___ **4.** The nuclear membrane forms around each group of daughter chromosomes during the telophase of mitosis.

___ **5.** In DNA, the two chains are joined by bonding between specific base pairs—adenine to thymine, guanine to cytosine.

___ **6.** Parts of the cell that are specialised for specific activities are called organelles.

___ **7.** The portion of the cell that controls its activities and contains hereditary material is the nucleus.

___ **8.** The five-carbon sugar in DNA is called ribose.

___ **9.** The mitochondria are called "powerhouses" of the cell because within them ATP is produced.

___ **10.** Water constitutes the most abundant single compound found in the human body.

Answer Sheet—Chapter 2

Exercise 2.1

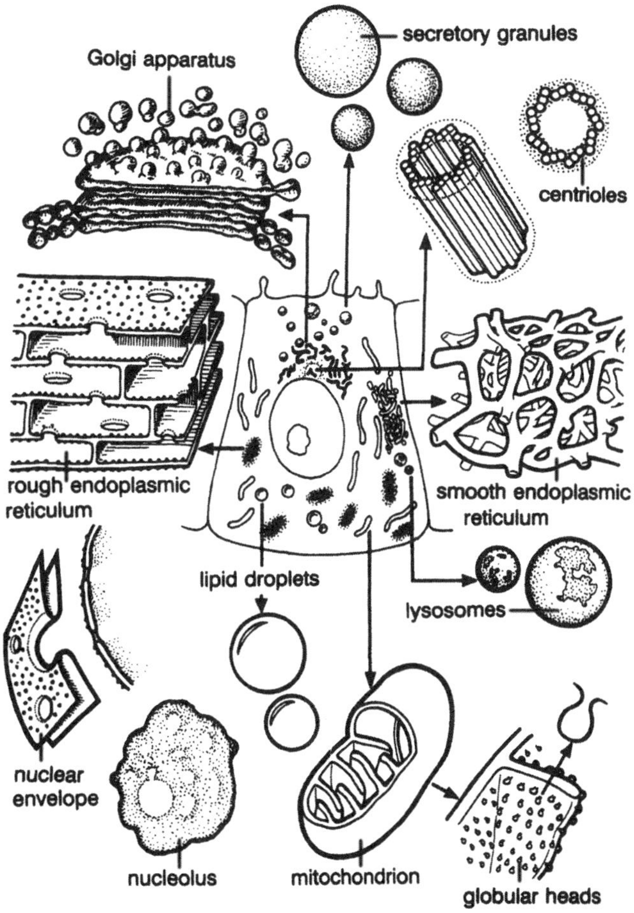

Figure 2.1 Cell (centre).

Exercise 2.2

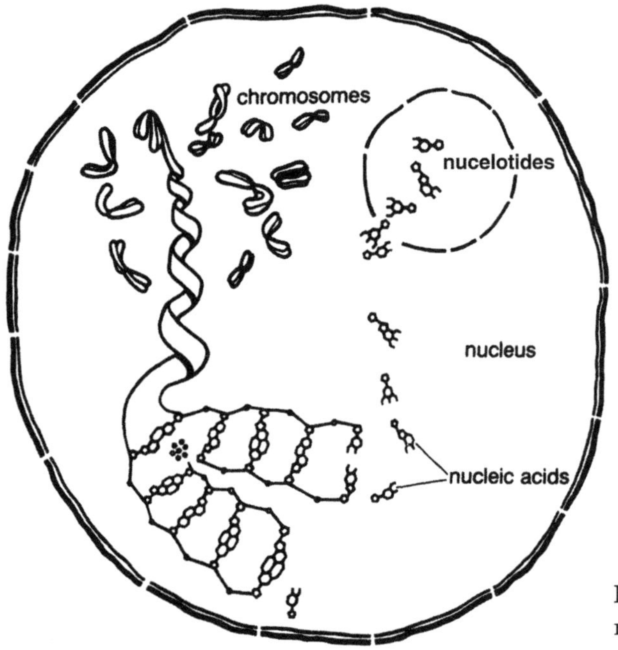

Figure 2.2 DNA molecule, showing replication in the nucleus.

Exercise 2.3

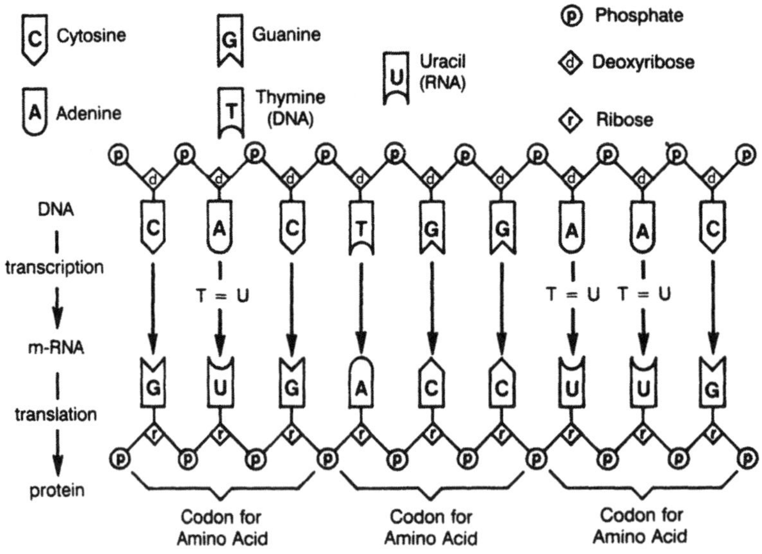

Figure 2.3 Transcription from one DNA strand to m-RNA showing codons that specify amino acids. Phosphates connect ribose molecules. Abbreviations: A, adenine; d, deoxyribose sugar; T, thymine; C, cytosine; r, ribose sugar; U, uracil; p, phosphate radicals.

Exercise 2.4

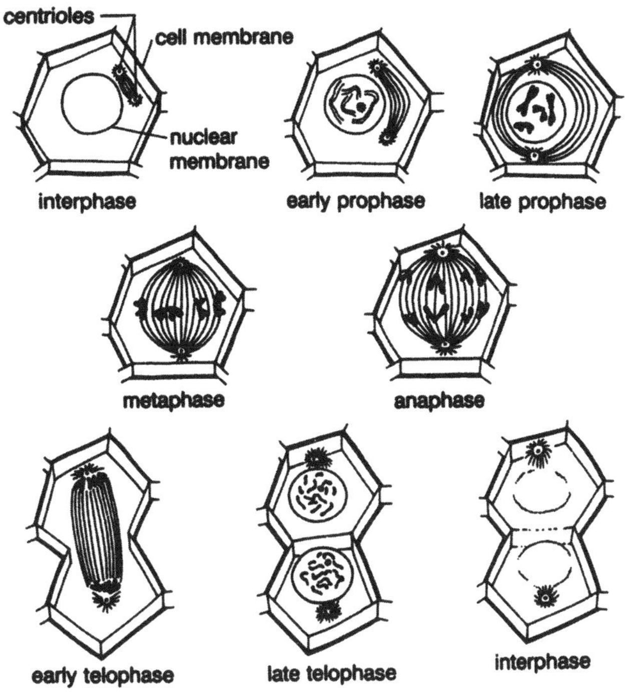

Figure 2.4 Schematic representation of mitosis of a cell. See text for an account of what happens during each of the various stages.

Test Items

A. 1. a, 2. d, 3. a, 4. a, 5. a, 6. a, 7. a, 8. d, 9. c, 10. b, 11. a, 12. b, 13. b, 14. b, 15. b, 16. a, 17. b, 18. a, 19. a, 20. b.

B. 1. c, 2. a, 3. g, 4. d, 5. f, 6. i, 7. k, 8. j, 9. h, 10. b.
1. d, 2. e, 3. b, 4. a, 5. c, 6. a.

C. 1. T, 2. F, 3. F, 4. T, 5. T, 6. T, 7. T, 8. F, 9. T, 10. T.

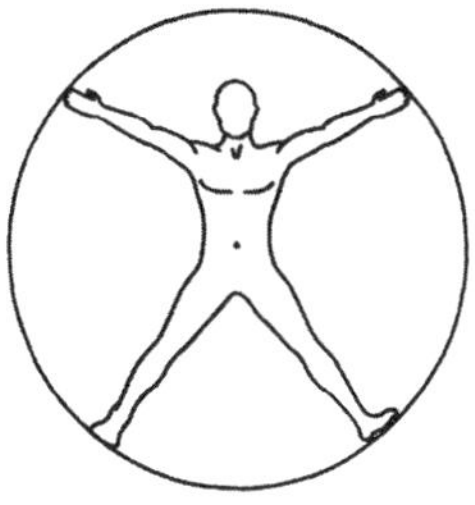

3

The Cell Membrane and Permeability

I. CHAPTER SYNOPSIS

The plasma cell membrane is a delicately balanced, functional organelle that separates the cell from its environment and allows materials to pass across it in both directions. By controlling ionic composition and water content, the membrane prevents the cell from swelling or shrinking and, therefore, is directly responsible for maintaining homeostasis.

The main barrier to substance exchange across the membrane is undoubtedly the lipid layer. A molecule must be able to pass through the small pores of the cell membrane or dissolve in the lipid layer and then diffuse through the membrane. Water passes readily through all membranes. Small, positively charged ions, however, move through the membrane very slowly due to the postulated positive charge of the lipid pores. Like charges repel each other. Negatively charged ions pass more easily.

II. OBJECTIVES

After reading the chapter, the student should be able to:

- Describe the molecular structure of a cell membrane.
- Define semipermeable membrane in terms of its role in governing the exchange of chemical compounds between cellular compartment and extracellular environment.
- Define diffusion and osmosis in terms of movement of particles or liquid in response to a concentration gradient.

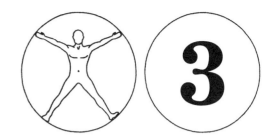

- Differentiate between facilitated diffusion and active transport.
- Define phagocytosis, pinocytosis, and exocytosis.
- Define isotonic, hypotonic, and hypertonic and their effects on cell volume.

III. IMPORTANT TERMS

Using your textbook, define the following terms:

active transport (ak′tiv trans-port′) ______________________________

____

Carrier proteins (kar-ee-er pro′teens) ______________________________

____

concentration gradient (kon-sun-tray′shun gray′dee-unt) ______________________________

____

crenation (kre-nay′shun) ______________________________

____

dehydration (de-hi-dray′-shun) ______________________________

____

dialysis (di-al′-i-sis) ______________________________

____

diffusion (di-fu′zhun) ______________________________

____

equilibrium (ee-kwi-lib′-ree-um) ______________________________

____

exocytosis (ek-soh-si-toh-sis) ______________________________

____

filtrate (fil-trate) ______________________________

____

filtration (fil-tray′-shun) ______________________________

____

glycocalyx (gli-ko-ka′lix) ______________________________

____

haemolysis (hee-mol′i-sis) ______________________________

____

homeostasis (ho-mee-o-sta′sis) ______________________________

____

hydrophilic (high-dro-fil′ik) ______________________________

____

hydrophobic (high-dro-fo′bik) ______________________________

____

hypertonic (hi-per-ton′ik) ______________________________

____

hypotonic (hi-po-ton′ik) ______________________________

____

isotonic (iso-ton′ik) ______________________________

____

lipid (phospho) (lip′id) ______________________________

____

lysis (lahy-sis) ______________________________

____

mosaic (mo-zay′ik) ______________________________

____

osmosis (oz-mo′sis) ______________________________

____

permeability (per-mee-ah-bil′-ity) ______________________________

____

permeable (per-mee-ah-bul) ______________________________

____

phagocytosis (fa-go-si-to′sis) ______________________________

____

pinocytosis (pi-no-si-to′sis) ______________________________

____

pore (pore) ______________________________

____

protein (pro′teen) ______________________________

____

semipermeable (se-mi-per′mee-ah-bul) ______________________________

____

solute (sol′yute) ______________________________

____

solvent (sol′vent) ______________________________

____

turgid (tur-jid) ______________________________

____

IV. EXERCISES

Complete the following exercises in the order given. A precise set of terms and structures has evolved to describe the cell membrane and permeability.

Exercise 3.1

Labelling. Write the name of each numbered part of the diagram in the space provided. Colour the different parts to identify their position in the membrane.

Key:

carbohydrate receptor sites (glycocalyx)
channel protein
hydrophilic layer
hydrophobic layer
phospholipid
protein molecules

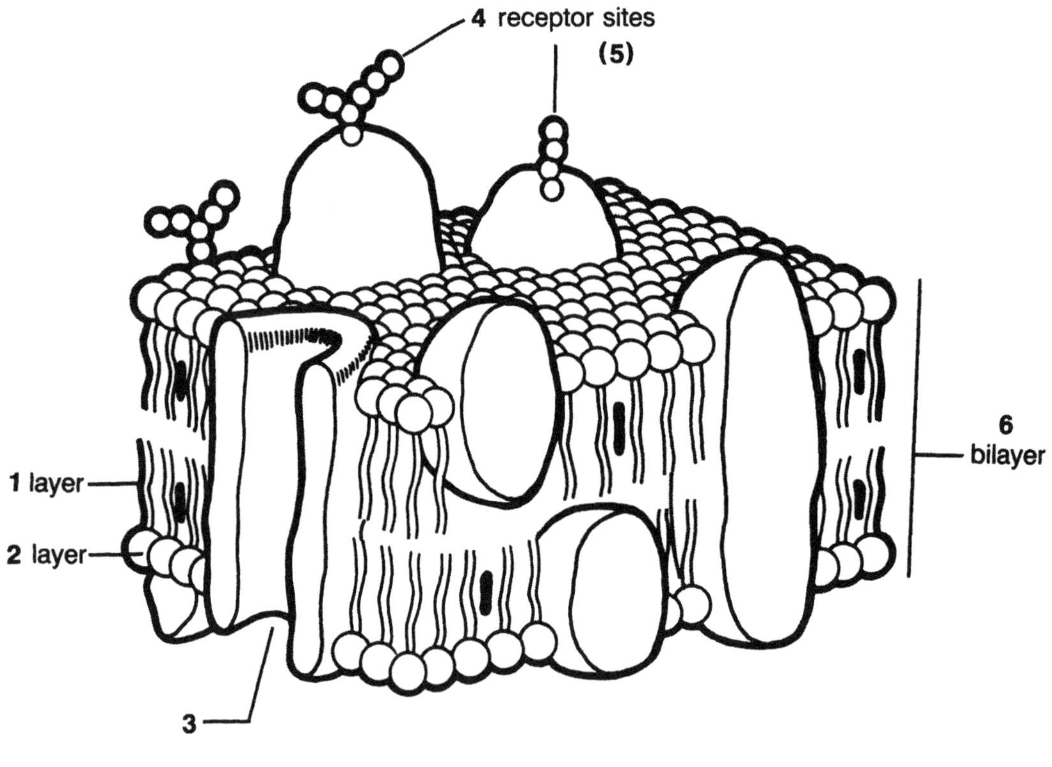

Figure 3.1 Fluid-mosaic model of the cell membrane.

1. ______________________
2. ______________________
3. ______________________
4. ______________________
5. ______________________
6. ______________________

Exercise 3.2

Labelling. Write the name of each numbered part of the diagram in the space provided. Colour the direction of flow in each instance. Terms may be used more than once.

Key:
active
ADP
ATP
carrier
facilitated
high
low

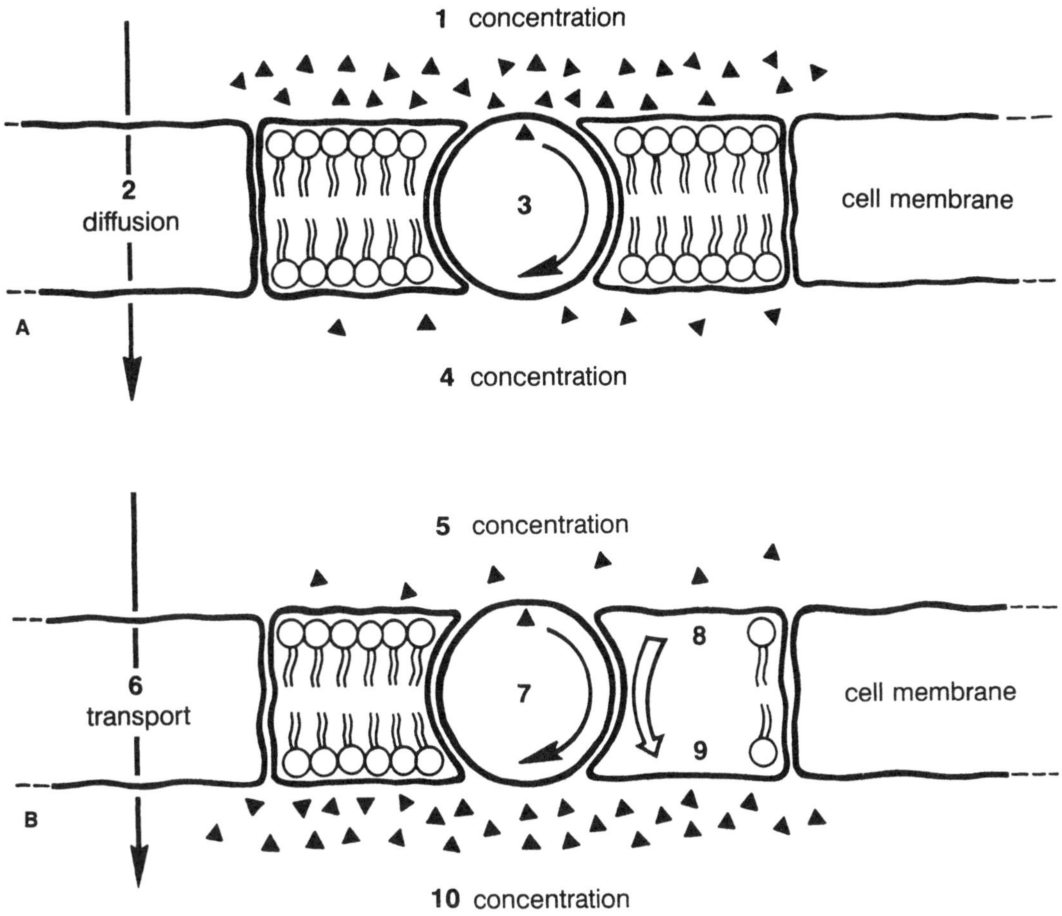

Figure 3.2 Two-carrier molecular system. **A.** Movement of a molecule across the membrane from higher to lower concentration of molecule. **B.** Movement of a molecule across a membrane from low to high concentration of molecule with the expenditure of energy to afford the transport.

1. ______________________
2. ______________________
3. ______________________
4. ______________________
5. ______________________
6. ______________________
7. ______________________
8. ______________________
9. ______________________
10. ______________________

V. TEST ITEMS

A. *Multiple Choice.* There is only one answer that is either correct or most appropriate. Circle the best answer for each question.

1. The movement of water through a membrane is dependent on
a. the concentration of solute
b. cholesterol
c. active transport
d. exocytosis

2. Carrier molecules are required for
a. diffusion
b. osmosis
c. facilitated transport
d. filtration

3. The cell membrane is composed of
a. cellulose
b. cellulose and protein
c. lipid
d. lipid and protein

4. Which of the following passes across the cell (plasma) membrane via simple diffusion?
a. carbon dioxide
b. glucose
c. amino acids
d. water

5. Which of these is absolutely necessary for diffusion to take place?
a. a semipermeable membrane
b. a true solution
c. a living cell
d. a concentration gradient

6. A blood cell will swell and burst (lysis) when placed in which kind of solution?
a. hypotonic
b. isotonic
c. hypertonic
d. homeostatic

7. When a substance moves from an area of low concentration to an area of high concentration,
a. diffusion has occurred
b. the cell bursts
c. energy is needed
d. osmotic pressure builds up

8. Proteins do not pass through cell membranes because
a. the membrane is made of protein
b. they contain nitrogen
c. they are very large molecules
d. they cause emulsification

9. If a 0.9% solution were isotonic to a cell, then
a. 0.9% would also be hypotonic
b. 0.9% would also be hypertonic
c. 1.0% would be hypertonic
d. 1.0% would be hypotonic

10. Isotonic means
a. the effective concentration of the dissolved substances in surrounding fluid is greater than the concentration in the cell
b. the effective concentration of the surrounding fluid is less than the concentration in the cell
c. the effective concentration of the dissolved substances in the surrounding fluid is the same as the concentration within the cell
d. all of these are true

11. A cell in a hypotonic solution
a. loses water
b. gains water
c. neither gains nor loses water
d. gains and loses water equally

12. Osmosis occurs when a membrane is
a. impermeable
b. differentially permeable (semi or selectively permeable)
c. permeable
d. both a and c

13. The process by which solid particulates such as bacteria are taken up by cells is termed
a. exocytosis
b. phagocytosis
c. pinocytosis
d. osmosis

14. Cells will shrink and show crenation in
a. a hypertonic solution
b. a hypotonic solution
c. an isotonic solution
d. none of the above

15. In which process is liquid forced through a semipermeable membrane or filter from an area of higher pressure into an area of lower pressure?
a. osmosis
b. active transport
c. filtration
d. diffusion

16. During diffusion, a substance always moves from a region
a. outside a cell to the inside of a cell
b. inside a cell to the outside of a cell
c. of higher concentration to a region of lower concentration
d. of lower concentration to a region of higher concentration

17. The separation of small molecules from large ones by diffusion of the smaller molecules through a semipermeable membrane is known as
   a. osmosis
   b. filtration
   c. active transport
   d. dialysis

18. In the body, the proper concentration and distribution of various inorganic salts is referred to as
   a. positive feedback
   b. inorganic equilibrium
   c. ionic stability
   d. electrolyte balance

19. If red blood cells are placed in a hypertonic solution of sodium chloride, what will happen to them?
   a. They will shrink and show crenation
   b. They will swell
   c. They will burst
   d. They will stick together

20. The plasma membrane
   a. is a semipermeable membrane
   b. surrounds the nucleus
   c. contains cellulose
   d. forms and excretes calcium

B. *Matching.* Each of the words or phrases in Column B refers to a term in Column A. Insert the letter of the word or phrase from Column B that best describes each term in Column A. Some words or phrases may be used more than once or not at all.

Column A	*Column B*
1. ___ solute	**a.** parts/volume
2. ___ solvent	**b.** greater to lesser
3. ___ concentration gradient	**c.** kinetic energy
4. ___ homeostasis	**d.** dissolved particle/molecule
5. ___ random movement	**e.** solution or vehicle
	f. relatively stable internal environment

Column A	*Column B*
1. ___ osmosis	**a.** carrier-assisted diffusion
2. ___ diffusion	**b.** energy-assisted transport
3. ___ filtration	**c.** particle/molecule from greater to lesser
4. ___ facilitated transport	**d.** water from a region of greater to lesser water concentration
5. ___ active transport	**e.** forced mechanical separation

C. *True or False.* Place a *T* or an *F* in the space provided to indicate true or false.

___ **1.** During diffusion there is a net movement of substances from low to high concentration of the diffusing substance.

___ **2.** During osmosis there is a net movement of water from the dilute to the more concentrated solution.

___ **3.** Osmosis refers to the scattering or spreading out of molecules.

___ **4.** In active transport, liquid is literally pushed through a semipermeable membrane from an area of higher pressure to an area of lower pressure.

___ **5.** Active transport involves movement of molecules against the concentration gradient.

___ **6.** Molecular size and solubility influence the transfer of molecules.

___ **7.** All the molecules of the same size diffuse through the membrane at the same rate.

___ **8.** The final equilibrium state reached by a molecule undergoing facilitated diffusion is the same as that for a molecule undergoing simple diffusion.

___ **9.** The principle of dialysis is employed in the operation of an artificial kidney.

___ **10.** In osmosis, the molecules of water pass through a membrane in only one direction.

Answer Sheet—Chapter 3

Exercise 3.1

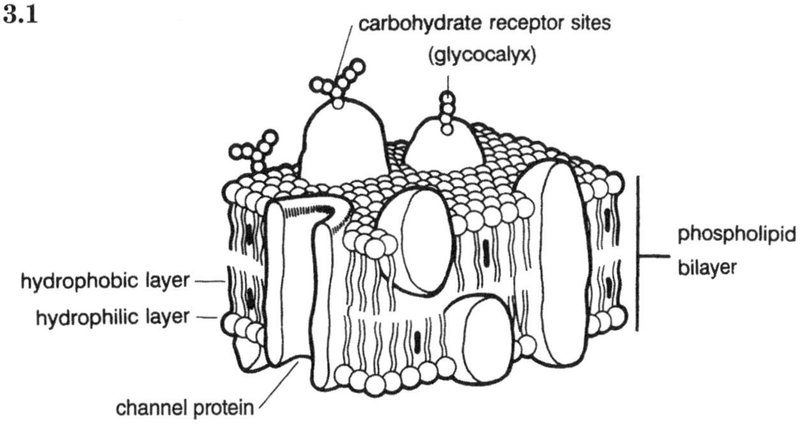

Figure 3.1 Fluid-mosaic model of the cell membrane.

Exercise 3.2

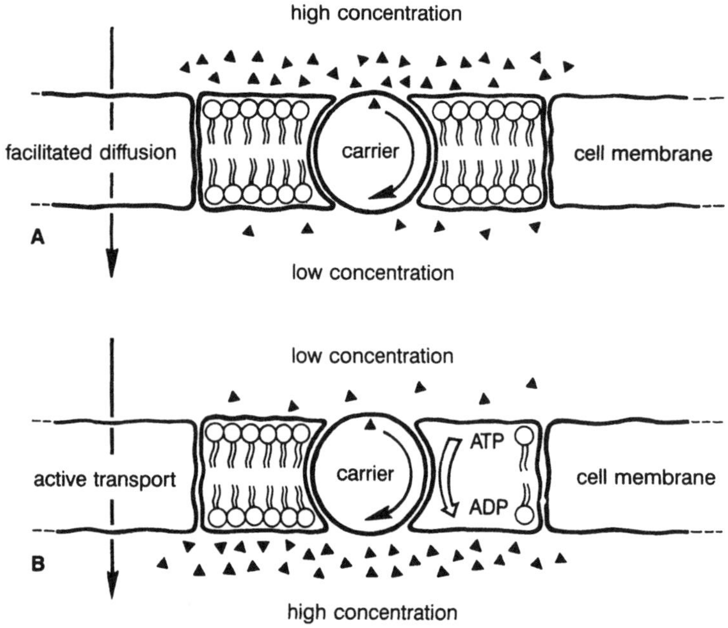

Figure 3.2 Two-carrier molecular system. **A.** Movement of a molecule across the membrane from higher to lower concentration of molecule. **B.** Movement of a molecule across a membrane from low to high concentration of molecule with the expenditure of energy to afford the transport.

Test Items

A. 1. a, 2. c, 3. d, 4. a, 5. d, 6. a, 7. d, 8. c, 9. c, 10. c, 11. b, 12. b, 13. b, 14. a, 15. c, 16. c, 17. a, 18. d, 19. a, 20. a.

B. 1. d, 2. e, 3. a, 4. f, 5. c.
1. d, 2. c, 3. e, 4. a, 5. b.

C. 1. F, 2. T, 3. F, 4. F, 5. T, 6. T, 7. F, 8. T, 9. T, 10. F.

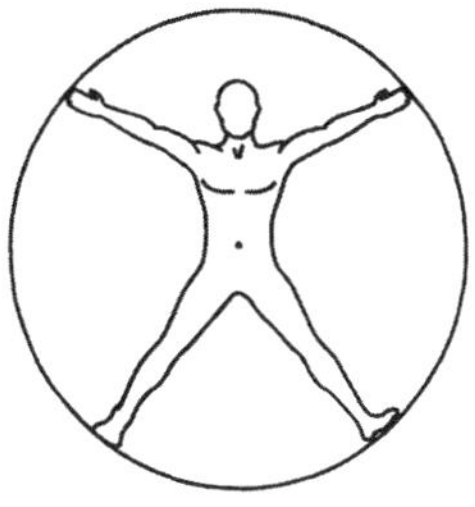

4

The Tissues and Integument

I. CHAPTER SYNOPSIS

The primary concern of this chapter is the organisation of cells into tissues. The structure, function, and location of the principal kinds of epithelial and connective tissues are examined. Throughout, the relationship of structure to function is emphasised. The student is introduced to the organ and the system levels of organisation by considering the structure and functions of the skin and its derivatives.

The integument, or skin, is a vital organ, serving as a protective barrier that responds to both internal and external challenges and contributes to the maintenance of homeostasis. Structurally, the skin is a complex combination of tissues that consists of two layers, the epidermis and dermis. The epidermis, a thin surface layer, is firmly cemented to the dermis, the deeper layer of skin that lies below it. The dermis, in turn, is attached through the subcutaneous tissue or superficial fascia to underlying structures such as bones and muscles. The appendages of the skin (the hair, cutaneous glands, and nails) develop embryologically from epidermal cells that grow down into the dermis. The blood supply to the skin is important in nourishment of the tissue cells and the regulation of body temperature. The nerve supply of the skin involves afferents from cutaneous receptors to the CNS and efferents to smooth muscle. The skin performs the essential functions of protection, temperature regulation, sensation of external stimuli, production of vitamin D, and a minor elimination of water and salts.

II. OBJECTIVES

After reading the chapter, the student should be able to:

- Differentiate between the kinds of epithelial and connective tissues.
- Explain the histological anatomy of the skin and its accessory structures.
- Identify the three types of skin burns with their respective skin strata.
- Detail the steps in wound healing.

III. IMPORTANT TERMS

Using your textbook, define the following terms:

Basement membrane (beys-muh′nt mem-breyn) ______________________________

____

benign (be-nine′) ______________________________

____

cancer (kan′sur) ______________________________

____

carcinoma (kar-si-no′mah) ______________________________

____

collagen (kol′ah-jen) ______________________________

____

connective (kuh-nek′tiv) ______________________________

____

corneum (kor′nee-um) ______________________________

____

dermis (der′mis) ______________________________

____

endocrine (en′do-krine) ______________________________

____

epidermis (epi-der′mis) ______________________________

____

epithelium (epi-the′lee-um) ______________________________

____

exocrine (ek′so-krine) ______________________________

____

gland (gland) ______________________________

____

integument (in-teg′-u-ment) ______________________________

____

keratin (ker′ah-tin) ______________________________

____

lacuna (lah-ku′nah) ______________________________

____

malignant (mah-lig′nant) ______________________________

____

matrix (may′triks) ______________________________

____

melanin (mel′ah-nin) ______________________________

____

neoplasm (neo′-plazm) ______________________________

____

papilla (pah-pil′ah) ______________________________

____

Pseudostratified (soo-doh-strat-uh-fahy) ______________________________

____

sarcoma (sar-ko′mah) ______________________________

____

Simple epithelium (sim-puh′l ep-uh-thee-lee-uh′m) ______________________________

____

Squamous (skwey-muh′s) ______________________________

____

Stratified epithelium (strat-uh-fahy ep-uh-thee-lee-uh′m) ______________________________

____

stratum (stra′tum) ______________________________

____

tissue (tish′u) ______________________________

____

IV. EXERCISES

Complete the following exercises in the order given. A precise set of terms and structures has evolved to describe the cell membrane and integument.

Exercise 4.1

Place the correct terms from the Key list into the appropriate blank space in the text on the right.

Key:
abut
basement
continuous
covers
lines
outside
sheet
stratified

EPITHELIUM

Epithelial tissue is a complex protective layer that ________ the body and ______________ all the cavities and organs having a direct connection to the ________________ of the body. To put it simply, epithelium is a kind of ________________ made up of a series of cells that ______________ each other. Epithelial cells are so closely joined together at these junctions that they form a ________________ barrier between the body parts they cover and the surrounding medium (water, air, or internal body fluids). Epithelial tissue may be composed of only one flat layer of cells, or it may be ____________ into different layers. When examined under a microscope, epithelial cells can be seen to have a supporting ______________ membrane, which appears in prepared sections as a fine line.

Key:
carbon dioxide
exchange
irregular
oxygen
scalelike
shapes
single

Types of Epithelial Tissues

Four distinct types of epithelia occur in the human body. Their classification is based on the ______________ and properties of the cells composing them.

1. *Squamous Epithelium.* Simple squamous epithelium is made up of scalelike flat cells arranged in a __________ layer. The term *squamous* means __________, and the cells of these tissues have __________ shapes like scales. Each cell contains a large, prominent nucleus at its centre. In its simplest form, squamous epithelial tissues line the small saclike structures of the lung (alveoli), which function in the ________ of ________ and __________ during breathing. Since squamous epithelium is thin and flat it is also known as pavement epithelium.

Key:
cube-shaped
glands
kidney
secretions

2. *Cuboidal Epithelium.* As its name suggests, cuboidal epithelium is made up of ______________ cells. This tissue lines the ducts of many ______________ and the tubules of the______________. The nuclei of its cells are spherical and usually are found in the centre of the cell. Some cuboidal cells are capable of forming ________________ and consequently are found in glands such as the thyroid, sweat glands, and salivary glands.

Key:
absorption
basement
columnlike
digestive
secretion
tall

3. *Columnar Epithelium.* Columnar epithelial cells are laterally compressed to form ______________ shapes. These ______________, thin cells have a nucleus that usually can be found near the ______________ membrane. Epithelial tissues made up of these cells occur in the ______________ tract, particularly in the intestines. Columnar epithelium is concerned primarily with the ______________ of digestive fluids and with the ______________ of food materials.

Key:
arranged
bronchi
cilia
currents
digestion
empty
flask
goblet
hairlike
layers
mucoid
mucus
passage
respiratory
shape
surface
tall
trachea
wavelike

4. *Pseudostratified Epithelium.* The fourth type of epithelium earned its name because on first glance it appears to be ______________ in ______________. This appearance is caused by variations in the ______________ of each cell making up the tissue. Although some of the cells in contact with the basement membrane do not reach the ______________ of the tissue, most of the cells are ______________ and do reach the surface. Pseudostratified epithelium is found most often in the ______________ tract, particularly in the ______________ and in the ______________ of the lung.

Two modifications occurring in the walls of epithelial tissues are worth considering here: ______________ cells and ______________. Goblet cells are ______________ shaped and contain ______________ secretion. Microscopically, they appear as open, ______________ cells in their tissues. Cilia are ______________ appendages of the cell. With their continuous ______________ motion, they produce ______________ in the fluids at the cell's surface. Both goblet cells and cilia occur in columnar and pseudostratified epithelium. Goblet cells aid ______________ by secreting ______________ for absorption of partially digested foods. Goblet cells and cilia are also essential in the respiratory tract, where goblet cells add moisture to the air taken in and cilia clean the air of foreign particles that could otherwise clog the alveoli of the lungs. This mechanism is referred to as the mucociliary escalator.

Key:
capillaries
circulatory
directly
endocrine
internal
no
passages

Glands

Some epithelial tissues are made up of cells specifically organised to enable secretion.

______________ glands are sometimes called glands of ______________ secretion because they are situated far beneath the epithelial surface and have ______________ ducts or ______________ by which their secretions can pass through the epithelium. Instead, they communicate ______________ with the ______________ system through the ______________, which permit the distribution of their secretions throughout the body. The thyroid is an example of an endocrine gland.

Key:
duct
ducts
endocrine
enzymes
exocrine
intestine
surface

Like the endocrine glands, ________________ glands are also located away from the epithelial surface. However, the exocrine glands are equipped with ________________ that carry their secretions to the tissue ____________. The salivary glands, for example, are exocrine glands. The pancreas is a gland that is both endocrine and exocrine. It produces digestive ___________ that are passed to the ______________ through the pancreatic ____________ (exocrine); but it also produces a hormone, insulin, which is transported through the body by the circulatory system (______________).

Key:
adjacent
binding
compositions
framework
matrix
physical
protection
separated
storage

CONNECTIVE TISSUES

Connective tissues are found throughout the body. As their name implies, the principal function of these tissues is __________________ the body parts together. They form a ________________ for the internal organs; they also perform a variety of other functions, ranging from ________________ against injury to _______________ of fat.

A fundamental difference between connective tissue and epithelial tissue can be seen in their cellular _______________. Epithelial cells are directly ________________ to one another, separated only by a very small amount of intercellular substance called _______________. On the other hand, connective tissue contains fewer cells, and these are widely ___________. The intercellular matrix is relatively abundant and usually determines the _______________ characteristics of a given connective tissue.

Key:
fibroblasts
fibrocyte
intercellular
lose
mesenchyme

Connective Tissue Cells

In their embryonic stage, typical connective tissue cells are large and star shaped, with many projections called processes. These cells are called __________, and they arise from an early embryonic tissue, the _______________. This tissue develops into many different forms, including blood cells and fat cells (adipocytes). As the connective tissues develop, the cells _____________ their star-shaped appearance and become widely separated by large amounts of ______________ material. The adult connective tissue cell, which is responsible for the formation of fibres, is the ________________. Other types of cells found in connective tissue are:

Key:
antibodies
anticoagulant
bacteria
defense
destroy
foreign
heparin
histamine
inflammatory/allergic
ingesting
phagocytosis
signet
store

1. *Histiocytes or Macrophages.* These cells move about through the connective tissue, ____________ ____________ materials, bacteria, and cellular debris (____________).

2. *Plasma Cells.* These small, irregular cells are associated with the formation of ____________, an important part of the body's ____________ against foreign substances.

3. *Mast Cells.* These are located near the blood vessels and are involved in the production of ____________, an ____________. They are also important in the production of ____________ in ____________ reactions.

4. *Blood Cells.* The white blood cells, such as lymphocytes, monocytes, and neutrophils, are often present in connective tissue, where their function is to ____________ ____________ by phagocytosis.

5. *Fat Cells (adipocytes).* These specialised cells ____________ fats and oils. Microscopically, a fat cell resembles a ____________ ring because the stored fat pushes the nucleus and the cytoplasm to one side of the cell.

Key:
bone
cartilage
cobweb
collagen
collagenous
elastic
elastic
fibres
glands
intercellular
ligaments
nonelastic
reticular
reticulum
yellow

Connective Tissue Fibres

The ____________ characteristic of connective tissue are found within the ____________ matrix. There are three general types:

1. ____________ fibres. These white fibres contain ____________, the principal structural protein of the body. This protein is synthesised by fibrocytes and is a major constituent of skin, ____________, ____________, and ____________. The fibres occur in bundles and are relatively nonelastic.

2. ____________ fibres. These fibres are ____________ and may occur singly or in bundles. They are highly ____________ and branch to unite with other fibres. Elastic fibres are both larger and straighter than collagenous fibres.

3. ____________ fibres. These short and very thin fibres branch freely, forming a ____________ network called a ____________. These fibres are ____________ and are usually found forming the internal framework of ____________.

Key:

adipose
areolar
fat
heat
insulate
loosely
padding
reserve
supply

Types of Connective Tissue

1. *Adipose Tissue.* __________ tissue beneath the dermis is commonly filled with __________ packed __________ cells held together in bundles by collagenous and elastic fibres. __________ (fat) tissue is found primarily as a kind of __________ around the joints, as soft pads between the organs, around the kidney and the heart, and in the yellow marrow of long bones. Its fat cells provide a __________ food __________ and also __________ the body against __________ loss.

Key:

aponeuroses
bones
cover
enclose
fascia
ligaments
muscle
muscles
restrain
separate
stronger
tendons

2. *Dense Connective Tissue.* Many parts of the body require a __________ type of connective tissue to __________, __________, or __________ functioning structures.

The basic forms of dense connective tissue are __________, which attach __________ to bone; __________, which connect the __________ that form joints; __________, which are thin, tendinous sheets attached to flat __________; and __________, the thin sheets of tissue that __________ muscles and hold them in place.

Key:

capsules
chondrocytes
covers
elastic
fibrous
hyaline
intervertebral
lacunae
modified
move
reinforces
rigid
skeletal template

3. *Cartilage.* Cartilage is a __________ form of connective tissue in which cartilage cells (__________) lie in small __________, the __________, which are surrounded by an irregular matrix made up of fibres and/or a gel.

__________ cartilage, the most common form of cartilage has a white or glossy appearance. It may contain any number of unevenly dispersed lacunae. Hyaline cartilage forms the __________ in the embryo and __________ the articulating surfaces of bones in the joint cavities. It also provides the structure for the nose and the connections of the ribs to the breastbone and, in the respiratory tract, forms the ring-like trachea and bronchi.

__________ cartilage contains many elastic fibres and is found wherever cartilage is required to __________, such as in the epiglottis and the auricle (pinna) of the external ear.

__________ cartilage is less __________ than hyaline, but contains heavy bundles of collagen fibres. It is found in the __________ disks, which absorb shocks between the vertebrae of the backbone. Fibrous cartilage also __________ the hyaline articular cartilages at the knee and hip.

Exercise 4.2

Labelling. Write the name of the structure of each numbered part of the skin on the line provided. Colour the different layers of the epidermis and dermis to highlight their structures.

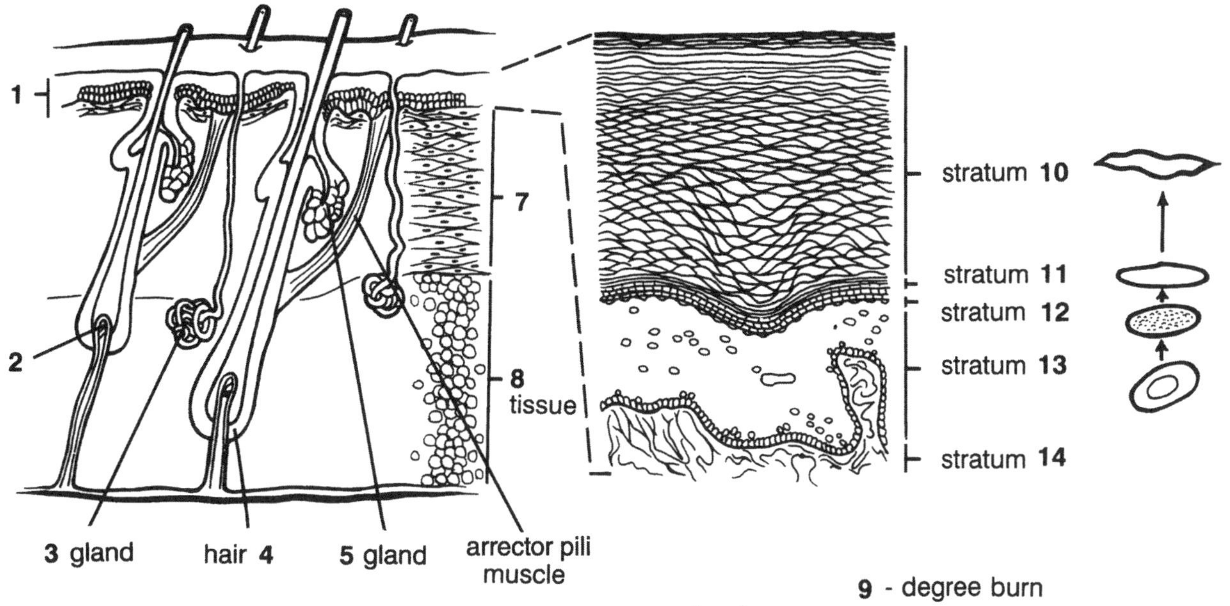

Key:

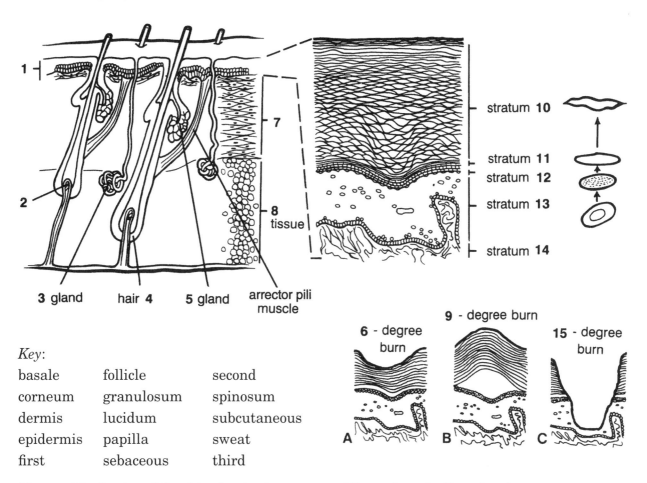

basale	follicle	second
corneum	granulosum	spinosum
dermis	lucidum	subcutaneous
epidermis	papilla	sweat
first	sebaceous	third

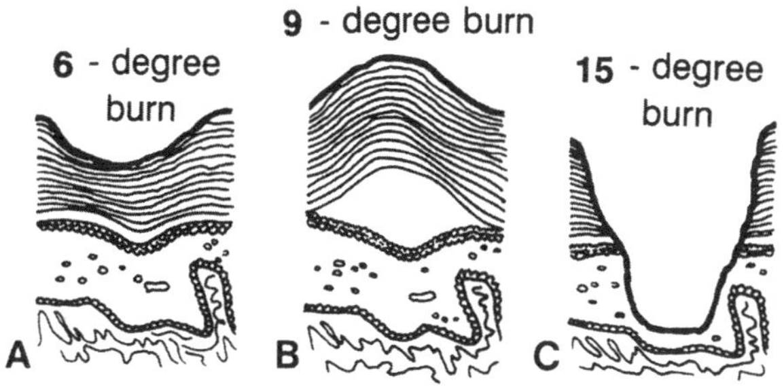

Figure 4.2 Section of the skin showing its structure. The nucleated cell produced by the stratum basale dies (granulates) as it is forced outward to become the dead, scaly stratum corneum. The number of layers of the epidermis affected by the three types of skin burns is also shown. **A.** Only corneum cells are involved in first-degree burns. **B.** Damage to the upper three layers occurs in second-degree burns, forming a blister between layers 3 and 4. **C.** A third-degree burn involves all epidermal layers and, therefore, usually requires a skin graft to replace the stratum basale.

1. ______________________
2. ______________________
3. ______________________
4. ______________________
5. ______________________
6. ______________________
7. ______________________
8. ______________________
9. ______________________
10. ______________________
11. ______________________
12. ______________________
13. ______________________
14. ______________________
15. ______________________

V. TEST ITEMS

A. *Multiple Choice.* There is only one answer that is either correct or most appropriate. Circle the best answer for each question.

1. Mucous membranes are located
- a. in joint cavities
- b. covering the heart
- c. lining the stomach
- d. covering the brain

2. The most external skin region is composed of
- a. simple columnar epithelium
- b. stratified squamous epithelium
- c. areolar connective tissue
- d. dense fibrous connective tissue

3. Skin colour is determined by
- a. amount of melanin in the skin
- b. pigments in the epidermis (melanin)
- c. the amount of keratin in the dermis
- d. the size of the blood vessels

4. The basal layer of the epidermis rests upon which membranous tissue?
- a. basilar membrane
- b. perineal membrane
- c. basement membrane
- d. reticular membrane

5. The ridges which make up finger, foot, and palm prints have their origin in which skin layer?
- a. dermis
- b. epidermis
- c. subcutaneous tissue
- d. deep fascia

6. Which tissue layer is rich in fat cells (adipocytes)?
- a. dermis
- b. epidermis
- c. subcutaneous layer (hypodermis)
- d. deep fascia

7. Which of the following represents the outer nonvascular layer of the skin?
- a. epidermis
- b. dermis
- c. fascia
- d. corium

8. Which cellular layer (stratum) of the epidermis is the only one capable of producing new cells?
- a. stratum corneum
- b. stratum lucidum
- c. stratum basale
- d. stratum granulosum

9. Which of the following constitutes a function of the skin?
- a. producing antibodies
- b. regulating body temperature
- c. integrating sensory activity
- d. producing haemoglobin

10. A melanoma is a malignant tumour that develops in the
a. skin
b. cartilage
c. muscle
d. epithelium

11. Cilia are
a. found in all epithelial structures
b. hairlike structures that move
c. hollow
d. secretory in function

12. A group of one or more cell types that work together for a common purpose is termed a (an)
a. organ
b. organism
c. tissue
d. system

13. Inadequate blood supply to the skin can cause
a. herpes
b. tanning
c. infections
d. ulcers

14. Which glands located adjacent to hair follicles secrete an oily substance functioning to keep the hair and skin soft and pliable?
a. sudoriferous glands
b. sebaceous glands
c. suprarenal glands
d. serous glands

15. The most abundant and strongest fibre in connective tissue is
a. reticular
b. collagen
c. elastic
d. spindle

16. Sebaceous glands are important for
a. production of keratin
b. keeping skin and hair soft
c. production of sweat
d. heat regulation of the body

17. The rule of nines is helpful clinically in
a. diagnosing skin cancer
b. estimating the extent of a burn
c. preventing acne
d. determining ulcers

18. What is the function of ligaments?
a. connect muscle to muscle
b. cover the ends of bones
c. connect muscle to bone
d. connect bone to bone

19. Glands, such as the thyroid, that secrete their products directly into the blood are classified as
a. exocrine
b. endocrine
c. sebaceous
d. ceruminous

20. Joe burned himself on a hot pipe. A blister formed. Joe's burn is likely a
a. first-degree burn
b. second-degree burn
c. third-degree burn
d. sunburn

B. *Matching.* Each of the words or phrases in Column B refers to a term in Column A. Insert the letter of the word or phrase from Column B that best describes each term in Column A. Some words may be used more than once or not at all.

Column A	*Column B*
1. ___ areolar connective tissue	a. lining of urinary bladder
2. ___ ciliated columnar epithelium	b. pleura (pleural membranes)
3. ___ fibrocartilage	c. beneath the skin, between muscles, underneath epithelial cells
4. ___ fibrous white connective tissue	d. framework of ear and epiglottis
5. ___ elastic cartilage	e. tendons and ligaments
6. ___ hyaline cartilage	f. ends of bones and tracheal rings
7. ___ irregular dense connective tissue	g. between vertebrae
8. ___ transitional epithelium	h. fallopian tubes
9. ___ squamous epithelium	i. dermis of the skin

Column A	*Column B*
1. ___ polyp	a. lack of skin pigment
2. ___ melanoma	b. under the skin
3. ___ albinism	c. under the epidermis
4. ___ subcutaneous	d. mucous membrane tumour
5. ___ dermis	e. corneum
	f. malignant skin tumour

C. *True or False.* Place a *T* or an *F* in the space provided to indicate true or false.

___ **1.** The colour of skin is due to the presence of a pigment called keratin.

___ **2.** Sweat glands of the skin are a type of simple coiled tubular gland.

___ **3.** Goblet cells are single-celled glands found in certain connective tissues.

___ **4.** The classification of epithelial tissues is based upon the shape and arrangement of cells.

___ **5.** Epithelial tissue can be distinguished from most connective tissue by sparseness of intercellular materials.

___ **6.** Cancer arises as a result of abnormal uncontrolled cell division.

___ **7.** Epithelial tissue has a rich blood supply.

___ **8.** A good example of elastic cartilage is found in the auricle (pinna) of the external ear.

___ **9.** All of the cells of the outer layer (stratum corneum) of the skin are dead.

___ **10.** A basement membrane seats or anchors epithelial tissue to underlying connective tissue.

Answer Sheet—Chapter 4

Exercise 4.1

EPITHELIUM

Epithelial tissue is a complex protective layer that covers the body and lines all cavities and organs having a direct connection to the outside of the body. To put it simply, epithelium is a kind of sheet made up of a series of cells that abut each other. Epithelial cells are so closely joined together at these junctions that they form a continuous barrier between the body parts they cover and the surrounding medium (water, air, or internal body fluids). Epithelial tissue may be composed of only one flat layer of cells, or it may be stratified into different layers. When examined under a microscope, epithelial cells can be seen to have a supporting basement membrane, which appears in prepared sections as a fine line.

Types of Epithelial Tissue

Four distinct types of epithelia occur in the human body. Their classification is based on the shapes and properties of the cells composing them.

1. *Squamous Epithelium.* Simple squamous epithelium is made up of scalelike flat cells arranged in a single layer. The term *squamous* means scalelike, and the cells of these tissues have irregular shapes like scales. Each cell contains a large, prominent nucleus at its centre. In its simplest form, squamous epithelial tissues line the small saclike structures of the lung (alveoli), which function in the exchange of oxygen and carbon dioxide during breathing.

2. *Cuboidal Epithelium.* As its name suggests, cuboidal epithelium is made up of cube-shaped cells. This tissue lines the ducts of many glands and the tubules of the kidney. The nuclei of its cells are spherical and usually are found in the centre of the cell. Some cuboidal cells are capable of forming secretions and consequently are found in glands such as thyroid, sweat glands, and salivary glands.

3. *Columnar Epithelium.* Columnar epithelial cells are laterally compressed to form column-like shapes. These tall, thin cells have a nucleus that usually can be found near the basement membrane. Epithelial tissues made up of these cells occur in the digestive tract, particularly in the intestine. Columnar epithelium is concerned primarily with the secretion of digestive fluids and with the absorption of food materials.

4. *Pseudostratified Epithelium.* The fourth type of epithelium earned its name because on first glance it appears to be arranged in layers. This appearance is caused by variations in the shape of each cell making up the tissue. Although some of the cells in contact with the basement membrane do not reach the surface of the tissue, most of the cells are tall and do reach the surface. Pseudostratified epithelium is found most often in the respiratory tract, particularly in the trachea and in the bronchi of the lung.

Two modifications occurring in the walls of epithelial tissues are worth considering here: goblet cells and cilia. Goblet cells are flask shaped and contain mucoid secretion. Microscopically, they appear as open, empty cells in their tissues. Cilia are hairlike appendages of the cell. With their continuous wavelike motion, they produce currents in the fluids at the cell's surface. Both goblet cells and cilia occur in columnar and pseudostratified epithelium. Goblet cells aid digestion by secreting mucus for absorption of partially digested foods. Goblet cells and cilia are also essential in the respiratory tract, where goblet cells add moisture to the air taken in and cilia clean the air of foreign particles that could otherwise clog the alveoli of the lungs. This mechanism is referred to as the mucociliary escalator.

Glands

Some epithelial tissues are made up of cells specifically organised to enable secretion. Endocrine glands are sometimes called glands of internal secretion because they are situated far beneath the epithelial surface and have no ducts or passages by which their secretions can pass through the epithelium. Instead, they communicate directly with the circulatory system through the capillaries, which permit the distribution of their secretions throughout the body. The thyroid is an example of an endocrine gland.

Like the endocrine glands, exocrine glands are also located away from the epithelial surface. However, the exocrine glands are equipped with ducts that carry their secretions to the tissue surface. The salivary glands, for example, are exocrine glands. The pancreas is a gland that is both endocrine and exocrine. It produces digestive enzymes that are passed to the intestine through the pancreatic duct (exocrine); but it also produces a hormone, insulin, which is transported through the body by the circulatory system (endocrine).

CONNECTIVE TISSUES

Connective tissues are found throughout the body. As their name implies, the principal function of these tissues is binding the body parts together. They form a framework for the internal organs; they also perform a variety of other functions, ranging from protection against injury to storage of fat.

A fundamental difference between connective tissue and epithelial tissue can be seen in their cellular compositions. Epithelial cells are directly adjacent to one another, separated only by a very small amount of intercellular substance called matrix. On the other hand, connective tissue contains fewer cells, and these are widely separated. The intercellular matrix is relatively abundant and usually determines the physical characteristics of a given connective tissue.

Connective Tissue Cells

In their embryonic stage, typical connective tissue cells are large and star shaped, with many projections called processes. These cells are called fibroblasts, and they arise from an early embryonic tissue, the mesenchyme. This tissue develops into many different forms, including blood cells and fat cells (adipocytes). As the connective tissues develop, the cells lose their star-shaped appearance and become widely separated by large amounts of intercellular material. The adult connective tissue cell, which is responsible for the formation of fibres, is the fibrocyte. Other types of cells found in connective tissue are:

1. *Histiocytes or Macrophages.* These cells move about through the connective tissue, ingesting foreign materials, bacteria, and cellular debris (phagocytosis).

2. *Plasma Cells.* These small, irregular cells are associated with the formation of antibodies, an important part of the body's defense against foreign substances.

3. *Mast Cells.* These are located near the blood vessels and are involved in the production of heparin, an anticoagulant. They are also important in the production of histamine in inflammatory/allergic reactions.

4. *Blood Cells.* The white blood cells, such as lymphocytes, monocytes, and neutrophils, are often present in connective tissue, where their function is to destroy bacteria by phagocytosis.

5. *Fat Cells (adipocytes).* These specialised cells store fats and oils. Microscopically, a fat cell resembles a signet ring because the stored fat pushes the nucleus and cytoplasm to one side of the cell.

Connective Tissue Fibres

The fibres characteristic of connective tissue are found within the intercellular matrix. There are three general types:

1. Collagenous fibres. These white fibres contain collagen, the principal structural protein of the body. This protein is synthesised by fibrocytes and is a major constituent of skin, ligaments, cartilage, and bone. The fibres occur in bundles and are relatively nonelastic.

2. Elastic fibres. These fibres are yellow and may occur singly or in bundles. They are highly elastic and branch to unite with other fibres. Elastic fibres are both larger and straighter than collagenous fibres.

3. Reticular fibres. These short and very thin fibres branch freely, forming a cobweb network called a reticulum. These fibres are nonelastic and are usually found forming the internal framework of glands.

Types of Connective Tissue

1. *Adipose Tissue.* Areolar tissue beneath the dermis is commonly filled with loosely packed fat cells and held together in bundles by collagenous and elastic fibres. Adipose (fat) tissue is found primarily as a kind of padding around the joints, as soft pads between the organs, around the kidney and heart, and in the yellow marrow of long bones. Its fat cells provide a reserve food supply and also insulate the body against heat loss.

2. *Dense Connective Tissue.* Many parts of the body require a stronger type of connective tissue to enclose, restrain, or separate functioning structures. The basic forms of dense connective tissue are tendons, which attach muscle to bone; ligaments, which connect the bones that form joints; aponeuroses, which are thin, tendinous sheets attached to flat muscles; and fascia, the thin sheets of tissue that cover muscles and hold them in place.

3. *Cartilage.* Cartilage is a modified form of connective tissue in which cartilage cells (chondrocytes) lie in small capsules, the lacunae, which are surrounded by an irregular matrix made up of fibres and/or a gel.

Hyaline cartilage, the most common form of cartilage has a white or glassy appearance. It may contain any number of unevenly dispersed lacunae. Hyaline cartilage forms the skeletal template in the embryo and covers the articulating surfaces of bones in the joint cavities. It also provides the structure for the nose and the connections of the ribs to the breastbone and, in the respiratory tract, forms the ringlike trachea and bronchi.

Elastic cartilage contains many elastic fibres and is found wherever cartilage is required to move, such as in the epiglottis and the auricle (pinna) of external ear. Fibrous cartilage is less rigid than hyaline, but contains heavy bundles of collagen fibres. It is found in the intervertebral disks, which absorb shocks between the vertebrae of the backbone. Fibrous cartilage also reinforces the hyaline articular cartilages at the knee and hip.

Exercise 4.2

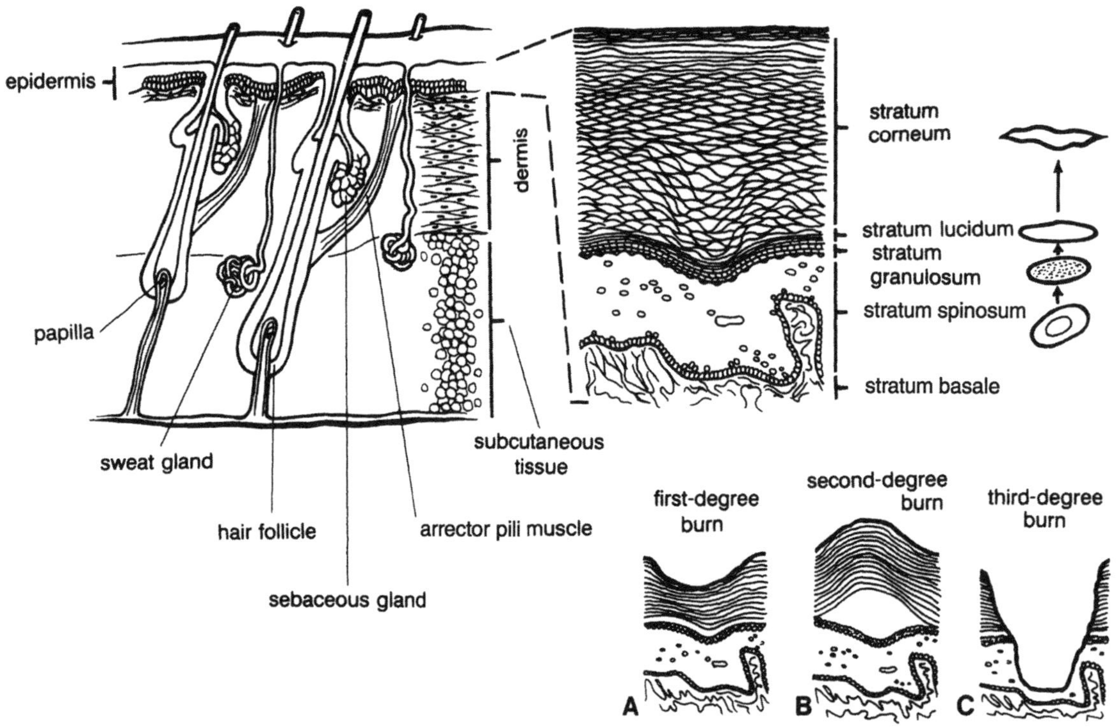

Figure 4.2 Section of the skin showing its structure. The nucleated cell produced by the stratum basale dies (granulates) as it is forced outward to become the dead, scaly stratum corneum. The number of layers of the epidermis affected by the three types of skin burns is also shown. **A.** Only corneum cells are involved in first-degree burns. **B.** Damage to the upper three layers occurs in second-degree burns, forming a blister between layers 3 and 4. **C.** A third-degree burn involves all epidermal layers and, therefore, usually requires a skin graft to replace the stratum basale.

Test Items

A. 1. c, 2. b, 3. c, 4. c, 5. b, 6. c, 7. a, 8. c, 9. b, 10. a, 11. b, 12. c, 13. d, 14. b, 15. b, 16. b, 17. b, 18. d, 19. b, 20. b.

B. 1. c, 2. h, 3. g, 4. e, 5. d, 6. f, 7. i, 8. a, 9. b.
1. d, 2. f, 3. a, 4. b, 5. c.

C. 1. F, 2. T, 3. F, 4. T, 5. T, 6. T, 7. F, 8. T, 9. T, 10. T.

5

The Skeletal System

I. CHAPTER SYNOPSIS

This chapter considers the major functions of the skeletal system, the histology of bone, intramembranous and endochondral ossification, and bone deposition and reabsorption as an example of the homeostasis of bone.

The student is introduced to the four principal kinds of bones, important bone markings, and the bones of the axial and appendicular skeletons.

The chapter includes a glossary of medical terminology associated with the skeletal system.

II. OBJECTIVES

After reading the chapter, the student should be able to:

- List the functions of the skeletal system.
- Describe the nature of red and yellow bone marrow.
- Describe the microscopic structure and composition of bone.
- Describe the gross anatomy of long and flat bones.
- Distinguish between the axial skeleton and the appendicular skeleton and name the components of each.
- Identify the bones that make up the pectoral and pelvic girdle.

III. IMPORTANT TERMS

Using your textbook, define the following terms:

appendicular (ap-en-dik′yoo-lur) ______________________

____

atlas (at′lus) ______________________

____

axial (ak′see-al) ______________________

____

axis (ak′sis) ______________________

____

calcification (kal-si-fi-kay′shun) ______________________

____

canal (can-ale) ______________________

____

cancellous (kan′se-lus) ______________________

____

cervical (ser′vi-kal) ______________________

____

compact (kom′-pakt) ______________________

____

diaphysis (di-af′i-sis) ______________________

____

epiphysis (e-pif′i-sis) ______________________

____

foramen (fo-ray′men) ______________________

____

fossa (fos′ah) ______________________

____

fracture (frak′shur) ______________________

____

lumbar (lum′bar) ______________________

____

ossification (osi-fi-kay′shun) ________________________________

____

osteocyte (os′tee-o-sight) ________________________________

____

periosteum (per-ee-os′tee-um) ________________________________

____

process (pro′sess) ________________________________

____

sesamoid (ses′ah-moid) ________________________________

____

spine (spine) ________________________________

____

suture (soo′cher) ________________________________

____

thoracic (tho-ras′ik) ________________________________

____

trabeculae (trah-bek′u-lah) ________________________________

____

vertebra (vur′te-bruh) ________________________________

____

IV. EXERCISES

Complete the following exercises in the order given. A precise set of terms and diagrams has been chosen to describe the skeletal system.

Exercise 5.1

Labelling. Write the name of the bone in the space provided. Colour the axial skeleton different from the appendicular skeleton.

Key:

carpal	ischium	ribs
clavicle	metacarpal	scapula
cranium	metacarpal	sternum
femur	patella	tarsals
fibula	phalanges	tibia
humerus	pubis	ulna
ilium	radius	vertebrae

1. ______________________
2. ______________________
3. ______________________
4. ______________________
5. ______________________
6. ______________________
7. ______________________
8. ______________________
9. ______________________
10. ______________________
11. ______________________
12. ______________________
13. ______________________
14. ______________________
15. ______________________
16. ______________________
17. ______________________
18. ______________________
19. ______________________
20. ______________________
21. ______________________

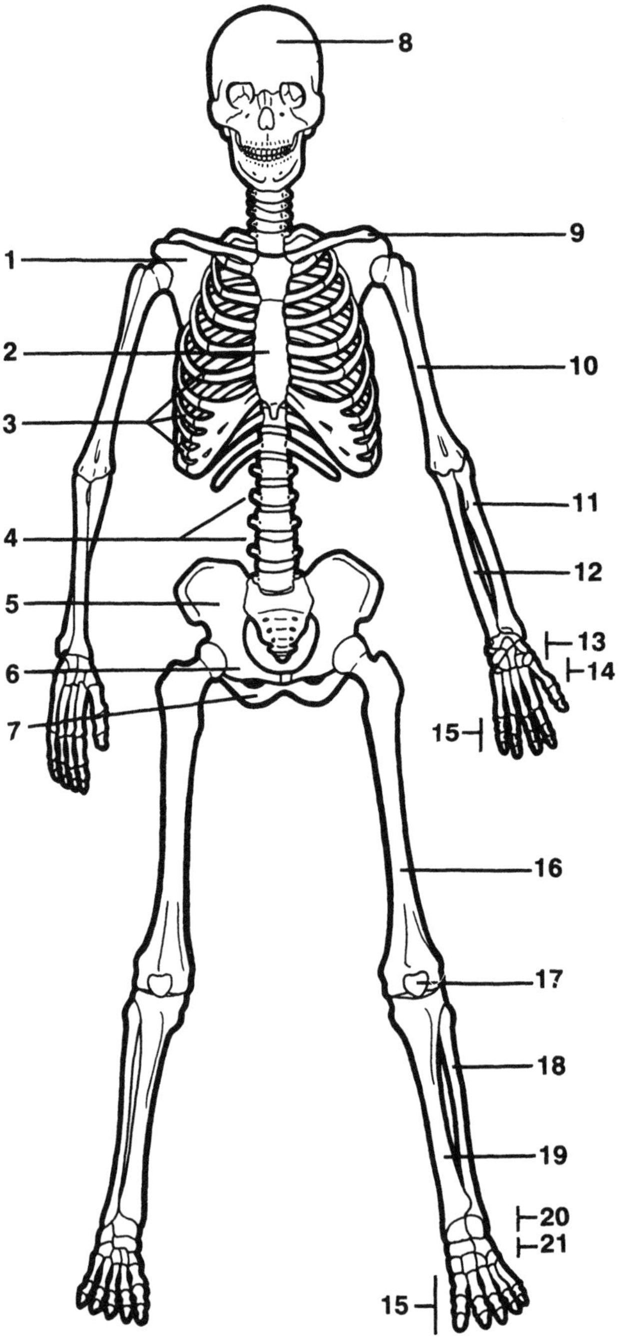

Figure 5.1 Human skeleton, anterior aspect.

Exercise 5.2

Labelling. Write the name of the structure of the bone in the space provided. Colour the total bone different from the canal network.

Key:
blood vessel
cancellous bone (spongy bone)
compact bone
diaphysis
distal epiphysis
epiphyseal line
Haversian canal
Haversian system
marrow
medullary cavity
periosteum
trabeculae
Volkmann's canal

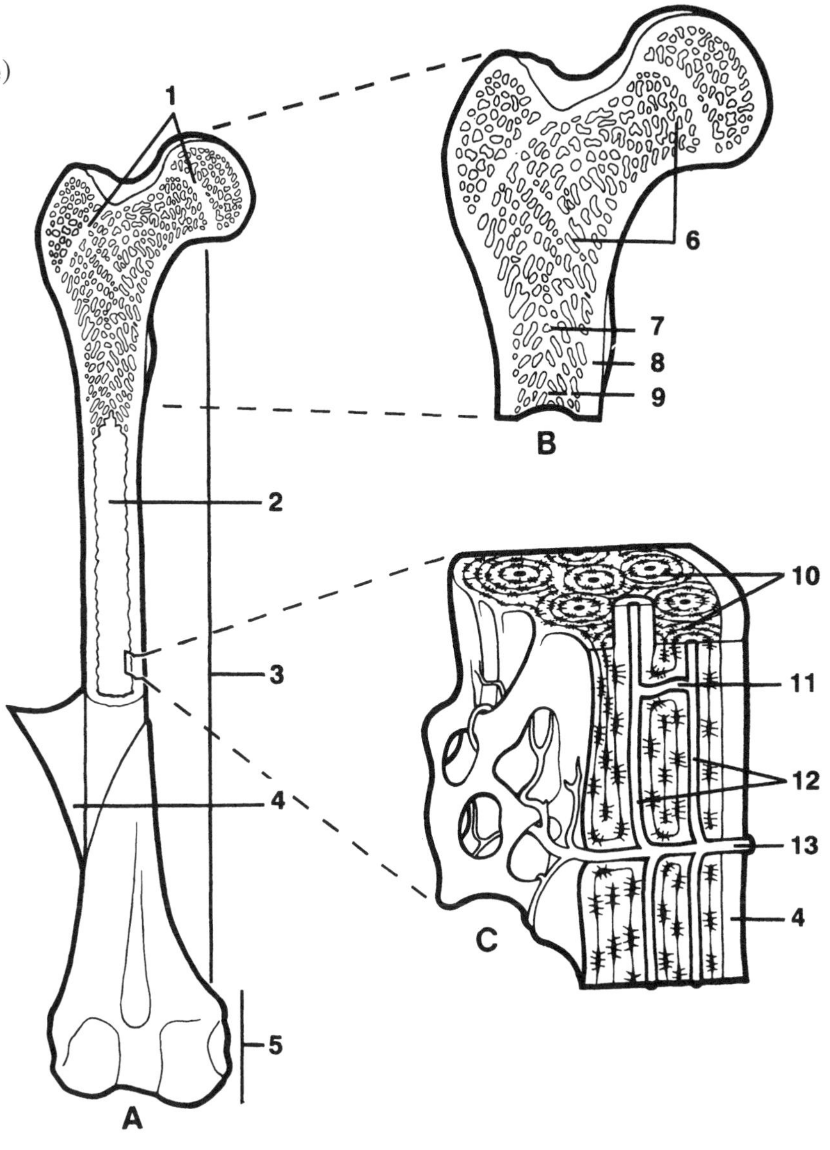

Figure 5.2 Schematic diagram of the structure of a typical long bone.
A. Longitudinal section.
B. Epiphyseal section.
C. Diaphyseal section.

1. ______________________
2. ______________________
3. ______________________
4. ______________________
5. ______________________
6. ______________________
7. ______________________
8. ______________________
9. ______________________
10. ______________________
11. ______________________
12. ______________________
13. ______________________

Exercise 5.3

Labelling. Write the name of the bone and its structures in the spaces provided. Colour each bone differently.

Key:
coronal structure
ethmoid
frontal
infraorbital foramen
mandible
mastoid process
maxillae
mental foramen
nasal
nasal conchae
optic foramen
parietal
sphenoid
squamous suture
temporal
vomer
zygomatic

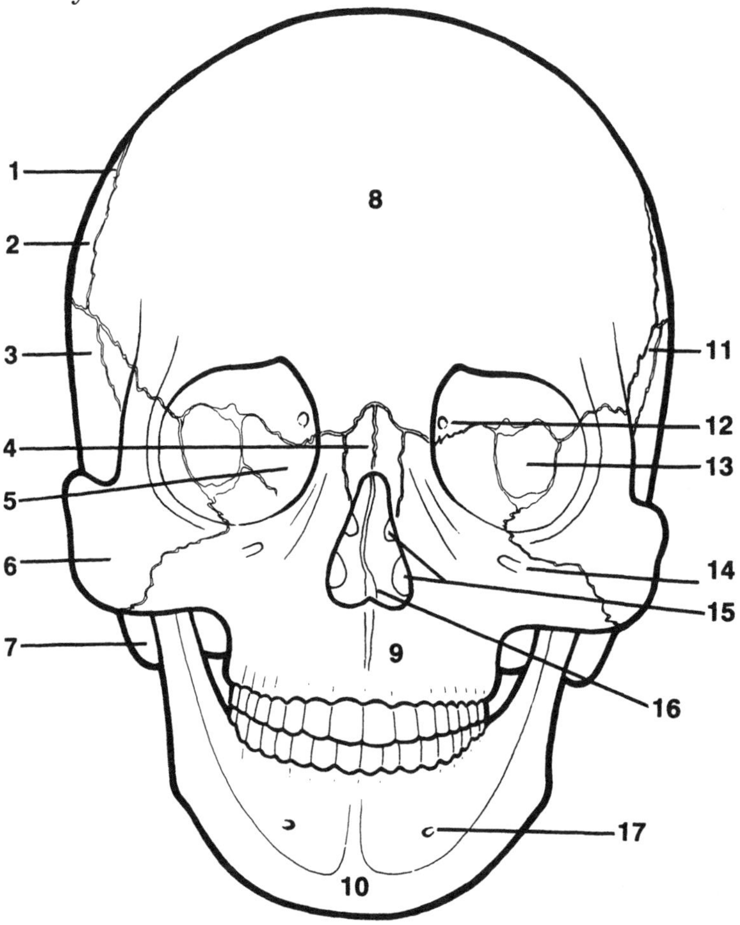

Figure 5.3 Frontal, lacrimal, zygomatic, maxillary, and nasal bones of the skull.

1. ______________________
2. ______________________
3. ______________________
4. ______________________
5. ______________________
6. ______________________
7. ______________________
8. ______________________
9. ______________________
10. ______________________
11. ______________________
12. ______________________
13. ______________________
14. ______________________
15. ______________________
16. ______________________
17. ______________________

Exercise 5.4

Labelling. Write the name of the bone and its structures in the spaces provided. Colour code this exercise with the frontal view (Exercise 5.3).

Key:
acoustic meatus
coronal suture
ethmoid
frontal
lacrimal
lacrimal fossa
lambdoid suture
mandible
mastoid process
maxilla
mental foramen
nasal
occipital
parietal
sphenoid
squamous suture
styloid process
temporal
zygomatic arch
zygomatic bone

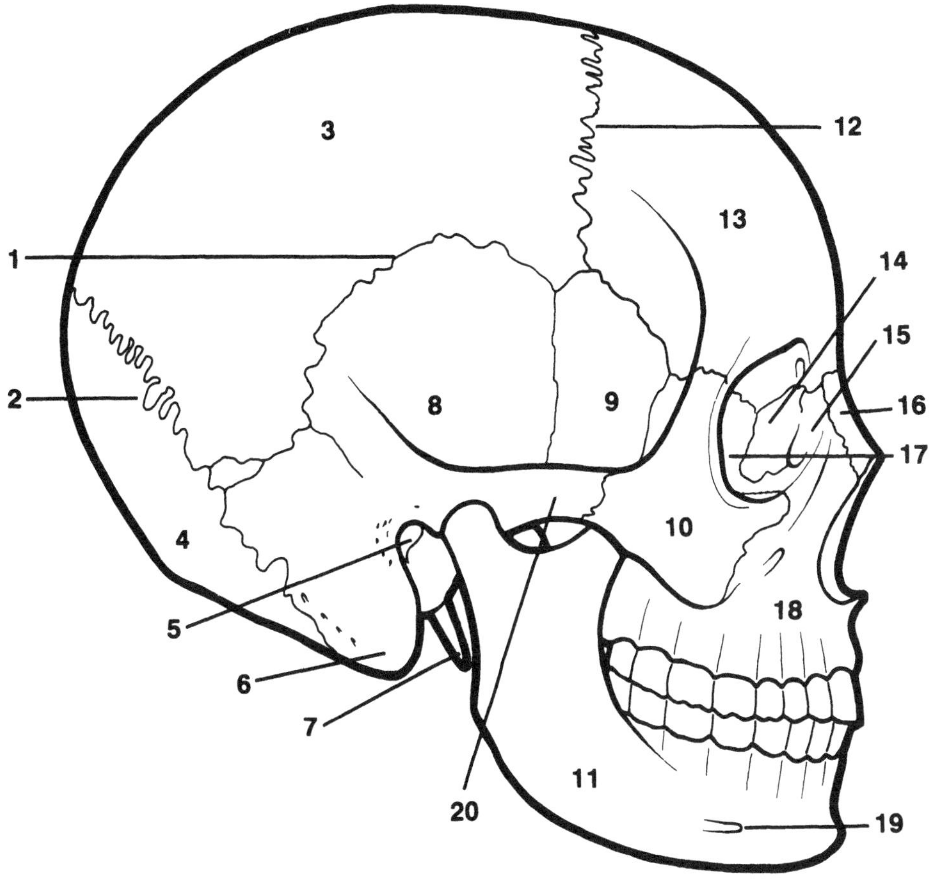

Figure 5.4 Skull, lateral aspect.

1. ______________________
2. ______________________
3. ______________________
4. ______________________
5. ______________________
6. ______________________
7. ______________________
8. ______________________
9. ______________________
10. ______________________
11. ______________________
12. ______________________
13. ______________________
14. ______________________
15. ______________________
16. ______________________
17. ______________________
18. ______________________
19. ______________________
20. ______________________

V. TEST ITEMS

A. *Multiple Choice.* There is only one answer that is either correct or most appropriate. Circle the best answer for each question.

1. Which one of the following is a bone-reabsorbing or -digesting cell?
   a. osteocyte
   b. osteoclast
   c. osteoblast
   d. bone cell

2. The major mineral component of human bone is
   a. calcium carbonate
   b. calcium hydroxide
   c. calcium phosphate
   d. calcium carbide

3. Yellow bone marrow is largely composed of
   a. blood
   b. cartilage
   c. collagen
   d. fat (adipose tissue)

4. A person with a fractured patella has sustained a break in which type of bone?
   a. short
   b. long
   c. sesamoid
   d. sutural

5. A vitamin D deficiency in an adult results in a condition called
   a. osteosarcoma
   b. osteomyelitis
   c. osteoma
   d. osteomalacia

6. The death of osseous tissue from the deprivation of blood supply is called
   a. osteomyelitis
   b. osteoarthritis
   c. necrosis
   d. osteoblastoma

7. The epiphyses of long bones are covered by
   a. periosteum
   b. endosteum
   c. Volkmann's canals
   d. articular cartilage

8. In adults the epiphysis of a typical long bone contains
   a. yellow bone marrow
   b. plasma
   c. red bone marrow
   d. serum

9. If you are told that a patient has a Pott's fracture, you know immediately that the bone involved is either the distal tibia or which other bone?
   a. humerus
   b. radius
   c. femur
   d. fibula

10. A patient with a lateral curvature of the spine to the left would have which of the following conditions?
   a. scoliosis
   b. kyphosis
   c. lordosis
   d. hunchback

11. Severe pain behind the external auditory meatus most likely involves the
    a. sphenoid bone
    b. mastoid process
    c. parietal bone
    d. zygomatic arch

12. A child exhibits the following symptoms: degeneration of epiphyseal cartilage, poor calcification, bowlegs, and malformations of the head and pelvic bones. It is likely that the individual is suffering from
    a. osteoporosis
    b. rickets
    c. osteomyelitis
    d. bone cancer

13. The remodeling of bone is a function of which cells?
    a. chondrocytes and osteocytes
    b. osteoblasts and osteocytes
    c. osteoblasts and osteoclasts
    d. chondroblasts and osteoclasts

14. A disorder of bones closely related to decreased activity of osteoblasts due to a hormone deficiency is
    a. osteomyelitis
    b. osteoporosis
    c. osteosarcoma
    d. osteomalacia

15. The growth of a long bone in length occurs at the
    a. epiphyseal plate
    b. articular cartilage
    c. medial diaphysis
    d. centre of the shaft

16. An incomplete fracture in which one side of the bone is broken and the other side bends is called
    a. comminuted
    b. transverse
    c. spiral
    d. greenstick

17. A Colles' fracture involves the
    a. radius
    b. tibia
    c. fibula
    d. femur

18. A compound fracture means
    a. the bone is fractured in several places
    b. the bone is splintered into several small fragments
    c. the broken end or ends of the bone protrude through the skin
    d. the broken ends of the bone are driven into each other

19. Lack of dietary calcium can result in
    a. heart disease
    b. thyroid disease
    c. stones
    d. osteoporosis

20. Metacarpal bones form the framework of the
    a. wrist
    b. ankle
    c. hand
    d. foot

B. *Matching.* Each of the phrases in Column B refers to a term in Column A. Insert the letter of the phrase from Column B that best describes each term in Column A. Some words may be used more than once or not at all.

Column A

1. ___ fossa

2. ___ tubercle

3. ___ spine

4. ___ foramen

5. ___ head

6. ___ crest

7. ___ condyle

8. ___ paranasal sinus

9. ___ meatus

10. ___ tuberosity

11. ___ groove

12. ___ trochanter

Column B

a. a rounded opening through which blood vessels, nerves, and ligaments pass

b. a prominent border or ridge on a bone

c. an air-filled cavity within a bone connected to the nasal cavity

d. a small, rounded process

e. a large, rounded, usually roughened process

f. a rounded projection supported on a neck

g. a sharp, slender process

h. a depression or hollow in or on a bone

i. a relatively large, convex knucklelike prominence

j. a very large, blunt projection found only on the femur

k. a tubelike passageway running within a bone

l. a furrow that accommodates soft tissues such as blood vessels, nerves, or tendons

C. *True or False.* Place a *T* or an *F* in the space provided to indicate true or false.

___ **1.** The flat bones of the skull develop via intramembranous ossification.

___ **2.** Lamellae are found only in cancellous bone.

___ **3.** The small passages connecting the lacunae are termed *Haversian canals*.

___ **4.** The spaces in cancellous bone are filled with red bone marrow.

___ **5.** Red bone marrow manufactures both white and red blood cells.

___ **6.** The greatest concentration of calcium in the body is in the blood.

___ **7.** Long bones are larger versions of short bones.

___ **8.** The humerus is an example of a long bone.

___ **9.** The styloid process is part of the ethmoid bone.

___ **10.** The three types of movable vertebrae are cervical, thoracic, and lumbar.

___ **11.** The axis is the second thoracic vertebra.

___ **12.** Hollowing of a bone is brought about by the action of osteoclasts.

___ **13.** In intramembranous bone formation, a scale model of hyaline cartilage is replaced by bone.

___ **14.** The sagittal suture joins the parietal bones of the skull.

___ **15.** The parietal bone articulates with the vertebral column.

___ **16.** The last five ribs are called false ribs.

___ **17.** The foramen at the base of the skull through which the spinal cord passes is called the foramen magnum.

___ **18.** The temporal bone contains the middle and inner ear.

___ **19.** The type of cartilage that serves as a model for the structure of all cartilage is elastic cartilage.

___ **20.** A periosteum surrounds bone.

Answer Sheet—Chapter 5

Exercise 5.1

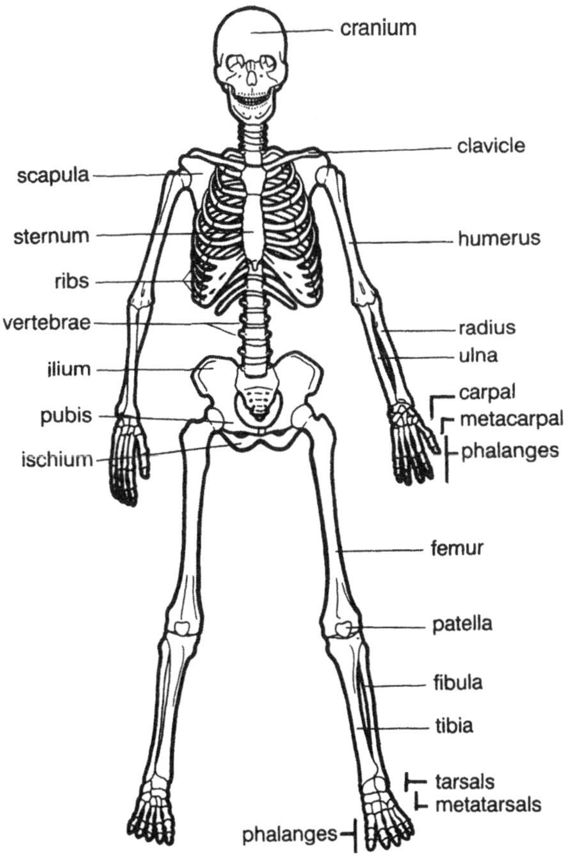

Figure 5.1 Human skeleton, anterior aspect.

Exercise 5.2

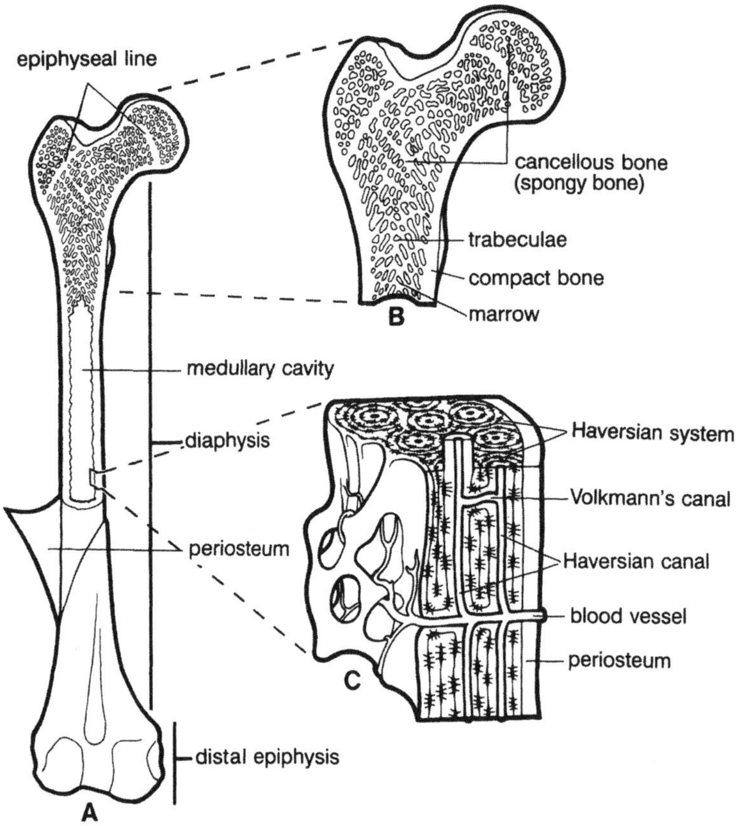

Figure 5.2 Schematic diagram of the structure of a typical long bone. **A.** Longitudinal section. **B.** Epiphyseal section. **C.** Diaphyseal section.

Exercise 5.3

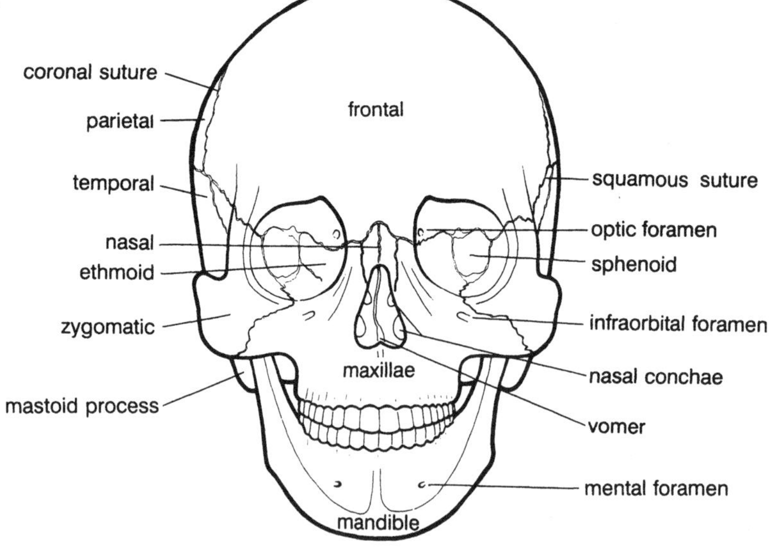

Figure 5.3 Frontal, lacrimal, zygomatic, maxillary, and nasal bones of the skull.

Exercise 5.4

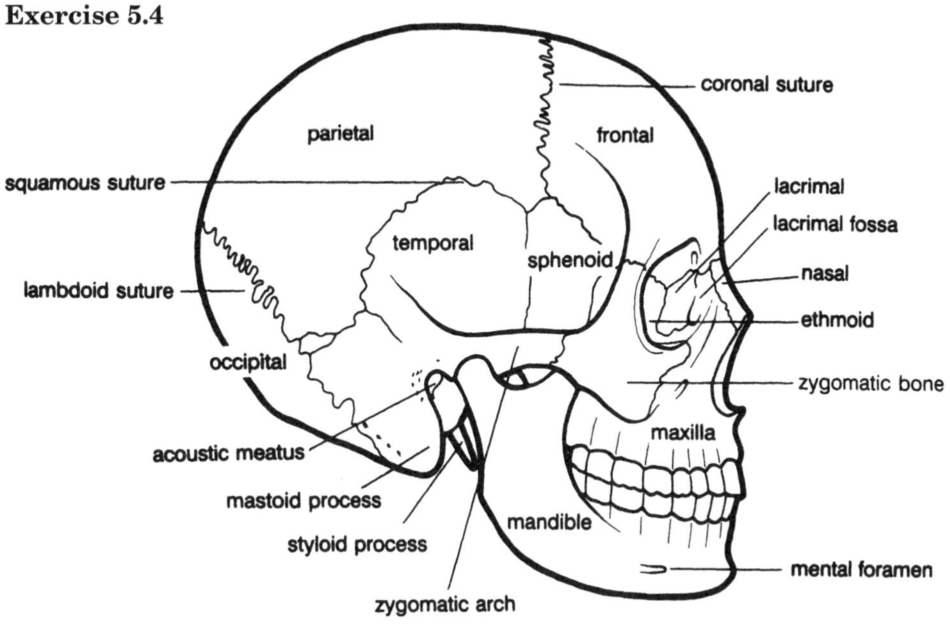

Figure 5.4 Skull, lateral aspect.

Test Items

A. 1. b, 2. c, 3. d, 4. c, 5. d, 6. c, 7. d, 8. c, 9. d, 10. a, 11. b, 12. b, 13. c, 14. b, 15. a, 16. d, 17. a, 18. c, 19. d, 20. c.

B. 1. h, 2. d, 3. g, 4. a, 5. f, 6. b, 7. i, 8. c, 9. k, 10. e, 11. l, 12. j.

C. 1. T, 2. F, 3. F, 4. T, 5. T, 6. F, 7. F, 8. T, 9. F, 10. T, 11. F, 12. T, 13. F, 14. T, 15. F, 16. T, 17. T, 18. T, 19. F, 20. T.

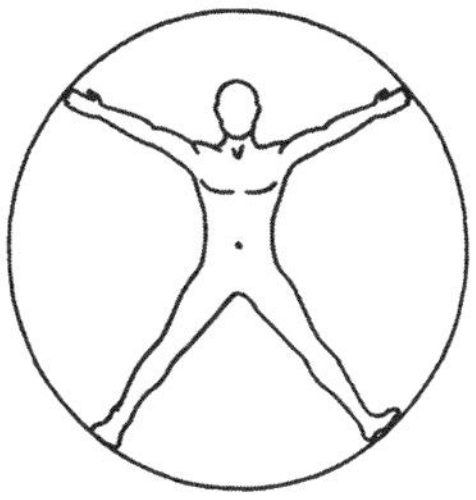

6

The Articular System

I. CHAPTER SYNOPSIS

The student is introduced to the various kinds of joints in the body. Articulations, or joints, can be divided into three classes: synarthroses, or immovable joints; amphiarthroses, or slightly movable joints; and diarthroses, or freely movable joints. The six subgroups of the diarthroses class are described along with the four types of angular movements and seven types of rotational movements that are possible at diarthrotic joints.

The most difficult part of the chapter deals with the planes of movement and axes of rotation. Some students grasp the idea almost intuitively, while others never seem to really understand it. For those who do, it makes muscle actions much easier to understand (and for instructors to explain) and reduces the amount of memorising required.

II. OBJECTIVES

After reading the chapter, the student should be able to:

- Classify body joints.
- Describe the distinguishing features of a synovial joint.
- Name the types of synovial joints and give an example of each.
- Describe the movements at synovial joints and give examples.

- Define arthritis and describe the different types.
- Define bursitis and relate, anatomically, its importance to joints.

III. IMPORTANT TERMS

Using your textbook, define the following terms:

abduction (ab-duk′shun) ______________________________

____

adduction (ah-duk′shun) ______________________________

____

amphiarthroses (am-fee-ahr-thro′sis) ______________________________

____

ankylosis (an-ki-lo′sis) ______________________________

____

arthritis (ar-thri′tis) ______________________________

____

articulate (ahr-tik′yoo-lut) ______________________________

____

articulation (ar-tik-u-lay′shun) ______________________________

____

bursitis (bur-si′tis) ______________________________

____

circumduction (ser-kum-duk′shun) ______________________________

____

diarthrosis (dye-ahr-thro′sis) ______________________________

____

dislocation (dis-lo-kay′shun) ______________________________

____

eversion (ee-ver′zhun) ______________________________

____

extension (ek-sten′shun) ______________________________

____

fibrositis (figh-bro-sigh′tis) ______________________________

____

flexion (flek′shun) ______

inversion (in-ver′zhun) ______

joint (joint) ______

ligament (lig′ah-ment) ______

pronation (pro-nay′shun) ______

protraction (pro-trak′shun) ______

retraction (ree-trak′shun) ______

rotation (ro-tay′shun) ______

sprain (sprayn) ______

supination (soo-pi-nay′shun) ______

symphysis (sim′fi-sis) ______

synarthrosis (sin-ahr-thro′sis) ______

synovia (sin-no′-vee-ah) ______

synovial (si-no′vee-al) ______

IV. EXERCISES

Complete the following exercises in the order given. A precise set of terms and diagrams has been chosen to describe the articular system.

Exercise 6.1

Labelling. Write the name of the type of joint or structure in the space provided. Colour each joint differently.

Key:
amphiarthrodial
cartilage
fibrocartilage
fibrous
intervertebral
pubic
suture
synarthrodial

Fill in the missing words in the corresponding blanks below.

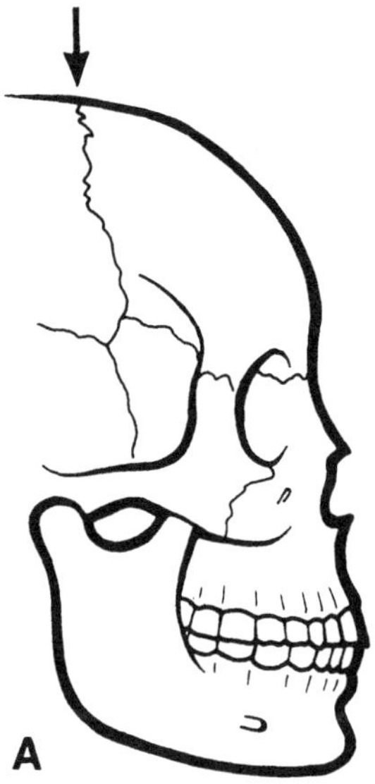

A

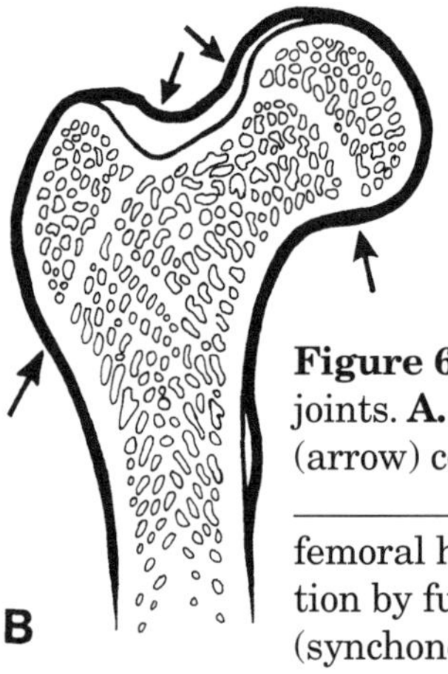

B

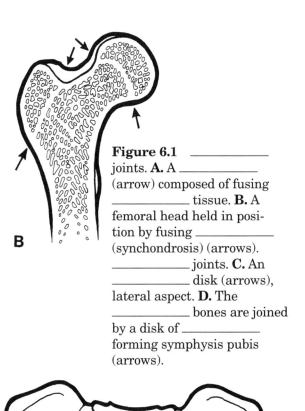

Figure 6.1 ____________ joints. **A.** A ____________ (arrow) composed of fusing ____________ tissue. **B.** A femoral head held in position by fusing ____________ (synchondrosis) (arrows). ____________ joints. **C.** An ____________ disk (arrows), lateral aspect. **D.** The ____________ bones are joined by a disk of ____________ forming symphysis pubis (arrows).

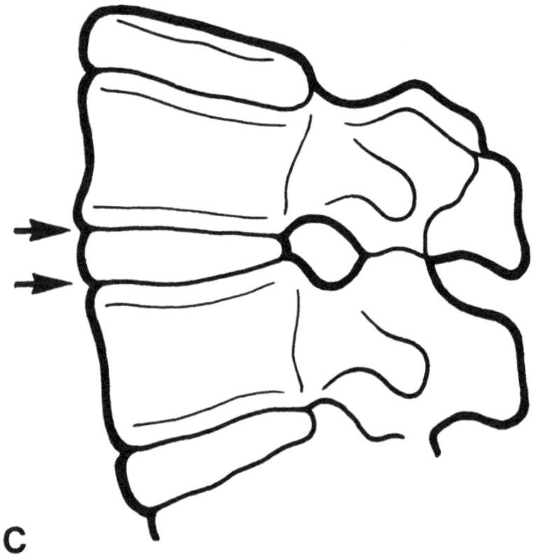

C

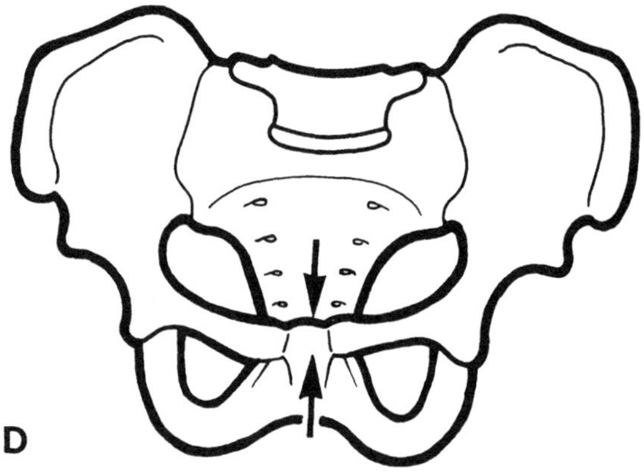

D

1. ______________________________
2. ______________________________
3. ______________________________
4. ______________________________
5. ______________________________
6. ______________________________
7. ______________________________
8. ______________________________

Exercise 6.2

Labelling. Identify the types of diarthrodial joints by placing the answer in the space provided. Colour each joint separately.

Key:
ball-and-socket
ellipsoidal
gliding
hinge
pivot
saddle

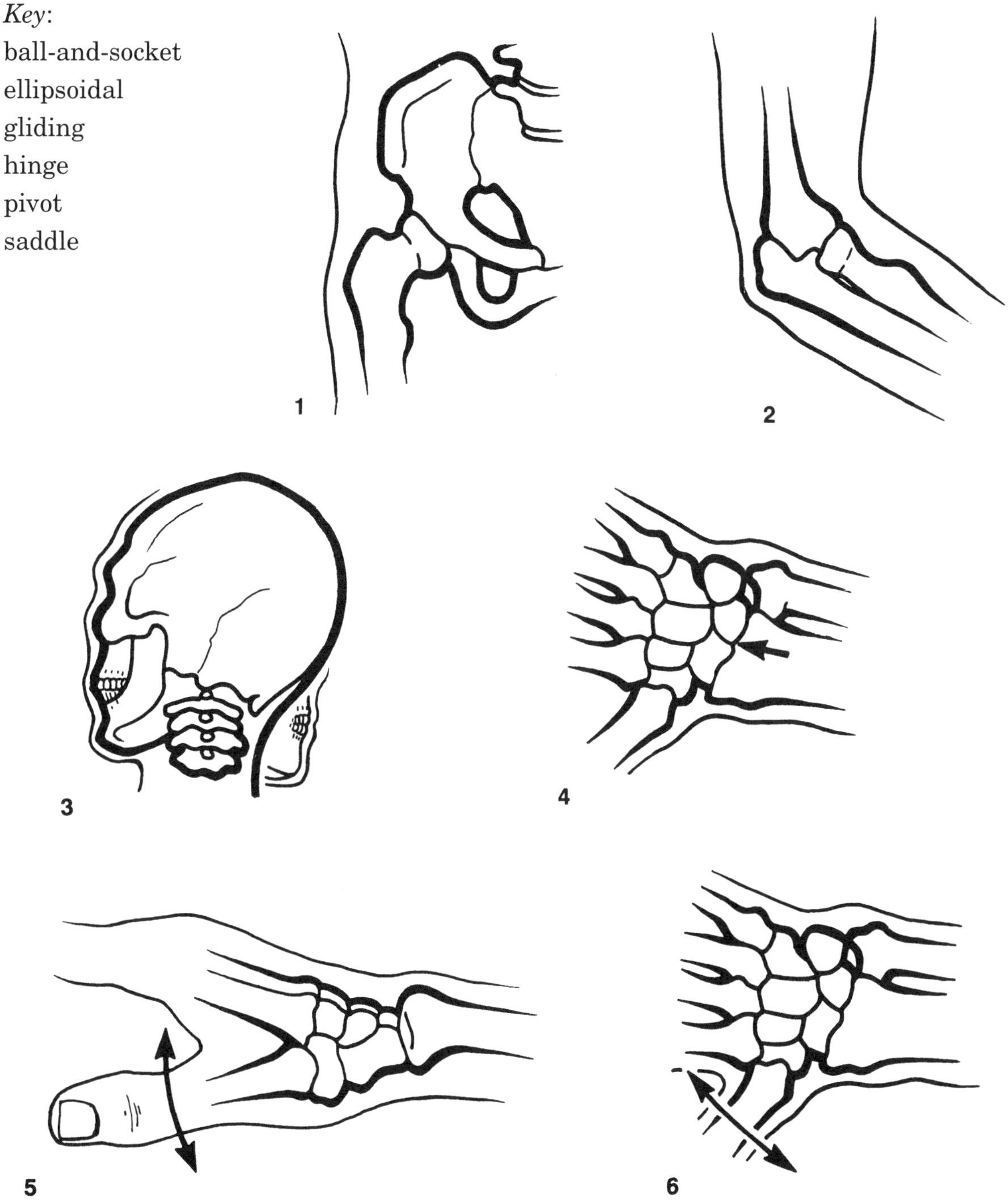

Figure 6.2 Types of diarthrodial joints.

1. ______________________________
2. ______________________________
3. ______________________________
4. ______________________________
5. ______________________________
6. ______________________________

Exercise 6.3

Labelling. Write the name of the movement at each joint on the space provided. Colour the arrows to indicate the motion.

Key:
abduction-adduction
circumduction
eversion-inversion
flexion-extension
protraction-retraction
rotation
supination-pronation

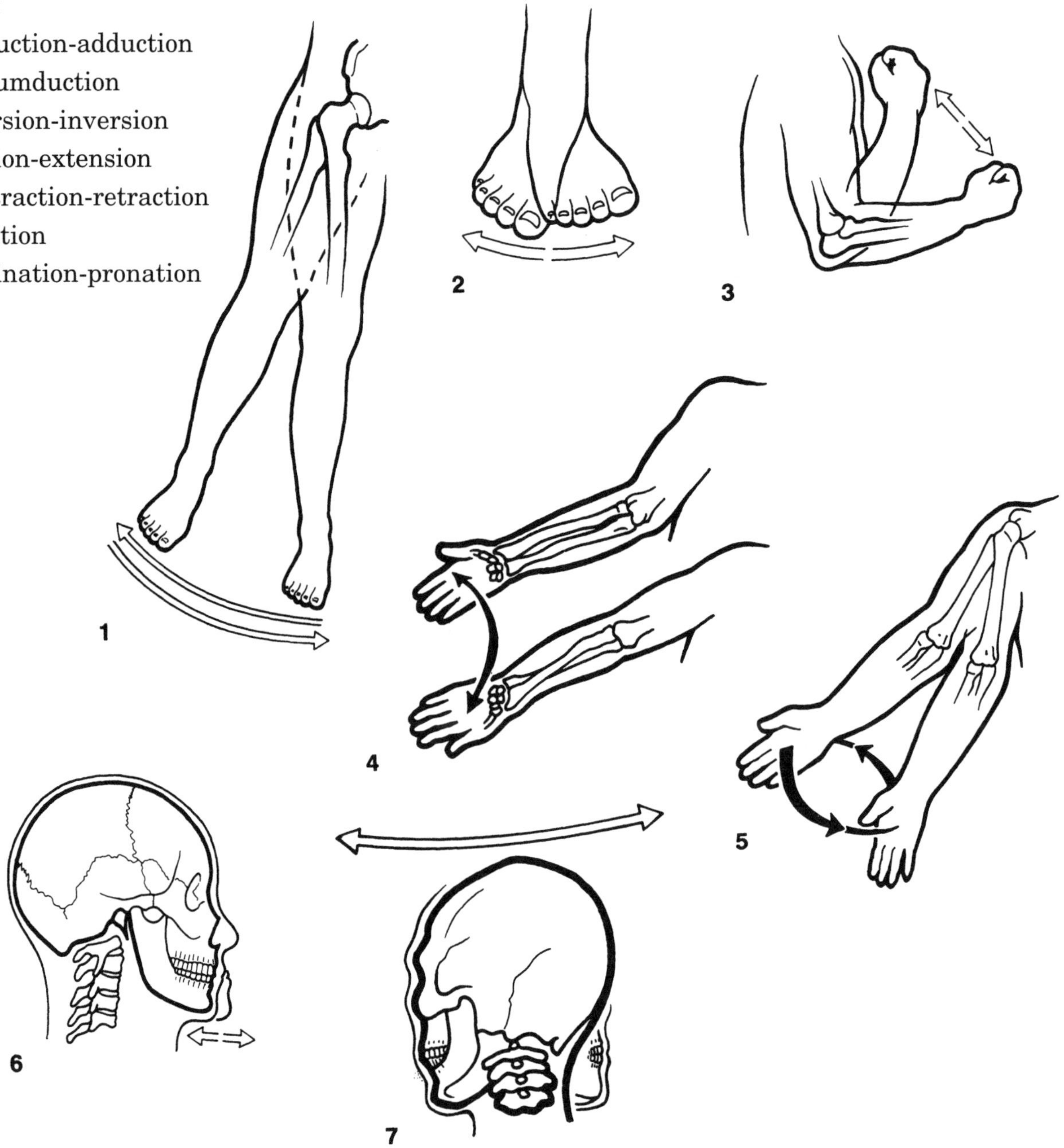

Figure 6.3 Movements of diarthrodial joints.

1. ______________________
2. ______________________
3. ______________________
4. ______________________
5. ______________________
6. ______________________
7. ______________________

Exercise 6.4

Labelling. Write the name of the structure of the true joint on the space provided. Colour the coronal section (B).

Key:

articular	joint	synovial
femur	ligament	tibia
fibula	patella	

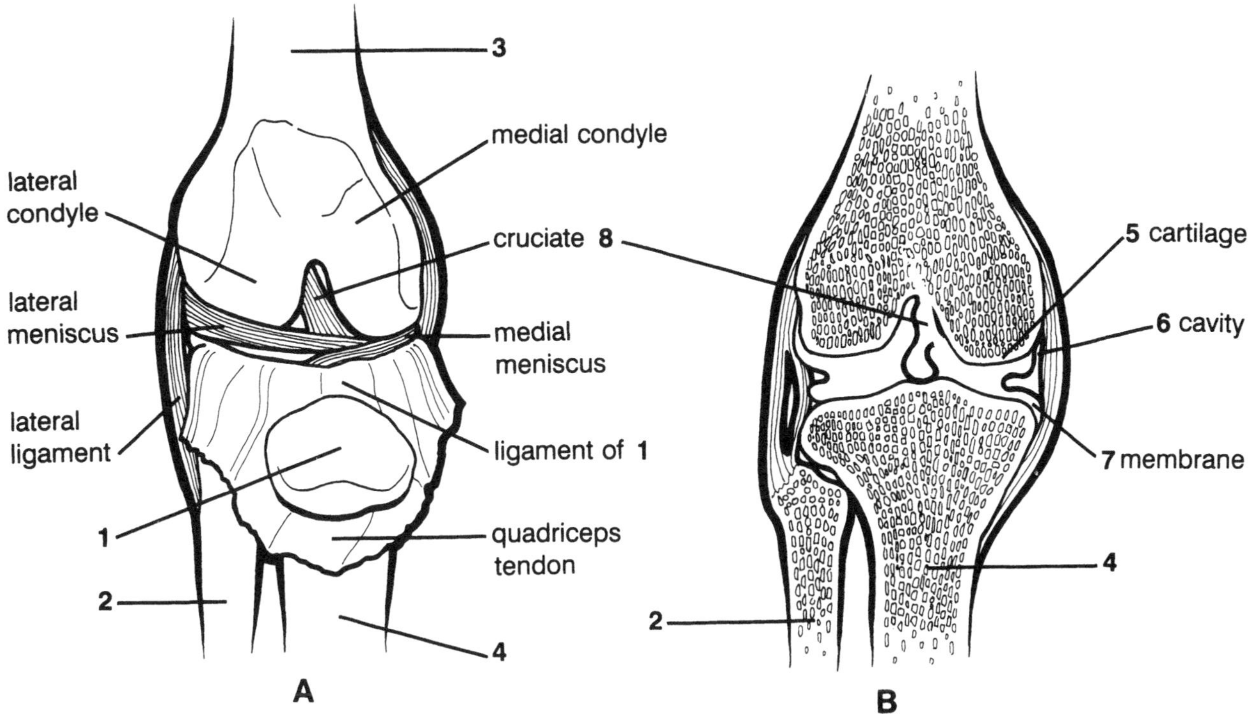

Figure 6.4 Right knee joint. **A.** Dissected from the front, with the patella resected and hanging down onto the tibia. **B.** Coronal section of the knee, exposing the joint cavity.

1. ______________________
2. ______________________
3. ______________________
4. ______________________
5. ______________________
6. ______________________
7. ______________________
8. ______________________

V. TEST ITEMS

A. *Multiple Choice.* There is only one answer that is either correct or most appropriate. Circle the best answer for each question.

1. What is the function of ligaments?
  a. bind bones at joints
  b. connect muscle to bone
  c. cover the ends of bones
  d. support bone growth

2. Freely movable joints are referred to as
  a. synarthrosis
  b. diarthrosis (synovial)
  c. amphiarthrosis
  d. sutures

3. When the angle between two bones is increased, the part is said to be
  a. adducted
  b. extended
  c. abducted
  d. flexed

4. Exaggeration of the posterior curvature of the thoracic vertebrae is called
  a. lordosis
  b. scoliosis
  c. kyphosis
  d. halitosis

5. The most common form of arthritis is called
  a. gout
  b. osteoarthritis
  c. rheumatoid
  d. lumbago

6. The hip and shoulder joints are examples of which type of joint?
  a. pivot
  b. ball and socket
  c. hinge
  d. rotation

7. The term used to describe overstretching or pulling of a part of muscle is
  a. sprain
  b. strain
  c. dislocation
  d. fracture

8. Which movements can you perform at both your hip and knee joints?
  a. abduction and extension
  b. abduction and adduction
  c. circumduction and rotation
  d. flexion and extension

9. The diarthrodial joint in which motion is limited to rotation is termed
  a. hinge
  b. flexor
  c. pivot
  d. condyloid

10. When the sole of the foot is turned toward the midline of the body, it is said to be
  a. extended
  b. pronated
  c. inverted
  d. everted

11. The common joint disorder that involves autoimmune reactions is
a. rheumatoid arthritis
b. osteoarthritis
c. septic arthritis
d. dislocation

12. A joint that affords three planes of movement is the
a. saddle
b. ellipsoidal
c. ball and socket
d. hinge

13. A movement in which the distal end of a bone moves in a circle while the proximal end remains relatively stable is called
a. rotation
b. circumduction
c. protraction
d. supination

14. Which of the following is *not* a synovial joint?
a. symphysis
b. pivot
c. gliding
d. ball and socket

15. Classification of joints is based on
a. location in the body
b. the presence or absence of tendons
c. movability
d. the length of the bones concerned

16. The clinical term applied to inflammation of a tendon and synovial membrane at a joint and commonly referred to as tennis elbow is
a. gout
b. osteitis
c. tendinitis
d. bursitis

17. The definition "to draw away laterally from the median plane of the body" best describes what word?
a. flexion
b. adduction
c. abduction
d. rotation

18. Extension of the foot at the ankle joint is known as
a. hyperextension
b. plantar flexion
c. dorsiflexion
d. abduction

19. The insertion of a plate, screw, or nail in a bone is called
a. open reduction
b. closed reduction
c. manipulation
d. internal fixation

20. Which of the following is true of osteoarthritis?
a. it is often referred to as a "wear and tear disorder"
b. it becomes more common with age
c. it commonly affects the knees
d. all of the above

B. *Matching.* Each of the words or phrases in Column B refers to a term or phrase in Column A. Insert the letter of the word or phrase from Column B that best describes each item in Column A. Some words may be used more than once or not at all.

Column A		*Column B*
1. ___	bursectomy	**a.** inflammation of a synovial membrane of a joint
2. ___	arthralgia	**b.** displacement of a bone from its natural position in a joint
3. ___	synovitis	**c.** removal of a bursa
4. ___	chondritis	**d.** inflammation of a cartilage
5. ___	arthrosis	**e.** severe or complete loss of movement at a joint
6. ___	dislocation	**f.** pain in a joint
7. ___	ankylosis	**g.** tearing of tendons and ligaments
8. ___	sprain	**h.** disease of a joint

Column A		*Column B*
1. ___	bunion	**a.** cone forming
2. ___	protraction	**b.** gouty arthritis
3. ___	tenosynovitis	**c.** toward the midline
4. ___	rotation	**d.** stiffening and immobility of a joint
5. ___	bony ankylosis	**e.** body part forward
6. ___	uric acid crystals	**f.** palm down
7. ___	adduction	**g.** foot turns in
8. ___	pronation	**h.** inflamed tendon sheath
9. ___	eversion	**i.** foot turns out
10. ___	circumduction	**j.** palm forward
		k. bony deformity of the big toe
		l. around central axis

C. *True or False.* Place a *T* or an *F* in the space provided to indicate true or false.

___ **1.** Synarthroses do not permit movement.

___ **2.** The synovial membrane is found only in diarthrodial joints and bursae.

___ **3.** Joint stability is provided by synovial fluids.

___ **4.** The saddle joint for the thumb refers to the joint between a metacarpal and a phalangeal bone.

___ **5.** Supination and pronation of the lower arm and hand occur when the radius rotates around the ulna.

____ **6.** All diarthroses permit free movement but not necessarily the same kinds of movements between articulating bones.

____ **7.** All diarthroses have a joint capsule and a joint cavity.

____ **8.** The term *synarthroses* is another name for synovial joints.

____ **9.** A large majority of joints in the body are synovial in type.

____ **10.** Most diarthroses are ball-and-socket–type joints.

____ **11.** Both the knee joint and the elbow joint are classified as hinge-type synovial joints.

____ **12.** Cartilaginous joints permit no movement between the articulating bones.

____ **13.** No diarthroses permit all of the following movements: flexion, extension, abduction, adduction, rotation, and circumduction.

____ **14.** Flexions are bending movements, whereas extensions are straightening movements.

____ **15.** Moving the forearm so as to turn the palm forward, as it is in the anatomical position, is called supination.

Answer Sheet—Chapter 6

Exercise 6.1

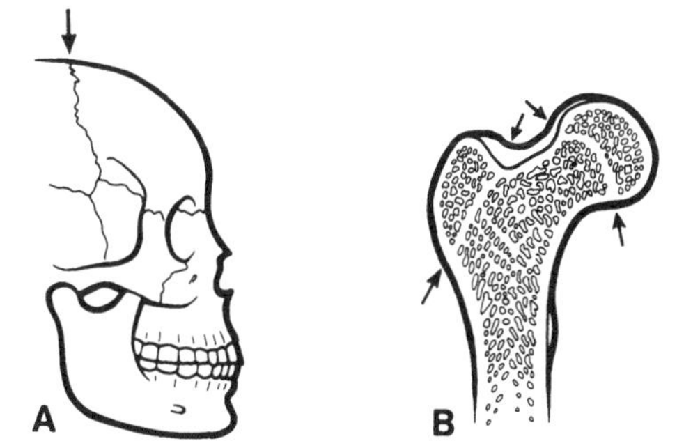

Figure 6.1 Synarthrodial joints. **A.** A suture (arrow) composed of fusing fibrous tissue. **B.** A femoral head held in position by fusing cartilage (synchondrosis) (arrows). Amphiarthrodial joints. **C.** An intervertebral disk (arrows), lateral aspect. **D.** The pubic bones are joined by a disk of fibrocartilage forming symphysis pubis (arrows).

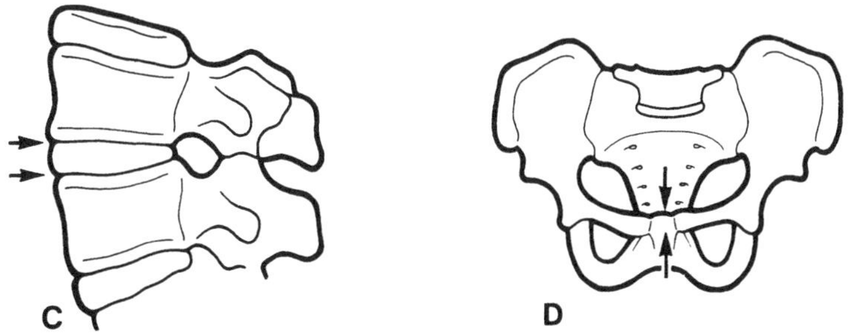

Exercise 6.2

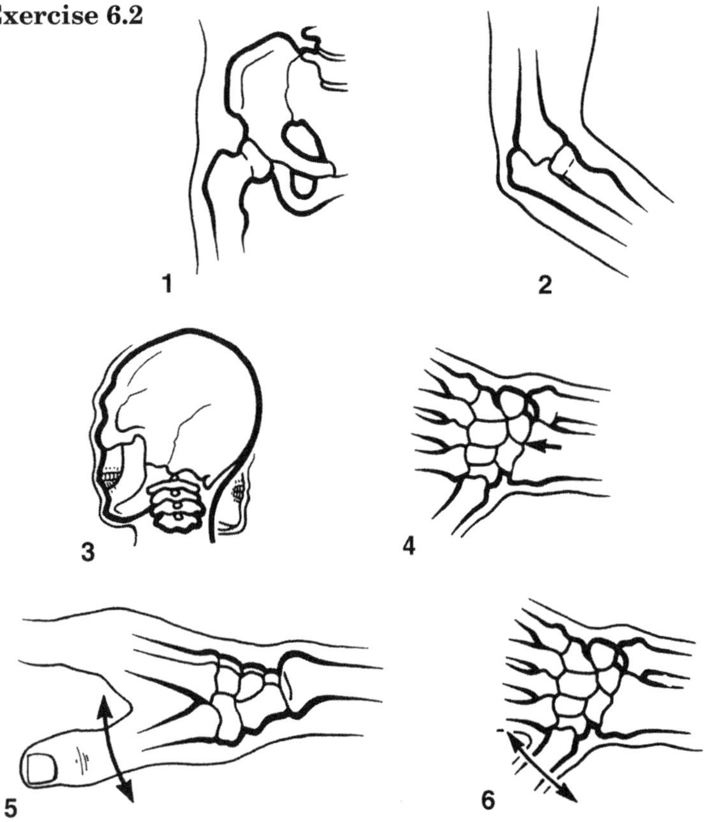

Figure 6.2 Types of diarthrodial joints. **1.** ball-and-socket. **2.** hinge. **3.** pivot. **4.** ellipsoidal. **5.** gliding. **6.** saddle.

Exercise 6.3

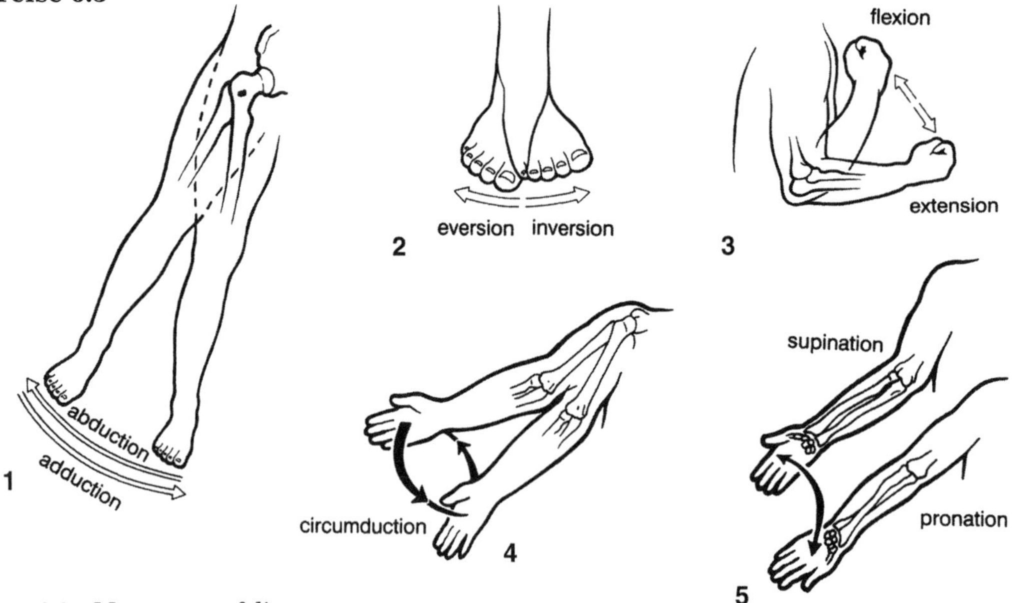

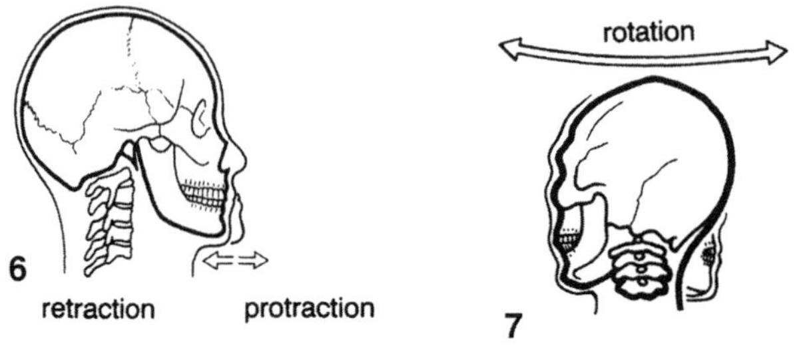

Figure 6.3 Movements of diarthrodial joints. **1.** abduction-adduction. **2.** eversion-inversion. **3.** flexion-extension. **4.** circumduction. **5.** supination-pronation. **6.** protraction-retraction. **7.** rotation.

Exercise 6.4

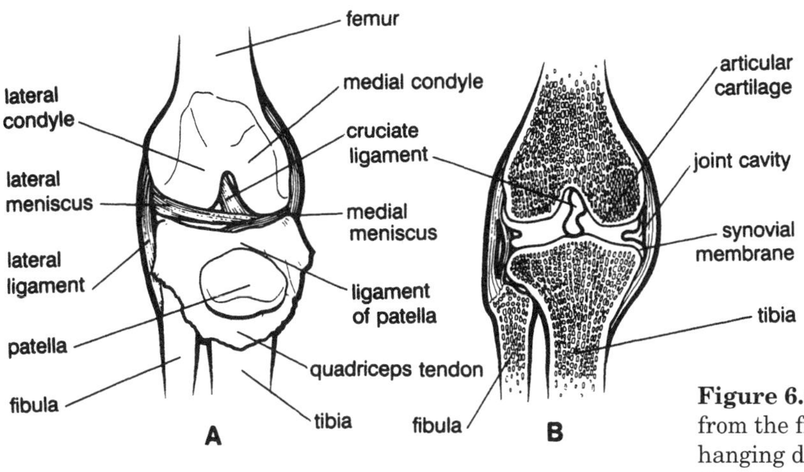

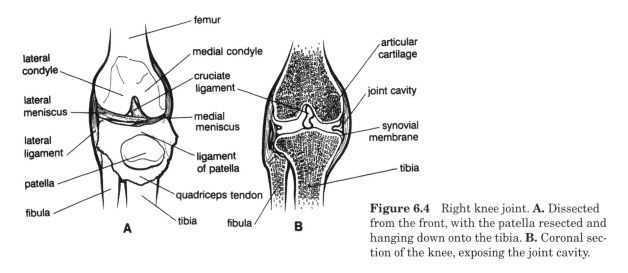

Figure 6.4 Right knee joint. **A.** Dissected from the front, with the patella resected and hanging down onto the tibia. **B.** Coronal section of the knee, exposing the joint cavity.

Test Items

A. 1. a, 2. b, 3. b, 4. c, 5. b, 6. b, 7. b, 8. d, 9. c, 10. c, 11. d, 12. c, 13. d, 14. a, 15. c, 16. c, 17. b, 18. b, 19. d, 20. b.

B. 1. c, 2. f, 3. a, 4. d, 5. h, 6. b, 7. e, 8. g.
1. k, 2. e, 3. h, 4. l, 5. d, 6. b, 7. c, 8. f, 9. i, 10. a.

C. 1. T, 2. T, 3. F, 4. F, 5. T, 6. T, 7. T, 8. F, 9. T, 10. F, 11. T, 12. F, 13. F, 14. T, 15. T.

7

The Muscles

I. CHAPTER SYNOPSIS

The end result of a control system is the activation of an effector organ that can produce a change in the environment. The two major effector organs in the body are muscle and glands.

Muscle tissue, owing to its ability to contract or shorten, thus producing movement of internal and external body parts, is responsible for such basic life processes as heartbeat, respiration, digestion, and production of body heat as well as for gross skeletal movements. There are three distinct types of muscle tissue: skeletal, cardiac, and smooth. Each type has a uniquely characteristic microscopic structure, gross structure, nerve supply, and blood supply, and each is designed for the performance of a certain type of work. Although all three types of muscle tissue have the same fundamental properties of excitability and contractility, certain differences are also present.

II. OBJECTIVES

After reading the chapter, the student should be able to:

- Describe the structure and control of three different types of muscles.
- Describe the microscopic anatomy of a contractile unit of muscle.
- Explain the sliding filament theory of muscle contraction.

- Detail a single muscle contraction.
- Analyse the major muscles according to their origin, insertion, and function.
- Distinguish between antagonistic and synergistic muscles.
- Draw and label a neuromuscular synapse (neuromuscular junction).
- Describe the motor end plate.

III. IMPORTANT TERMS

Using your textbook, define the following terms:

acetylcholine (ase-til-ko′leen) ______________________________

____

actin (ak′tin) ______________________________

____

adenosine triphosphate (a-den′uh-seen try-fos′fate) ______________________________

____

antagonist (an-tag′uh-nist) ______________________________

____

aponeuroses (ap-o-new-ro′sis) ______________________________

____

axon (acks′on) ______________________________

____

contraction (kon-trak′shun) ______________________________

____

cross-bridge (kros bridj) ______________________________

____

elasticity (ee-las-tis′i-tee) ______________________________

____

energy (en′er-jee) ______________________________

____

fascia (fash-ee-uh) ______________________________

____

fatigue (fa-teeg′) ______________________________

____

fibrillation (fi-bri-lay′shun) ______________________________

hypertrophy (high-per′truh-fee) ______________________________

insertion (in-sur′shun) ______________________________

muscle (mus′ul) ______________________________

myalgia (my-al′juh) ______________________________

myofibril (migh-o-figh′bril) ______________________________

myosin (my′o-sin) ______________________________

origin (or′i-jin) ______________________________

peristalsis (per-i-stal′sis) ______________________________

sarcomere (sahr′ko-meer) ______________________________

spasm (spaz′um) ______________________________

synergist (sin′ur-jist) ______________________________

tendon (ten′dun) ______________________________

vesicle (ves′i-kul) ______________________________

IV. EXERCISES

Complete the following exercises in the order given. A precise set of terms and diagrams has been chosen to describe the muscular system.

Exercise 7.1

Labelling. Write the name of the structure of a muscle fibre on the space provided. Colour the bands differently.

Key:
A-band
cross-bridges
energy
H-zone
I-band
sarcomere
Z-line

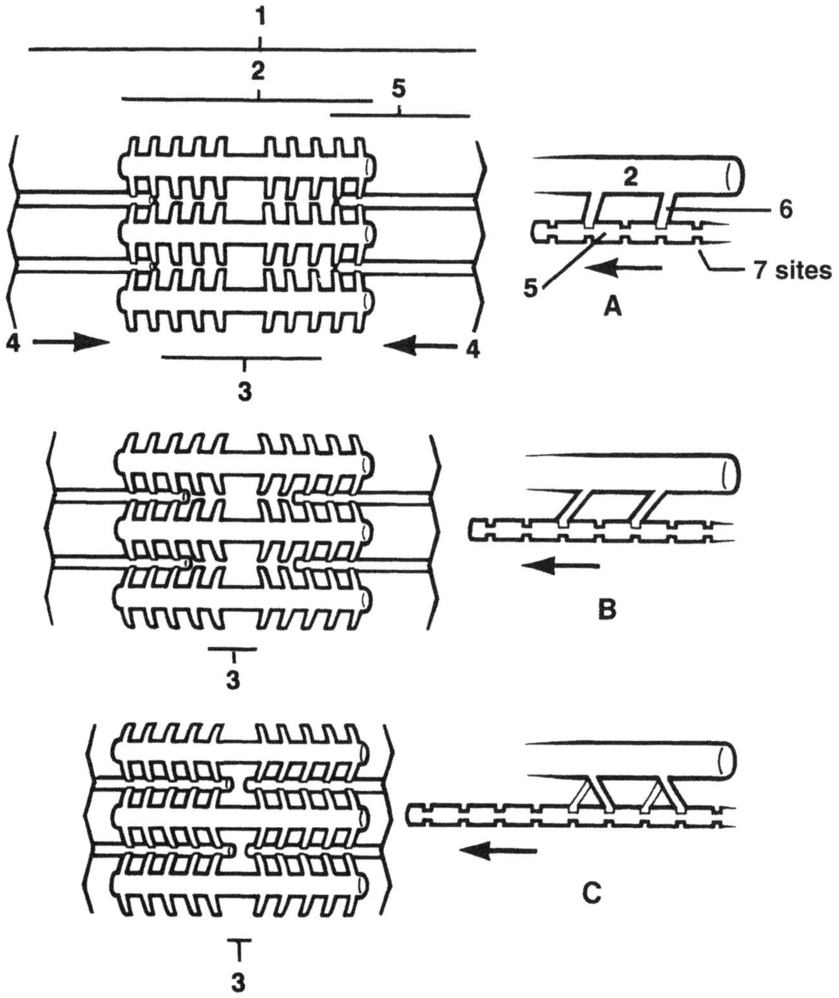

Figure 7.1 Contraction of a muscle. **A.** Sliding filament theory proposes that the —2— contain flexible —6— that come in contact with —7— sites on the more numerous —5—. **B.** and **C.** With the availability of —7—, the —6— pull the active filament a short distance (**B**), release it, and attach to another site (**C**), resulting in the shortening of the —3— between the —5—: contraction.

1. ______________________
2. ______________________
3. ______________________
4. ______________________
5. ______________________
6. ______________________
7. ______________________

Exercise 7.2

Labelling. Write the name of the structure in the space provided. Colour the nerve fibre one colour and the muscle fibre another.

Key:
acetylcholine
axon
muscle
myelin
Schwann
terminal

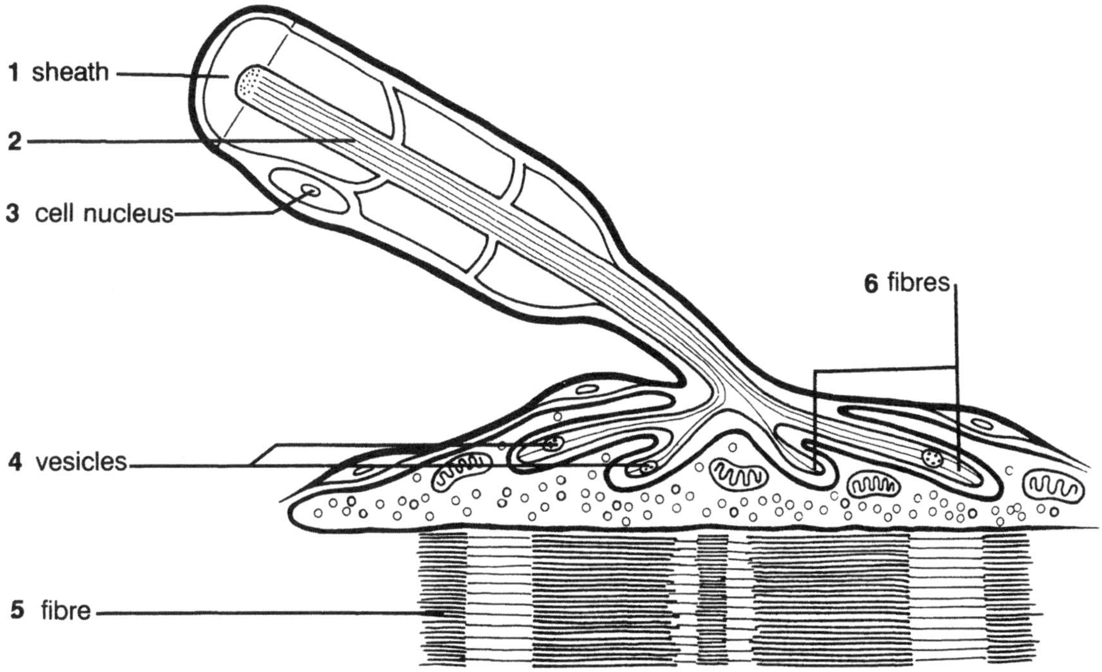

Figure 7.2 Cross-section of a motor end plate on a skeletal muscle, showing the actual connection between the muscle and the terminal branch of the nerve fibre.

1. ______________________
2. ______________________
3. ______________________
4. ______________________
5. ______________________
6. ______________________

Exercise 7.3

Labelling. Write the name of the muscle on the space provided. Colour the muscle mass, leaving the tendons white.

Key:
adductor
biceps
deltoid
extensor
external
flexor
frontalis
gastrocnemius
gracilis
oculi
orbicularis
pectoralis
rectus
sartorius
serratus
sternocleidomastoid
tibialis
trapezius
vastus
zygomaticus

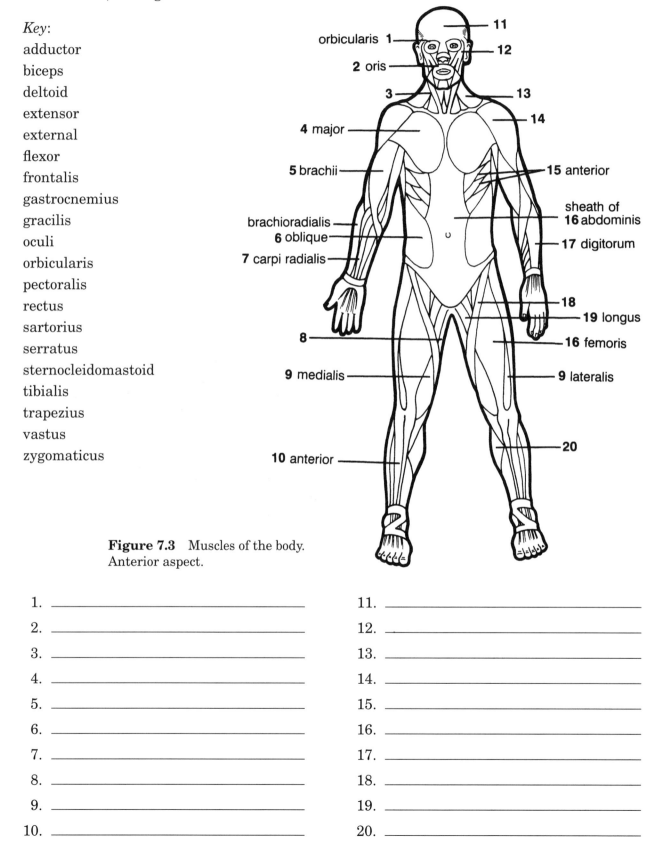

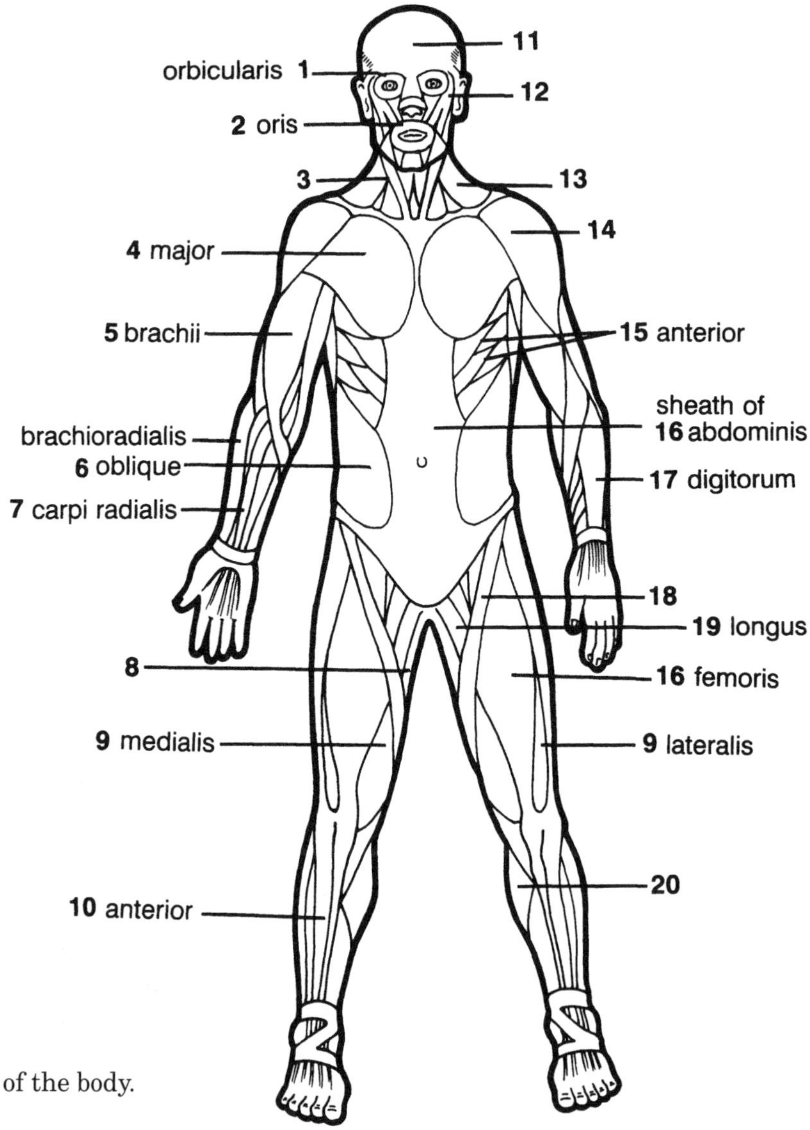

Figure 7.3 Muscles of the body. Anterior aspect.

1. ______________________
2. ______________________
3. ______________________
4. ______________________
5. ______________________
6. ______________________
7. ______________________
8. ______________________
9. ______________________
10. ______________________
11. ______________________
12. ______________________
13. ______________________
14. ______________________
15. ______________________
16. ______________________
17. ______________________
18. ______________________
19. ______________________
20. ______________________

Exercise 7.4

Labelling. Write the name of the muscle on the space provided. Colour the muscle mass, leaving the tendons white.

Key:
Achilles
biceps
deltoid
gastrocnemius
gluteus
infraspinatus
latissimus
occipitalis
plantaris
semimembranosus
semitendinosus
soleus
teres
trapezius
triceps

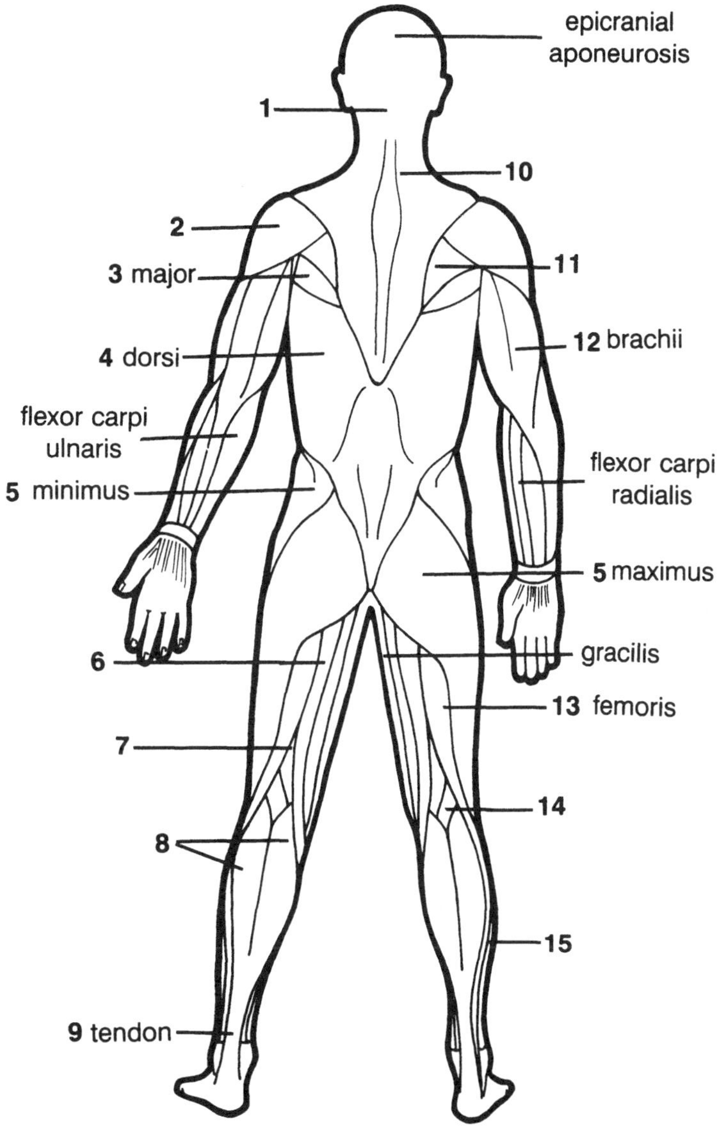

Figure 7.4 Muscles of the body. Posterior aspect.

1. ______________________
2. ______________________
3. ______________________
4. ______________________
5. ______________________
6. ______________________
7. ______________________
8. ______________________
9. ______________________
10. ______________________
11. ______________________
12. ______________________
13. ______________________
14. ______________________
15. ______________________

V. TEST ITEMS

A. *Multiple Choice.* There is only one answer that is either correct or most appropriate. Circle the best answer for each question.

1. What functional characteristic of muscle is displayed after being stimulated by an electric shock?
a. extensibility
b. contractility
c. selectivity
d. elasticity

2. The connective tissue component of skeletal muscle that surrounds fasciculi is called the
a. perimysium
b. epimysium
c. endomysium
d. tendomysium

3. The ability of muscle tissue to receive and respond to a stimulus is referred to as
a. contractility
b. irritability
c. elasticity
d. extendability

4. The location at which a nerve actually joins a muscle is called a
a. motor neuron
b. neuromuscular synapse (neuromuscular junction)
c. myofibril
d. sarcomere

5. A sarcolemma is present in
a. epithelial cells
b. striated muscle tissue
c. adipose tissue
d. blood

6. According to the sliding filament model of muscle contraction,
a. cross-bridges are lateral extensions of thick filaments, but temporarily attach to thin ones
b. cross-bridges are on thin filaments, but temporarily attach to thick ones
c. cross-bridges are on both thick and thin filaments
d. only filaments of the same size are interconnected

7. When muscle fibres contract, the H zone
a. increases as the actin moves
b. decreases as the filaments slide
c. increases as the myosin disappears
d. decreases as the myosin enlarges

8. Skeletal muscle is also commonly known as:
a. involuntary muscle
b. smooth muscle
c. striated muscle
d. cardiac muscle

9. Microscopically, muscle fibres are seen to contain parallel myofibrils, banded by repeating units. Each unit is called
a. an actin
b. a myosin
c. a sarcomere
d. a myofibril

10. The breakdown of which high-energy molecule is believed to provide immediate energy for muscle work?
a. adenosine diphosphate (ADP)
b. glycogen
c. adenosine triphosphate (ATP)
d. glucose

11. Which of these gives the correct order from large to small?
a. muscle, muscle cells, myofibrils, sarcomeres, myosin filaments, actin filaments
b. muscle, muscle fibres, myofibrils, myosin filaments, actin filaments
c. muscle, sarcolemma, myofibrils, myosin filaments, actin filaments
d. muscle cells, myofibrils, sarcoplasm, filaments

12. Sarcopaenia is a term that describes
a. significant muscle growth
b. significant muscle atrophy
c. muscle spasms
d. muscle paralysis

13. During muscle fatigue, the production of lactic acid
a. indicates lack of O_2
b. accompanies alcohol formation
c. is responsible for carbon dioxide formation
d. is necessary for glucose formation

14. An increase in muscle size is called
a. atrophy
b. myositis
c. hypertrophy
d. myalgia

15. At the neuromuscular synapse (neuromuscular junction),
a. acetylcholine is released from the muscle cell in response to an action potential
b. curare prevents the release of acetylcholine in response to an action potential
c. acetylcholine is rapidly broken down by an enzyme present in the end-plate membrane
d. the end-plate potential results in the inside of the membrane at the end plate becoming positive and the outside positive

16. According to the sliding-filament hypothesis,
a. potassium ions are necessary for contraction
b. Z lines move away from the A band
c. actin filaments move toward each other
d. myosin filaments move toward each other

17. The following clinical symptoms—degeneration of muscle fibres, muscle atrophy, weakening of skeletal muscles, and fat deposition—are associated with
a. muscular dystrophy
b. fatigue
c. convulsions
d. myositis

18. Myofibrils are stacked in definite compartments partitioned by separations called Z-lines. Such compartments are known as
a. sarcoplasm
b. sarcoplasm reticulum
c. triads
d. sarcomeres

19. Calcium prevents the inhibitory effect of
a. myosin
b. troponin
c. actin
d. sodium

20. Glucose is stored in muscle in the form of
a. lactic acid
b. glycerol
c. glycogen
d. amino acids

B. *Matching.* Each of the words or phrases in Column B refers to a word or phrase in Column A. Insert the letter of the word or phrase from Column B that best describes each word or phrase in Column A. Some words or phrases may be used more than once or not at all.

Column A	*Column B*
1. ___ myofilaments make up a	**a.** actin
2. ___ contain the protein myosin	**b.** troponin
3. ___ attached to the Z-line	**c.** myofibril
4. ___ a regulatory protein	**d.** smooth muscle
5. ___ a single muscle cell	**e.** recruitment
6. ___ the combination of the motor neuron and a muscle fibre	**f.** cardiac muscle
	g. norepinephrine (adrenaline)
7. ___ the process of increasing the number of motor neurons	**h.** myocyte
	i. A-band
8. ___ lacks a well-developed	**j.** motor unit
9. ___ located in the myocardium	
10. ___ a neurotransmitter	

Column A	*Column B*
1. ___ deltoid	**a.** extends thigh and flexes leg
2. ___ hamstring group	**b.** flexes leg and extends foot
3. ___ triceps	**c.** extends leg and flexes thigh
4. ___ gastrocnemius	**d.** flexes and adducts arm
5. ___ quadriceps femoris group	**e.** extends forearm
6. ___ pectoralis major	**f.** abducts arm

C. *True or False.* Place a *T* or an *F* in the space provided to indicate true or false.

___ **1.** The thin filaments of a myofibril are composed of the protein myosin.

___ **2.** The motor unit is the basic unit of contraction.

___ **3.** The A-band contains myosin and is light.

___ **4.** The Z-line is located in the central region of the I band.

___ **5.** Muscle tone results from a constant stream of stimuli to the skeletal muscles.

___ **6.** Acetylcholine also plays an important role in ATP synthesis.

___ **7.** A muscle fibre is made up of myofibrils, which in turn are made up of overlapping thick and thin protein filaments.

___ **8.** When skeletal muscle contracts, the A band decreases in length.

___ **9.** Injuring your biceps brachii muscle will impair your ability to flex your forearm.

___ **10.** The point of attachment of a muscle to the bone that is moved as the muscle contracts is called the insertion of the muscle.

___ **11.** With the vertebrae, ribs, and pelvis fixed, contraction of the latissimus dorsi will extend and abduct the arm.

___ **12.** Smooth muscle is found primarily in the musculature of the extremities.

___ **13.** Smooth muscle is often arranged in sheets and layers.

___ **14.** A disorder in which the muscle shortens in length is hypertrophy.

___ **15.** Myalgia refers to pain in the muscular tissue.

___ **16.** Synergists are muscles that assist the agonist.

___ **17.** According to the all-or-none principle, muscle fibres contract all the way or they do not contract at all.

___ **18.** On a myogram of a twitch contraction, the relaxation period is indicated as an upward tracing.

___ **19.** Fibrositis of the lower back is called myopathy.

___ **20.** The biceps is a flexor and the triceps is an extensor; therefore, they are antagonists.

Answer Sheet—Chapter 7

Exercise 7.1

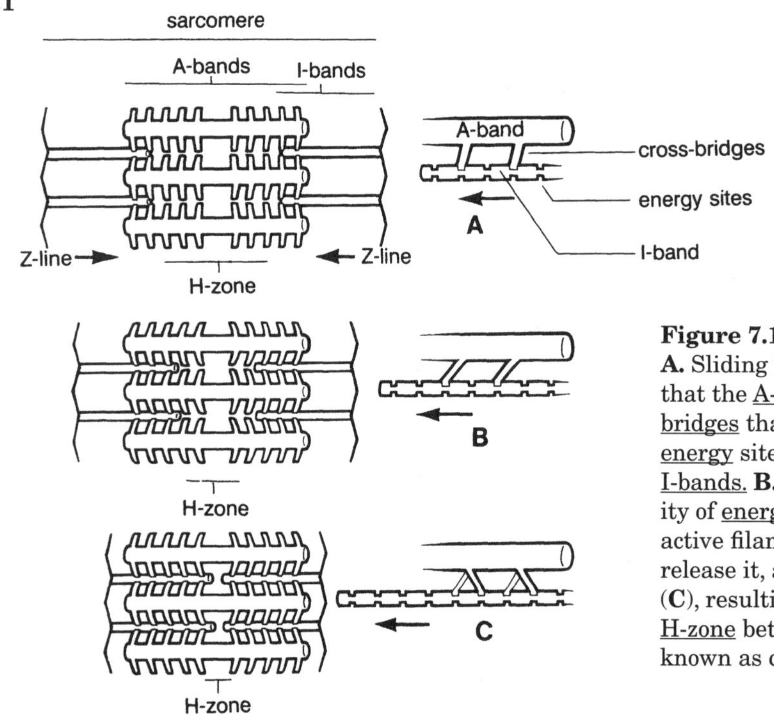

Figure 7.1 Contraction of a muscle. **A.** Sliding filament theory proposes that the A-bands contain flexible cross-bridges that come in contact with energy sites on the more numerous I-bands. **B.** and **C.** With the availability of energy, the cross-bridges pull the active filament a short distance (**B**), release it, and attach to another site (**C**), resulting in the shortening of the H-zone between the I-bands, which is known as contraction.

Exercise 7.2

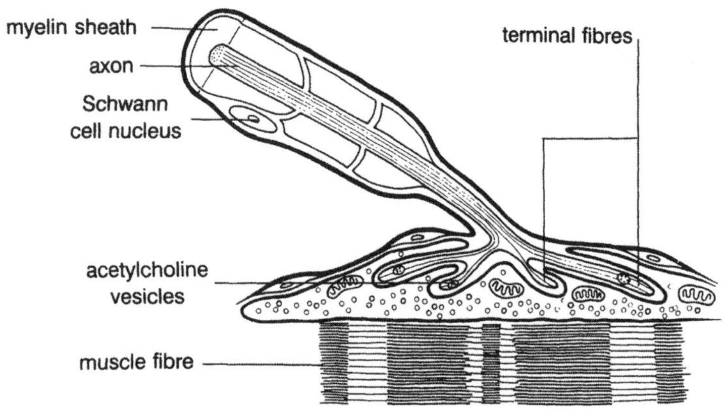

Figure 7.2 Cross-section of a motor end plate on a skeletal muscle, showing the actual connection between the muscle and the terminal branch of the nerve fibre.

Exercise 7.3

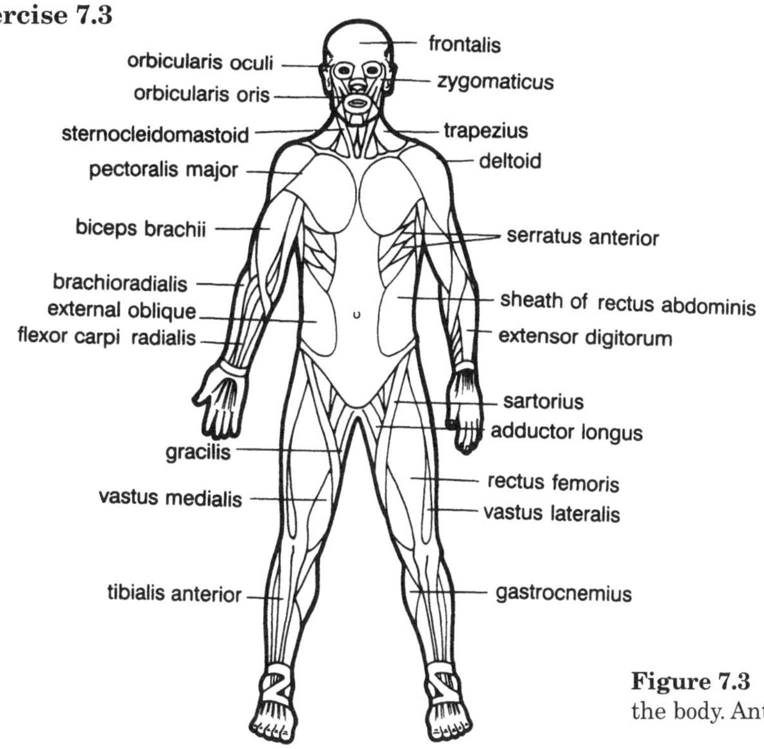

Figure 7.3 Muscles of the body. Anterior aspect.

Exercise 7.4

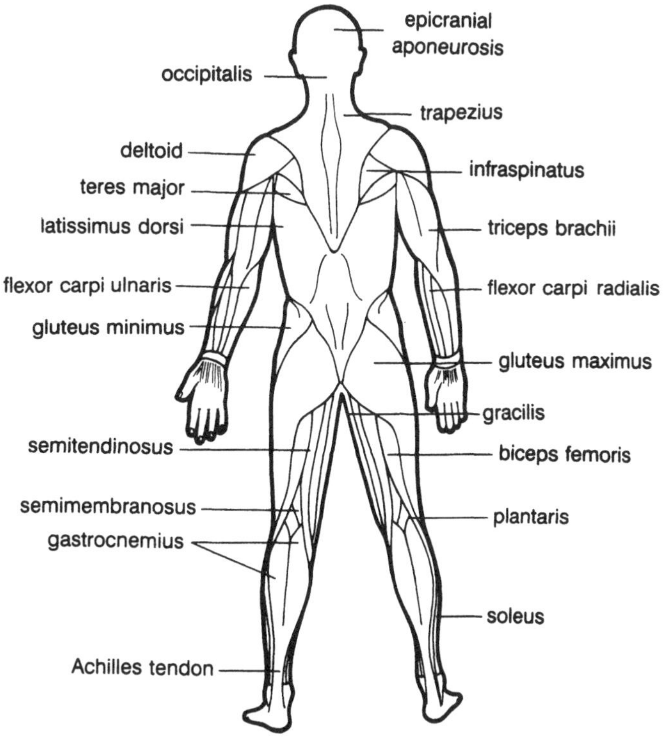

Figure 7.4 Muscles of the body. Posterior aspect.

Test Items

A. 1. b, 2. a, 3. b, 4. b, 5. b, 6. b, 7. b, 8. c, 9. c, 10. c, 11. b, 12. b, 13. a, 14. c, 15. c, 16. c, 17. a, 18. d, 19. b, 20. c.

B. 1. c, 2. i, 3. a, 4. b, 5. h, 6. j, 7. e, 8. d, 9. f, 10. g.
1. f, 2. a, 3. e, 4. b, 5. c, 6. d.

C. 1. F, 2. T, 3. F, 4. T, 5. T, 6. F, 7. T, 8. F, 9. T, 10. T, 11. F, 12. F, 13. T, 14. F, 15. T, 16. T, 17. T, 18. F, 19. F, 20. T.

8

The Voluntary Nervous System

I. CHAPTER SYNOPSIS

The general plan of the nervous system involves mechanisms of correlation and coordination similar to a central nervous system (CNS) switchboard that connects a network of peripheral nerves. The divisions of the nervous system involve the CNS and the peripheral nervous system (PNS). The structural features of nervous tissue are described for nerve cells and supporting neurological cells. Neurons are classified functionally as afferent, efferent, or central in relation to the CNS.

The nervous system is divided into two parts: the CNS and the PNS. The CNS consists of the brain inside the skull and the spinal cord, which runs up inside the vertebral column and expands into the brain. Communicating centres within the CNS and various nerve tracts make possible the appropriate unconscious or conscious response to sensory stimulus. The PNS is made up of a network of nerves and sense organs that gathers information from the rest of the body and feeds it into the brain.

Once some of the body systems have been studied, it becomes fairly obvious that not one of these systems is capable of functioning alone. The systems are interdependent. All must work together as one functioning unit so that homeostasis may be maintained within the body. The mechanism that ensures that the organs and systems operate in smooth coordination is the nervous system. Conditions within and outside the body are constantly changing, and one purpose of the nervous system is to respond to these internal and external changes so that the body may adapt itself.

II. OBJECTIVES

After reading the chapter, the student should be able to:

- Describe the structure of a neuron.
- Classify neurons according to their structure, function, and position.
- Explain a simple reflex.
- Distinguish between simple and complex reflexes.
- Differentiate between the white and grey matter of nerve tissue.
- Describe the cerebrum and identify the lobes by their location and function.
- List the organs of the hind brain and relate their functions to the brain and spinal cord.
- Identify the 12 cranial nerves by their number, function, and distribution.

III. IMPORTANT TERMS

Using your textbook, define the following terms:

afferent (af′ur-ent) ____________________

____

arc (ark) ____________________

____

association (a-so-see-ay′shun) ____________________

____

axon (aks′on) ____________________

____

conduction (kun-duk′shun) ____________________

____

cortex (kor′teks) ____________________

____

dendrite (den′drite) ____________________

____

dorsal (dor′sul) ____________________

____

efferent (ef′ur-ent) ____________________

____

epineurium (ep-i-new′ree-um) ____________________

____

fissure (fish′ur) ______________________________

grey (gray) ______________________________

gyrus (jye′rus) ______________________________

internuncial (in-ter-nun′see-ul) ______________________________

medulla (me-dool′uh) ______________________________

motor (mo′tur) ______________________________

myelin (my′e-lin) ______________________________

neuralgia (new-ral′juh) ______________________________

neuritis (new-ry′tis) ______________________________

neurofibril (new-ro-fy′bril) ______________________________

neurilemma (new-ruh-lem′uh) ______________________________

plexus (plek′sus) ______________________________

receptor (re-sep′tur) ______________________________

reflex (ree′fleks) ______________________________

sensory (sen′suh-ree) ______________________________

spinal (spy′nul) ______________________________

ventral (ven′trul) ______________________________

white (white) ______________________________

IV. EXERCISES

Complete the following exercises in the order given. A precise set of terms and diagrams has been chosen to describe the nervous system.

Exercise 8.1

Labelling. Write the name of the structure on the space provided. Colour the three types of neuron differently.

Key:

axon	neurilemma
cell body	neurofibril
dendrite	Nissl
epineurium	nucleus
fasciculus	perineurium
muscle	Ranvier
myelin	receptor
myoneural	Schwann
nerve	

1. ____________
2. ____________
3. ____________
4. ____________
5. ____________
6. ____________
7. ____________
8. ____________
9. ____________
10. ____________
11. ____________
12. ____________
13. ____________
14. ____________
15. ____________
16. ____________
17. ____________

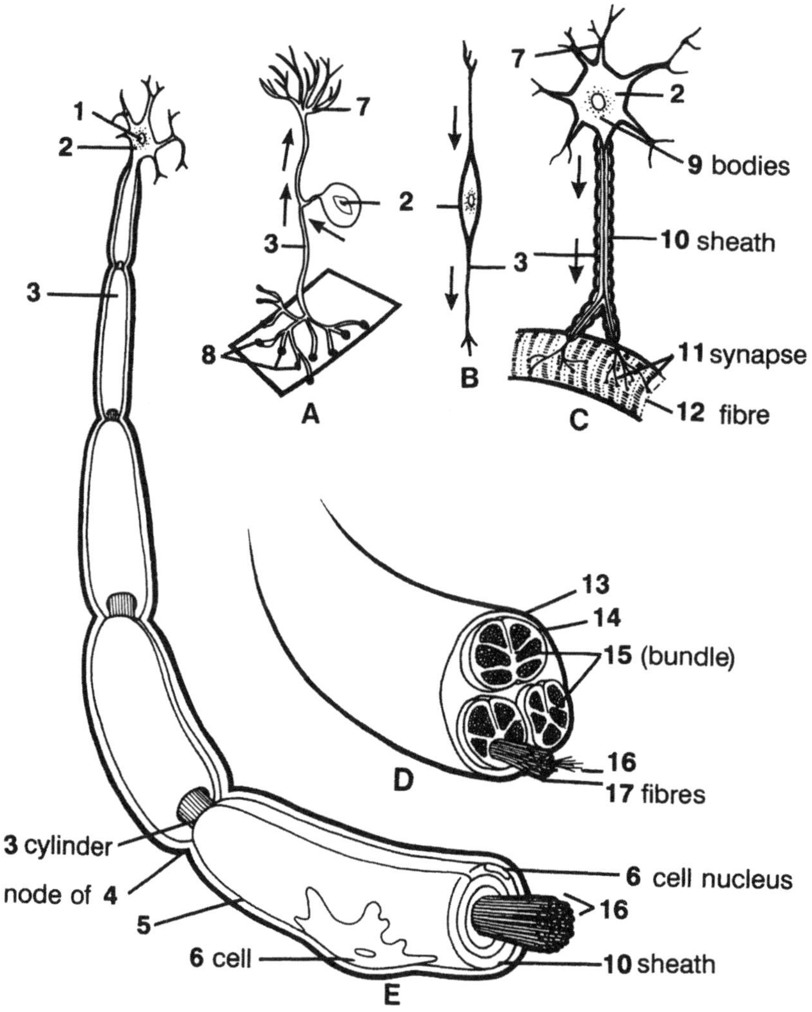

Figure 8.1 The structure of a neuron. **A.** Unipolar sensory neuron. **B.** Bipolar retinal neuron in the eye. **C.** Multipolar neuron, showing a muscle-nerve synapse. **D.** Structure of a typical nerve. **E.** An enlarged extension of an axon, showing its protective myelin sheath and neurilemma.

Exercise 8.2

Labelling. Write the name of the glial cells in the space provided. Colour the different structures of each cell.

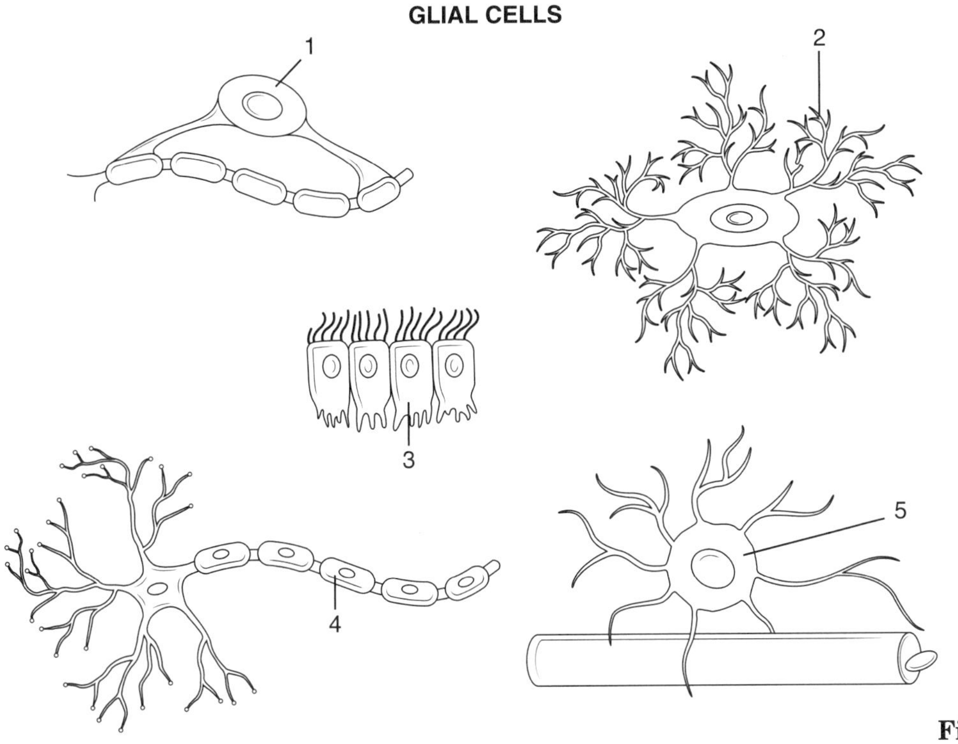

Figure 8.2 Glial cells.

1. ______________________
2. ______________________
3. ______________________
4. ______________________
5. ______________________

Exercise 8.3

Labelling. Write the name of the structure in the space provided. Colour the white matter different from the grey matter.

Key:

dorsal	internuncial	sensory
effector	motor	ventral
grey	receptor	white

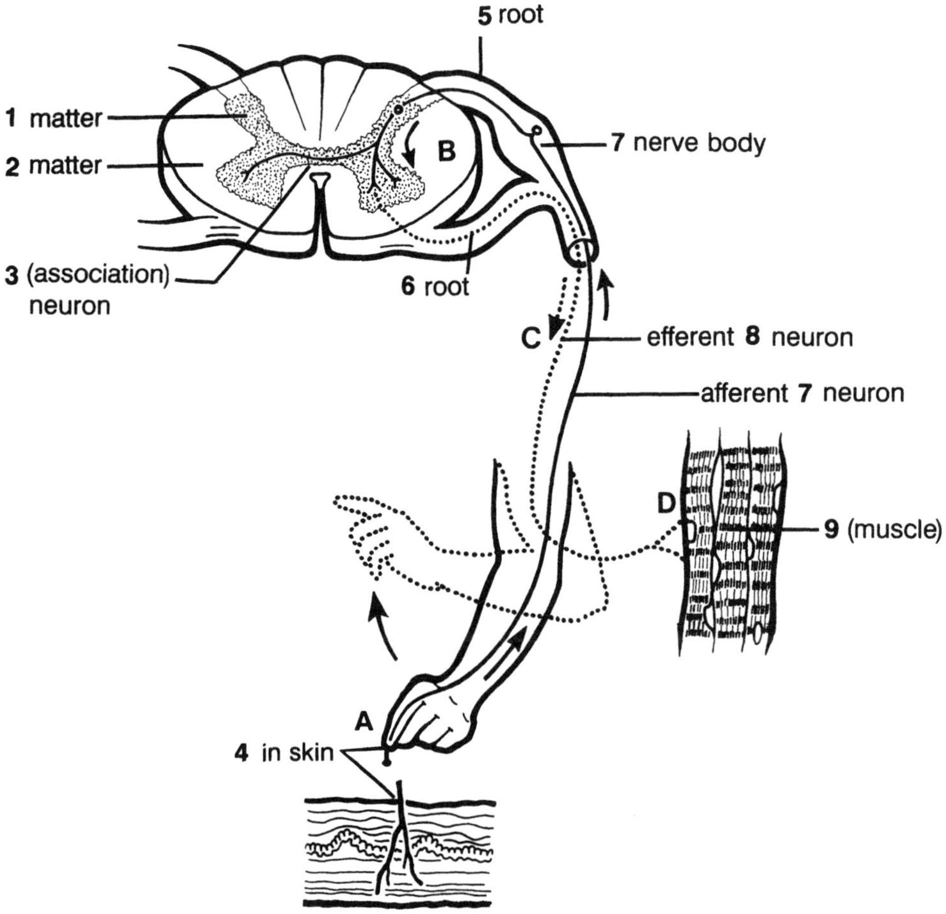

Figure 8.3 A simple reflex arc. An impulse is initiated at the finger by a receptor (**A**) in the skin. The impulse travels over a sensory afferent neuron to the spinal cord, where it is transmitted via the interneuron (**B**) to the efferent motor neuron. The impulse travels via the efferent motor neuron (**C**) to the muscle (**D**), which effects a response.

1. ______________________
2. ______________________
3. ______________________
4. ______________________
5. ______________________
6. ______________________
7. ______________________
8. ______________________
9. ______________________

Exercise 8.4

Labelling. Write the name of the structure or function on the space provided. Colour each lobe separately; correlate A and B.

Key:
association
auditory
central
cerebellum
cerebrum
frontal
lateral sulcus
medulla
motor
motor speech
occipital
parietal
pons
sensory
speech
spinal cord
taste
visual

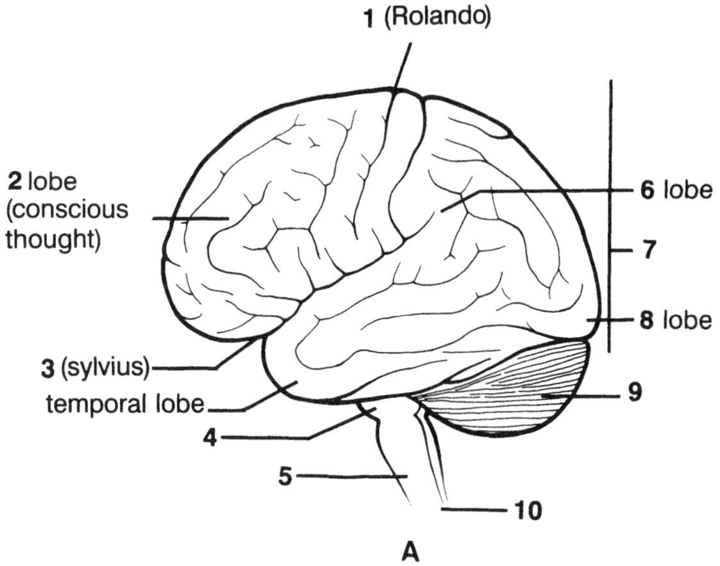

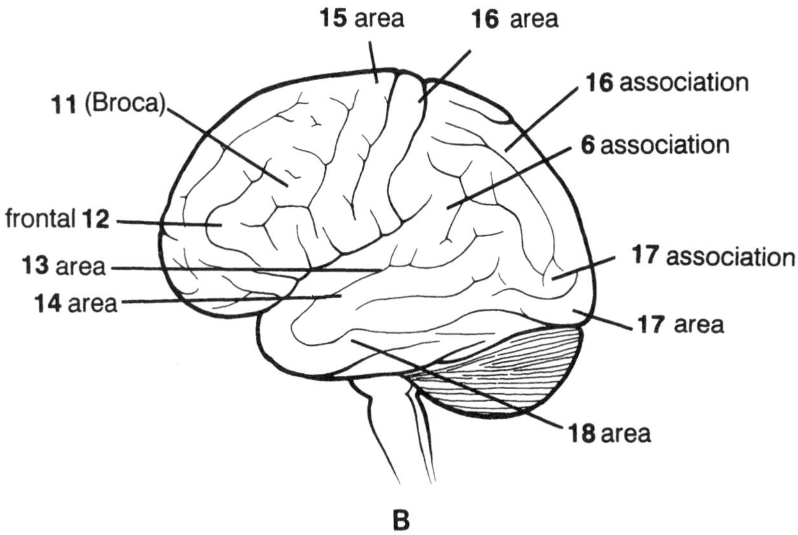

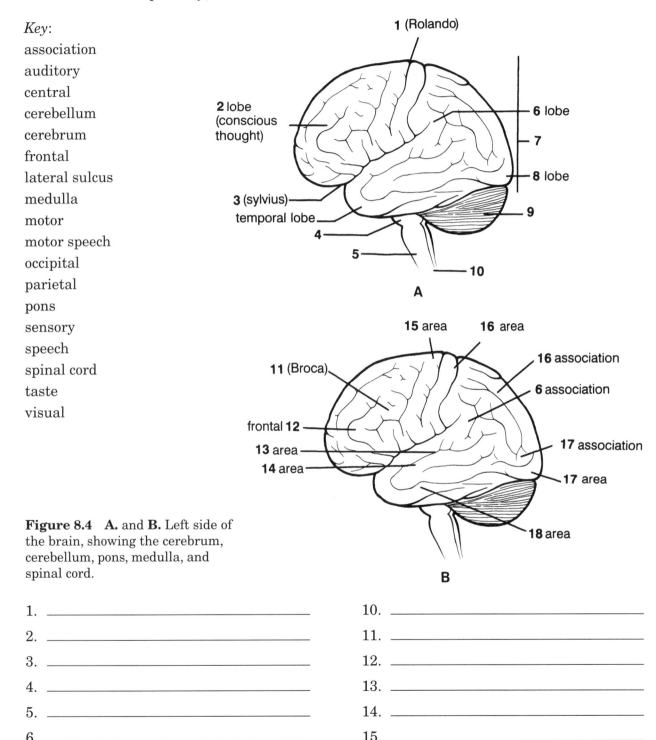

Figure 8.4 A. and **B.** Left side of the brain, showing the cerebrum, cerebellum, pons, medulla, and spinal cord.

1. ______________________
2. ______________________
3. ______________________
4. ______________________
5. ______________________
6. ______________________
7. ______________________
8. ______________________
9. ______________________
10. ______________________
11. ______________________
12. ______________________
13. ______________________
14. ______________________
15. ______________________
16. ______________________
17. ______________________
18. ______________________

Exercise 8.5

Labelling. Write the name of the cranial nerve in the space provided.
Colour the nerves according to their functions.

Key:

abducens	oculomotor
accessory	olfactory
acoustic	optic
facial	trigeminal
glossopharyngeal	trochlear
hypoglossal	vagus

Figure 8.5 Cranial nerves. Twelve pairs of nerves arise from the undersurface of the brain to supply the head and neck and most viscera. They may be sensory (s), motor (m), or mixed in function.

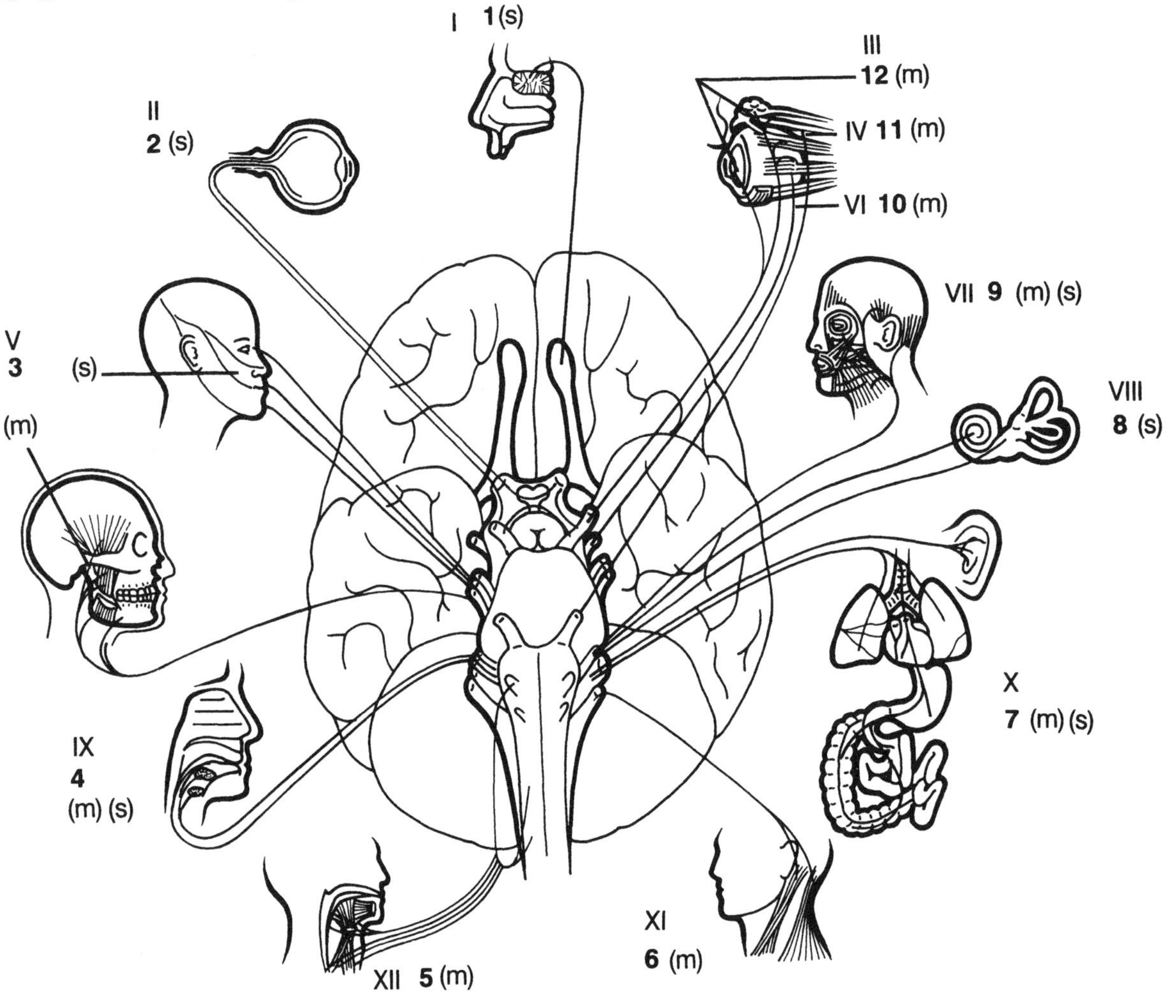

1. ______________________
2. ______________________
3. ______________________
4. ______________________
5. ______________________
6. ______________________
7. ______________________
8. ______________________
9. ______________________
10. ______________________
11. ______________________
12. ______________________

V. TEST ITEMS

A. *Multiple Choice.* There is only one answer that is either correct or most appropriate. Circle the best answer for each question.

1. At a synapse, impulse transmission is accomplished by means of
  a. inactivators
  b. neurotransmitters
  c. inhibitors
  d. enzymes

2. The medulla obongata has centres for
  a. sexual development
  b. metabolism and hunger
  c. control of heartbeat, respiration, and blood vessels
  d. taste and smell

3. In an axon of a motor neuron, the impulse travels
  a. to the cell body
  b. away from the cell body
  c. toward the brain
  d. away from the brain

4. Destruction of the motor area of the right cerebrum results in loss of
  a. left body reflexes
  b. left voluntary motion
  c. left body sensations
  d. right voluntary motion

5. A lumbar puncture is best performed between which two lumbar vertebrae?
  a. 1 and 2
  b. 2 and 3
  c. 3 and 4
  d. 4 and 5

6. If your body had to immediately react to a stress, which system would assume control?
  a. nervous
  b. circulatory
  c. endocrine
  d. integumentary

7. Which of the following is not part of a neuron?
  a. cell body
  b. dendrite
  c. axon
  d. neuroeffector junction

8. If the anterior root of a spinal nerve were cut, what would be the result in the regions supplied by that spinal nerve?
  a. complete loss of sensation
  b. complete loss of movement
  c. complete loss of sensation and movement
  d. complete loss of sensation, movement, and autonomic control of blood vessels and sweat glands

9. A neuron that transmits a nerve impulse to the central nervous system is called a(n)
  a. motor neuron
  b. sensory neuron
  c. bipolar neuron
  d. association neuron

10. A physician informs you that a patient has a disorder of the central nervous system. Which part of the nervous system is involved?
   a. nerves in the forearm
   b. nerves to the heart
   c. brain and spinal cord
   d. sympathetic neurons

11. Neurons that conduct impulses to the spinal cord or brain stem are called
   a. afferent neurons
   b. efferent neurons
   c. interneurons
   d. visceral neurons

12. The distal ends of sensory neuron dendrites are called
   a. effectors
   b. Nissl bodies
   c. receptors
   d. synapses

13. The part of a neuron that conducts impulses away from its cell body is called
   a. an axon
   b. a dendrite
   c. an effector
   d. a neurilemma

14. Which one of the following fissures separates the temporal lobe from the frontal and parietal lobes of the centrum?
   a. longitudinal
   b. lateral (fissure of Sylvius)
   c. central
   d. parieto-occipital

15. The lobe of the cerebrum most associated with voluntary action is the
   a. frontal lobe
   b. occipital lobe
   c. parietal lobe
   d. temporal lobe

16. Control of the peripheral nervous system appears to be centred in the
   a. spinal cord
   b. thalamus
   c. cerebellum
   d. hypothalamus

17. Abnormal body movements, such as uncontrollable shaking and involuntary movements of the skeletal muscles, indicate damage to the
   a. sensory areas of the cerebrum
   b. basal ganglia (cerebral nuclei)
   c. association areas of the cortex
   d. primary olfactory areas

18. A patient with a tumour of the cerebellum would probably exhibit
  a. absence of the patellar reflex
  b. unconsciousness
  c. the inability to execute smooth, precise movements
  d. the inability to perform voluntary movements

19. The peripheral nervous system consists of
  a. brain and spinal cord
  b. cranial and spinal nerves
  c. spinal nerves only
  d. brain nerves only

20. The reason that the motor areas of the right cerebral cortex control voluntary movements on the left side of the body is that the
  a. cerebrum contains projection fibres
  b. cerebellum controls voluntary movements
  c. medulla contains decussating pyramids
  d. pons connects the spinal cord with the brain

B. *Matching.* Each of the phrases in Column B refers to a term in Column A. Insert the letter of the phrase from Column B that best describes each term in Column A. Some phrases may be used more than once or not at all.

Column A	*Column B*
1. ___ coma	**a.** acute inflammation of the brain caused by a virus
2. ___ analgesia	**b.** abnormality of one or more vertebral arches in which part of the spinal cord may be exposed
3. ___ sciatica	**c.** inflammation of a nerve
4. ___ paralysis	**d.** attacks of pain along a peripheral nerve
5. ___ torpor	**e.** abnormally deep unconsciousness with an absence of voluntary response to stimuli
6. ___ shingles	**f.** diminished or complete loss of ability to comprehend and/or express spoken or written words
7. ___ neuritis	**g.** abnormal inactivity or no response to normal stimuli
8. ___ anaesthesia	**h.** severe pain along the sciatic nerve and its branches
9. ___ bacterial meningitis	**i.** loss of feeling
10. ___ viral encephalitis	**j.** insensibility to pain
11. ___ spina bifida	**k.** acute inflammation of the meninges caused by a bacterium
12. ___ neuralgia	**l.** diminished or total loss of motor function resulting from damage to nervous or muscular tissue
13. ___ aphasia	**m.** inflammation caused by a virus that attacks sensory cell bodies of dorsal root ganglia and produces a characteristic line of skin blisters

Match the following malfunctions with the most probable cranial nerves. For each defect, you should pick a *single* most likely nerve. Some nerves may be used more than once.

Body Malfunctions

1. ____ loss of hearing and the sense of equilibrium
2. ____ inability to roll the eyeball upward
3. ____ blindness
4. ____ inability to move the tongue
5. ____ inability to move the shoulder and turn the head
6. ____ loss of smell
7. ____ inability to focus and partial loss of eye movement
8. ____ inability to move the eyeball laterally
9. ____ difficulty in swallowing
10. ____ inability to masticate and lack of senses of the face
11. ____ inability to smile
12. ____ gastrointestinal problems
13. ____ no sense of taste from the posterior portion of the tongue

Cranial Nerves

a. olfactory
b. optic
c. oculomotor
d. trochlear
e. trigeminal
f. abducens
g. facial
h. vestibulocochlear
i. glossopharyngeal
j. vagus
k. accessory
l. hypoglossal

C. *True or False.* Place a *T* or an *F* in the space provided to indicate true or false.

____ **1.** The nervous and endocrine systems play the major role in regulation and coordination of the body.

____ **2.** The efferent pathway in a physiological control system is the path from the integrating centre to an effector.

____ **3.** The posterior columns of grey matter contain ventral horn cells.

____ **4.** The lateral grey columns contain cell bodies of the axons that pass out to sympathetic ganglia.

____ **5.** The anterior division of the thoracic spinal nerves form the thoracic plexus.

____ **6.** The spinal cord of the adult extends the entire length of the vertebral canal.

____ **7.** The posterior and anterior columns of the central grey matter, together with the core, follow the general form of an H.

____ **8.** A reflex is a voluntary response to a harmful stimulus.

___ **9.** Transection of the spinal cord results in a release of functions normally inhibited by the higher centres.

___ **10.** The myelin sheath forms the continuous covering of a neuron.

___ **11.** Some neurons are specialised for the secretion of hormonal substances.

___ **12.** The neurons of the peripheral ganglia are true bipolar cells.

___ **13.** Both bipolar and multipolar neurons have single axons.

___ **14.** All cells have membrane potentials.

___ **15.** All action potentials within any one cell obey the all-or-none law.

___ **16.** The irritable and conducting units of the nervous system are called neurons.

___ **17.** The Nissl bodies in the cytoplasm of neurons are prominent areas of rough endoplasmic reticulum.

___ **18.** Motor nerve cells and interneurons are multipolar.

___ **19.** Neurological cells are conducting units.

___ **20.** Nerve endings for pain and for posture have a short period of adaptation.

Answer Sheet—Chapter 8

Exercise 8.1

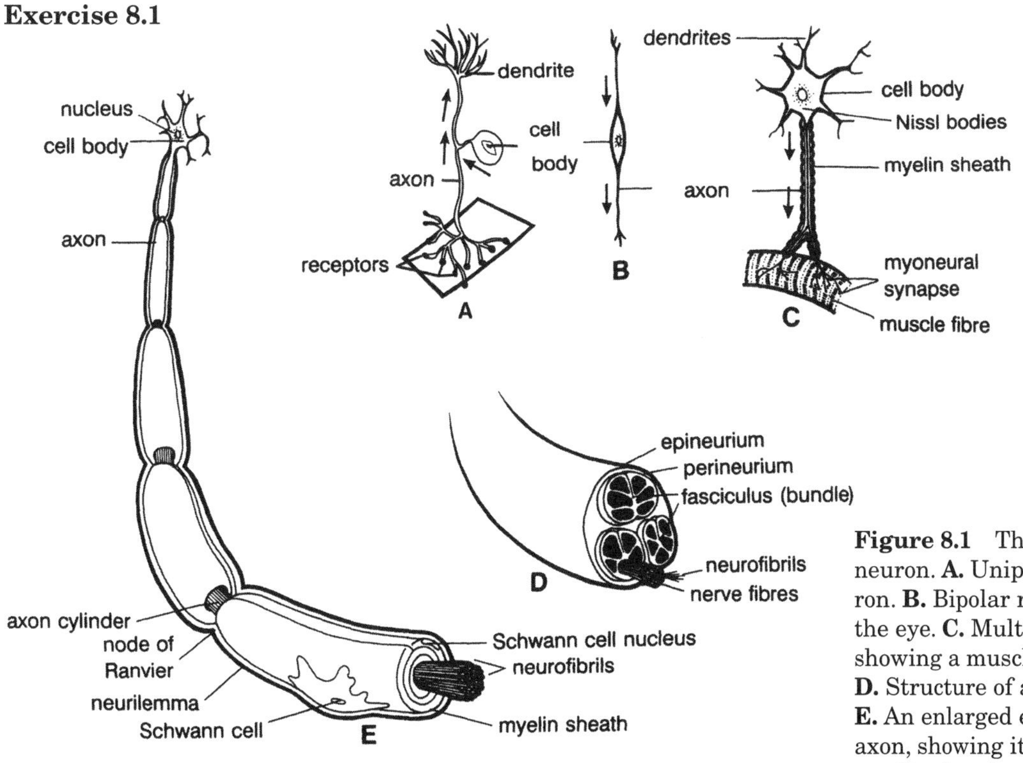

Figure 8.1 The structure of a neuron. **A.** Unipolar sensory neuron. **B.** Bipolar retinal neuron in the eye. **C.** Multipolar neuron, showing a muscle-nerve synapse. **D.** Structure of a typical nerve. **E.** An enlarged extension of an axon, showing its protective myelin sheath and neurilemma.

Exercise 8.2

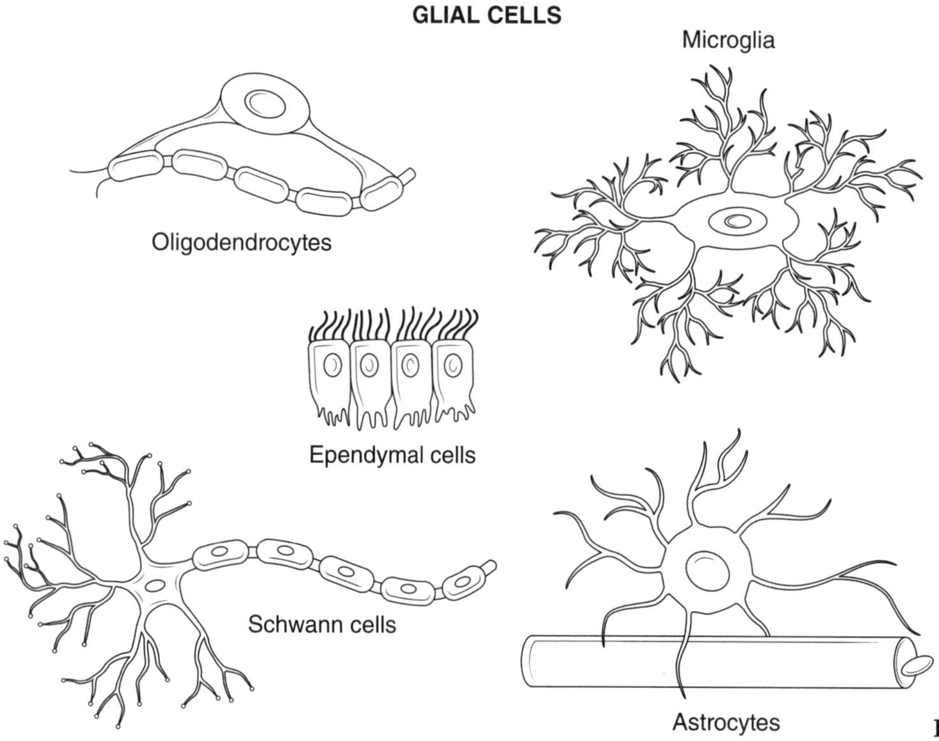

Figure 8.2 Glial cells.

Exercise 8.3

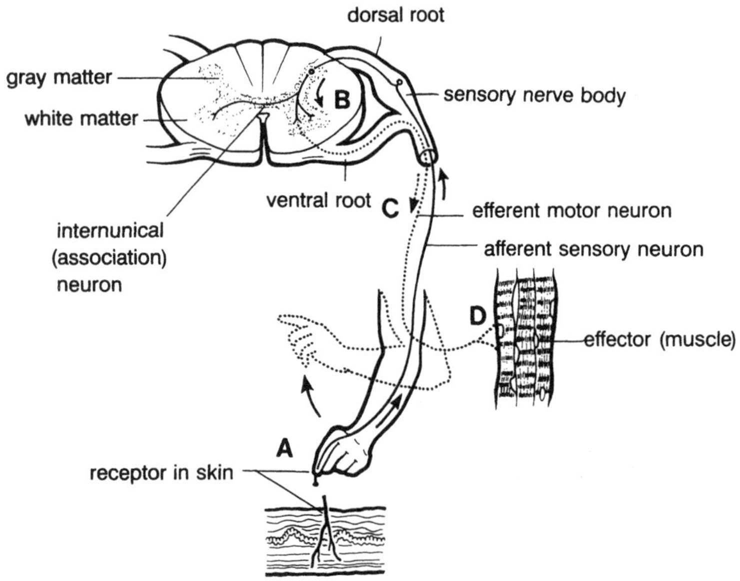

Figure 8.3 A simple reflex arc. An impulse is initiated at the finger by a receptor (**A**) in the skin. The impulse travels over a sensory afferent neuron to the spinal cord, where it is transmitted via the interneuron (**B**) to the efferent motor neuron. The impulse travels via the efferent motor neuron (**C**) to the muscle (**D**), which effects a response.

Exercise 8.4

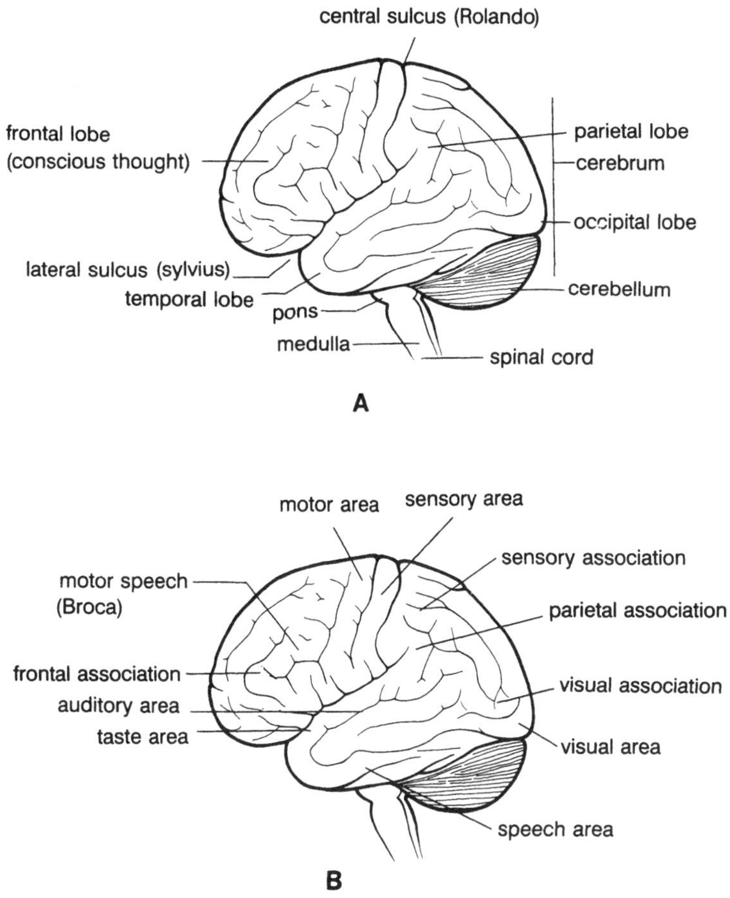

Figure 8.4 **A.** and **B.** Left side of the brain, showing the cerebrum, cerebellum, pons, medulla, and spinal cord.

Exercise 8.5

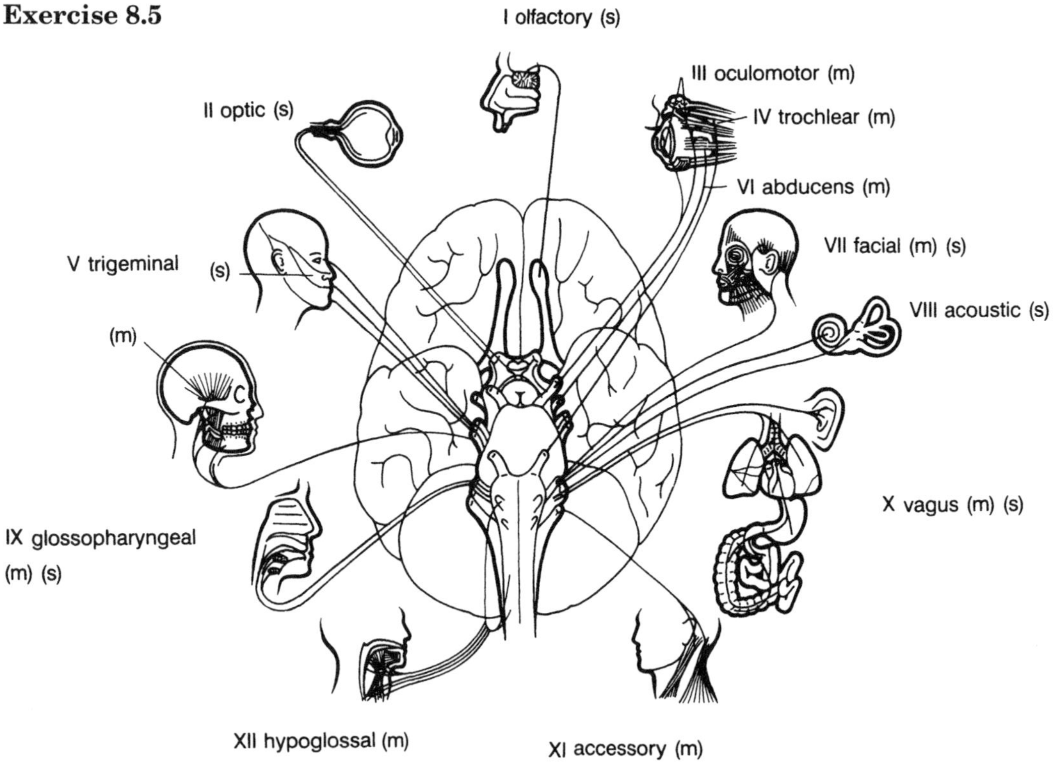

Figure 8.5 Cranial nerves. Twelve pairs of nerves arise from the undersurface of the brain to supply the head and neck and most viscera. They may be sensory (s), motor (m), or mixed in function.

Test Items

A. 1. b, 2. c, 3. b, 4. b, 5. c, 6. a, 7. d, 8. b, 9. b, 10. c, 11. a, 12. c, 13. a, 14. b, 15. a, 16. d, 17. b, 18. c, 19. b, 20. c.

B. 1. e, 2. j, 3. h, 4. l, 5. g, 6. m, 7. c, 8. i, 9. k, 10. a, 11. b, 12. d, 13. f.
1. h, 2. d, 3. b, 4. l, 5. k, 6. a, 7. c, 8. f, 9. i, 10. e, 11. g, 12. j, 13. l.

C. 1. T, 2. T, 3. F, 4. T, 5. F, 6. F, 7. T, 8. F, 9. T, 10. F, 11. T, 12. F, 13. T, 14. T, 15. T, 16. T, 17. T, 18. T, 19. F, 20. F.

9

The Involuntary Nervous System

I. CHAPTER SYNOPSIS

Students are introduced to the autonomic nervous system (ANS), and the structure and physiology of this system are described in detail. The autonomic system is the portion of the nervous system that regulates the activities of smooth muscle, cardiac muscle, and glands. Structurally, the system consists of visceral efferent neurons organised into nerves, ganglia, and plexuses. Functionally, it usually operates without conscious control. The autonomic nervous system consists of two principal divisions: the sympathetic and the parasympathetic. Both divisions are compared in terms of structure, physiology, and chemical transmitters released.

Physiologically, both divisions of the ANS contribute to the maintenance of homeostasis through their regulation of visceral activities. Most visceral effectors have a dual autonomic nerve supply from each division of the ANS. The parasympathetic division is concerned with activities of restoration and conservation of bodily energy and with the elimination of wastes. The sympathetic division is influenced by changes in external environment and is best known for the initiation of a widespread response to physical danger. Although visceral structures have a degree of functional independence, they are constantly monitored and regulated by cortical and subcortical areas, primary the hypothalamus. Biofeedback is a term applied to techniques used to gain conscious control over visceral responses.

Acetylcholine is released by cholinergic fibres that include all preganglionic fibres and the postganglionic fibres of the parasympathetic division. Norepinephrine (noradrenaline) is released by most postganglionic fibres of the sympathetic division, and fibres that release this neurotransmitter are called adrenergic fibres.

II. OBJECTIVES

After reading the chapter, the student should be able to:

- Describe the anatomy of the autonomic nervous system.
- Differentiate between a white and grey ramus and their contents.
- Integrate the autonomic nervous system with the central nervous system.
- Describe the sympathetic trunk and its preganglionic and postganglionic fibres.
- Explain the chemical action of both the sympathetic and parasympathetic divisions.
- Identify adrenergic and cholinergic fibres and their receptors.
- Define antagonism.

III. IMPORTANT TERMS

Using your textbook, define the following terms:

adrenaline (add-ren-a-lin) ____________________

____

adrenergic (a-dre-nur′jik) ____________________

____

autonomic (aw-to-nom′ik) ____________________

____

celiac (see′lee-ak) ____________________

____

cholinergic (ko-lin-ur′jick) ____________________

____

cholinesterase (ko-lin-es′tur-ace) ____________________

____

collateral (kuh-lat′ur-ul) ____________________

____

communicans (kom-yoo′ni-kanz) ____________________

____

enteric (en-terr′ik) ____________________

____

epinephrine (ep-i-nef′rin) ______________________________

ganglion (gang′glee-un) ______________________________

grey ramus (gray ray′mus) ______________________________

hypogastric (high-po-gas′trik) ______________________________

hypothalamus (hi-po-thuh-la′mus) ______________________________

inhibit (in-hib′it) ______________________________

involuntary (in-vol′un-terr-ee) ______________________________

medulla (me-dul′uh) ______________________________

neurotransmitter (new-ro-tranz-mit′ur) ______________________________

noradrenalin (nor-add-ren-a-lin) ______________________________

norepinephrine (nor-ep-i-nef′rin) ______________________________

parasympathetic (par-uh-sim-puh-thet′ik) ______________________________

peripheral (pe-rif′e-rul) ______________________________

plexus (plek′sus) ______________________________

postganglionic (pohst-gang-glee-on′ick) ______________________________

preganglionic (pree-gang-glee-on′ik) ______________________________

spinal (spy′nul) ______________________________

sympathetic (sim-puh-thet′ik) ______________________________

____

synoptic (si-nop-ti′k) ______________________________

____

target (tahr′get) ______________________________

____

vasoconstriction (vay-zo-kun-strik′shun) ______________________________

____

vasodilatation (vay-zo-dye-lat-tay-shun) ______________________________

____

vasodilation (vay-zo-dye-lay-shun′) ______________________________

____

vasomotor (vay-zo-mo′tur) ______________________________

____

white ramus (white ray′mus) ______________________________

____

IV. EXERCISES

Complete the following exercises in the order given. A precise set of terms and diagrams has been chosen to describe the involuntary nervous system.

Exercise 9.1

Labelling. Write the name of the structure on the space provided. Colour the spinal cord and visceral cord differently.

Key:

bladder	parasympathetic	preganglionic
ganglion	pelvic	spinal
hypogastric	postganglionic	sympathetic

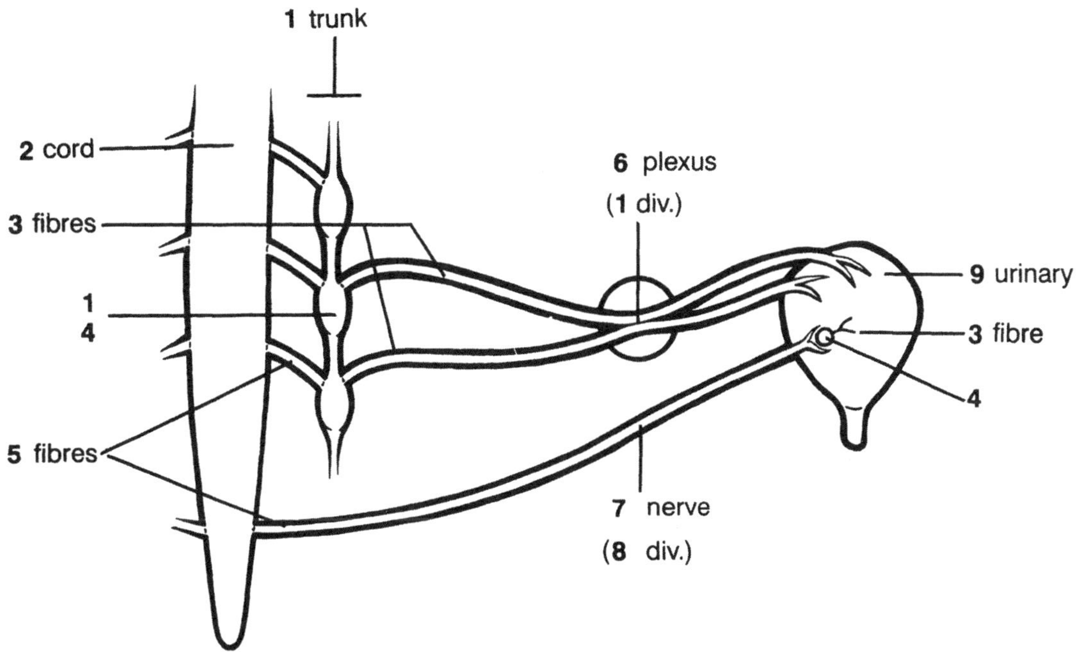

Figure 9.1 The lumbosacral segment of the autonomic nervous system, showing the arrangement of the ganglia, preganglionic fibres of both the sympathetic and parasympathetic divisions to the spinal cord, and visceral organs.

1. ______________________
2. ______________________
3. ______________________
4. ______________________
5. ______________________
6. ______________________
7. ______________________
8. ______________________
9. ______________________

Exercise 9.2

Labelling. Write the name of the structure on the space provided. Colour the spinal cord, trunk, and visceral organ differently.

Key:

collateral	ganglion	root	trunk
communicans	grey	spinal	ventral
dorsal	postganglionic	sympathetic	white

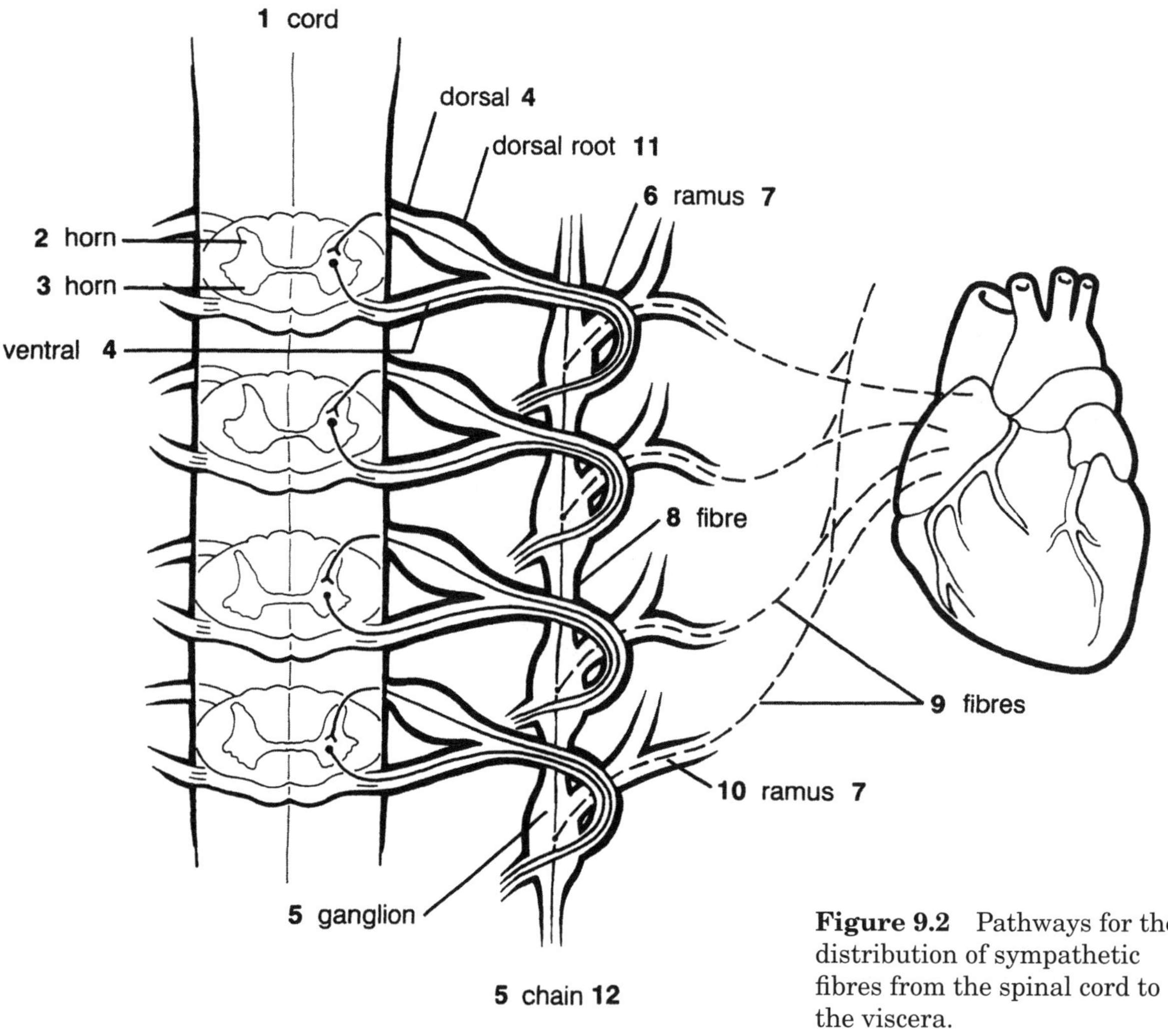

Figure 9.2 Pathways for the distribution of sympathetic fibres from the spinal cord to the viscera.

1. ______________________
2. ______________________
3. ______________________
4. ______________________
5. ______________________
6. ______________________
7. ______________________
8. ______________________
9. ______________________
10. ______________________
11. ______________________
12. ______________________

Exercise 9.3

Fill in the Blanks. Fill in the blanks with the appropriate terms. Some terms may be used more than once.

Key:

adrenal
adrenergic
autonomic
bloodstream
chemical
epinephrine (adrenaline)
excitation
grey
medulla
neurons
norepinephrine (noradrenaline)
peripheral
postganglionic
spinal
stimulate
sympathetic
terminal
viscera

CHEMICAL TRANSMITTERS

Adrenergic Fibres

The ______________ filaments of most ______________ postganglionic ______________ produce chiefly ______________. This substance is also secreted by the ______________ of the ______________ gland, and therefore these fibres are classified as ______________. Exceptions are the sympathetic fibres to sweat glands, to the blood vessels of the skin, and to the arrector muscles that elevate the hair. These ______________ fibres enter the ______________ nerves through the ______________ communicans and reach the skin incorporated in the ______________ nerves.

The effects of ______________ also secreted by the adrenal medulla, and ______________ can be widespread because these ______________ substances, which result from ______________ of the ______________ postganglionic fibres, are carried by the ______________. ______________ transmitters ______________ the ______________ controlled by the sympathetic division of the ______________ nervous system.

Key:

acetic acid
acetylcholine
acts
biochemistry
bloodstream
both
choline
cholinesterase
depolarising
destroys
ganglia
hyperpolarisation
inhibit
inhibition
not
parasympathetic
preganglionic
synaptic
target

Cholinergic Fibres

______________ fibres also produce a chemical substance, ______________, which is promptly converted to ______________ and ______________ by the action of the enzyme ______________. Acetylcholine is a ______________ substance that ______________ aids transmission at the ______________ terminals in ______________ sympathetic and parasympathetic ______________. At the postganglionic terminal of the parasympathetic or craniosacral division, secretion of ______________ ______________ to ______________ the organ. The ability of acetylcholine to excite at the first synapse and inhibit at the second synapse is due to differences in the ______________ of the ______________ cells. In the heart, for example, parasympathetic stimulation is followed by ______________ of the cardiac cells and ______________ of the heartbeat. The enzyme ______________ quickly ______________ acetylcholine, which therefore has effects only locally, where it is secreted. Unlike norepinephrine (noradrenaline), it probably is ______________ carried by the ______________.

V. TEST ITEMS

A. *Multiple Choice.* There is only one answer that is either correct or most appropriate. Circle the best answer for each question.

1. Myelinisation of nerve fibres in the PNS is the job of
a. neurons
b. pia mater
c. epithelial cells
d. Schwann cells

2. A spinal nerve root has
a. motor pathways
b. both motor and sensory pathways
c. sensory pathways
d. ganglia cells

3. Preparing the body for fight or flight is the role of the
a. sympathetic nervous system
b. cerebrum
c. parasympathetic nervous system
d. cerebellum

4. Which statement concerning the autonomic nervous system is *not* true?
a. It usually operates without any conscious control
b. It regulates visceral activities
c. All of its axons are afferent fibres
d. It contains rami and ganglia

5. Terminal ganglia receive
a. postganglionic fibres from the parasympathetic division
b. postganglionic fibres from the sympathetic division
c. preganglionic fibres from the parasympathetic division
d. preganglionic fibres from the sympathetic division

6. When the sympathetic nervous system is stimulated, which of the following occurs?
a. Vessels in the skeletal muscles constrict
b. Blood pressure increases
c. Respirations decrease
d. Peristalsis increases

7. When the parasympathetic nervous system is stimulated, which of the following occurs?
a. Digestive processes are increased
b. Bronchioles dilate
c. Pupils dilate
d. Vessels in the skin constrict

8. The most abundant chemical that aids in transmission of nerve impulses across synapses is
a. strychnine
b. monamine oxidase
c. cholinesterase
d. acetylcholine

9. Autonomic nerve fibres supply
   a. skeletal muscle, cardiac muscle, and glands
   b. visceral muscle, cardiac muscle, and glands
   c. skeletal muscle, visceral muscle, and cardiac muscle
   d. skeletal muscle, visceral muscle, and glands

10. Sympathetic responses generally have widespread effects on the body because
   a. preganglionic fibres are short and postganglionic fibres are long
   b. myoneural junctions contain a substance that inactivates acetylcholine
   c. preganglionic fibres synapse with several postsynaptic fibres
   d. they reach visceral effectors faster than parasympathetic impulses

11. The cell bodies of preganglionic neurons of the parasympathetic division of the autonomic nervous system are located in the
   a. lateral grey horns of the thoracic cord
   b. nuclei in the brain stem and lateral grey horns of the sacral cord
   c. lateral grey horns of the cervical cord
   d. lateral grey horns of the lumbar cord

12. Autonomic ganglia located on either side of the vertebral column from the base of the skull to the coccyx are called
   a. prevertebral ganglia
   b. collateral ganglia
   c. terminal ganglia
   d. sympathetic trunk ganglia

13. Axons from preganglionic neurons of the parasympathetic division of the autonomic nervous system are known as
   a. synapse in sympathetic chain ganglia
   b. synapse in prevertebral ganglia
   c. synapse in terminal ganglia
   d. part of the thoracolumbar outflow

14. In their course from vertebral rami to the sympathetic trunk, sympathetic preganglionic fibres are contained in structures called
   a. white rami communicans
   b. meningeal branches
   c. dorsal rami
   d. grey rami communicans

15. Diminished or total loss of motor function from damage to nervous tissue or a muscle is called
   a. paralysis
   b. sciatica
   c. neuralgia
   d. aphasia

16. Which of these is *not* a component of the sympathetic nervous system?
   a. white rami communicans
   b. inferior cervical ganglion
   c. ciliary ganglion
   d. grey rami communicans

17. One sympathetic response is
 a. dilatation of the bronchial tubes
 b. normal or excessive lacrimal secretion
 c. increased intestinal motility
 d. increased pancreatic secretion

18. The autonomic nervous system
 a. is made up of motor neurons only
 b. has preganglionic and postganglionic fibres
 c. has cell bodies in both the cord and in ganglia
 d. all of the above

19. Which of the following is not generally associated with the autonomic system?
 a. speaking
 b. digestion
 c. heartbeat
 d. body temperature

20. When a person's heart races
 a. the parasympathetic effect is more influential than that of the sympathetic
 b. the sympathetic effect is more influential than that of the parasympathetic
 c. there is a perfect balance between the parasympathetic and the sympathetic effects
 d. voluntary control is in effect

B. *Matching.* Each of the terms in Column B refers to a term in Column A. Insert the letter of the term from Column B that best describes the term in Column A. Some terms in Column B may be used more than once or not at all.

	Column A		*Column B*
1. ___	preganglionic	**a.**	thoracolumbar
2. ___	postganglionic	**b.**	cholinergic
3. ___	epinephrine (adrenaline)	**c.**	craniosacral
4. ___	autonomic	**d.**	heart
5. ___	enteric plexus	**e.**	involuntary
6. ___	sympathetic trunk	**f.**	voluntary
7. ___	parasympathetic	**g.**	grey ramus
8. ___	acetylcholine	**h.**	digestive tract
9. ___	solar plexus	**i.**	adrenergic
10. ___	cardiac plexus	**j.**	white ramus
		k.	stomach
		l.	kidneys

Place in each blank the letter corresponding to the word that describes the change in activity produced by strongly stimulating the sympathetic or thoracolumbar division of autonomics. The letters may be used more than once.

	Column A		*Column B*
1. ___	blood vessels in skin	**a.**	constricted
2. ___	blood vessels in abdominal viscera	**b.**	dilated
3. ___	blood vessels in skeletal muscle	**c.**	decreased
4. ___	blood pressure	**d.**	increased
5. ___	blood sugar level		
6. ___	bronchioles of the lung		
7. ___	flow of watery saliva		
8. ___	peristalsis of digestive tube		
9. ___	perspiration		
10. ___	pupil of eye		
11. ___	rate of heartbeat		
12. ___	rate of breathing		
13. ___	secretion of epinephrine (adrenaline)		

C. *True or False.* Place a *T* or an *F* in the space provided to indicate true or false.

___ **1.** The adrenal medulla is part of the sympathetic nervous system.

___ **2.** Stimulation of the parasympathetic system will cause the release of epinephrine (adrenaline) from the adrenal medulla.

___ **3.** The primary function of the autonomic nervous system is the involuntary regulation of the internal environment.

___ **4.** In general, norepinephrine (noradrenaline) is released from postganglionic sympathetic nerve endings.

___ **5.** Acetylcholine is the transmitter agent released from postganglionic parasympathetic fibres.

___ **6.** All preganglionic sympathetic axons leave the spinal cord via the ventral root and then pass to a paravertebral ganglion via the white ramus.

___ **7.** The autonomic nervous system innervates skeletal muscles and glands.

___ **8.** Regulation of the autonomic nervous system occurs primarily in the medulla and hypothalamus of the brain.

___ **9.** A spinal nerve is formed by the junction of the dorsal and ventral roots.

___ **10.** Spinal shock may depress visceral reflexes controlling the emptying of the bladder and rectum.

____ **11.** The parasympathetic division of the autonomic nervous system consists of nerve fibres that arise from cells in the brain stem and sacral region of the spinal cord.

____ **12.** As a rule, the two divisions of the autonomic nervous system function in an antagonistic fashion.

____ **13.** Nerve impulse (action potential) conduction can be compared to a self-propagating wave of negativity passing along a neuron's membrane.

____ **14.** Grey matter consists of a series of myelinated nerve fibres.

____ **15.** The hypothalamus has centres for initiating sympathetic and parasympathetic responses.

Answer Sheet—Chapter 9

Exercise 9.1

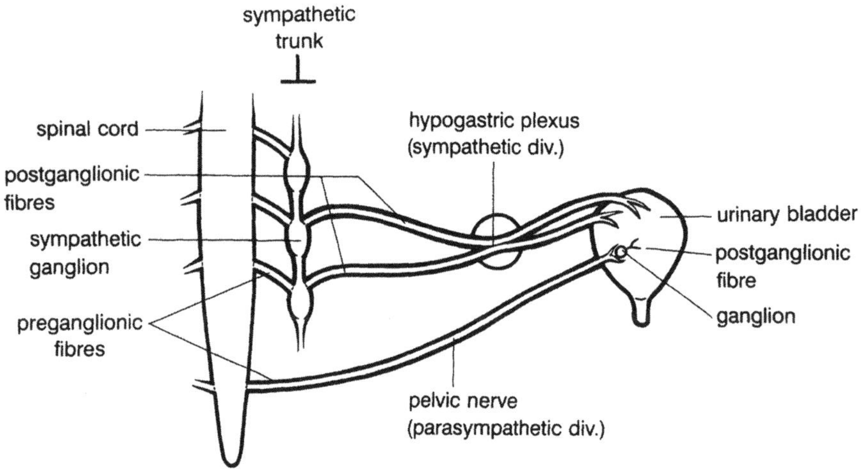

Figure 9.1 The lumbosacral segment of the autonomic nervous system, showing the arrangement of the ganglia, preganglionic fibres of both the sympathetic and parasympathetic divisions to the spinal cord, and visceral organs.

Exercise 9.2

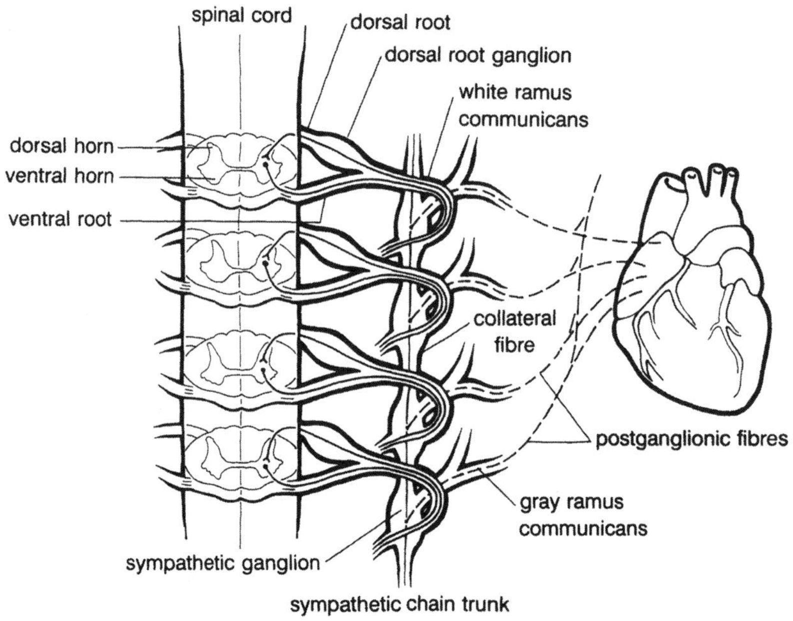

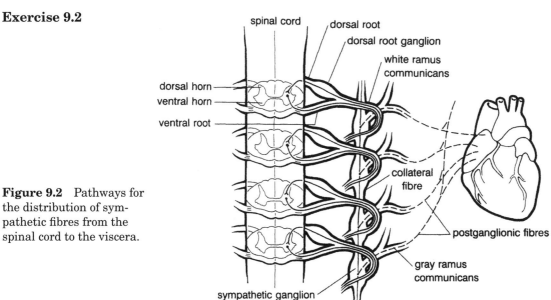

Figure 9.2 Pathways for the distribution of sympathetic fibres from the spinal cord to the viscera.

Exercise 9.3

CHEMICAL TRANSMITTERS

Adrenergic Fibres

The terminal filaments of most sympathetic postganglionic neurons produce chiefly norepinephrine. This substance is also secreted by the medulla of the adrenal gland, and therefore these substances are classified as adrenergic. Exceptions are the sympathetic fibres to sweat glands, to the blood vessels of the skin, and to the arrector muscles that elevate the hair. These postganglionic fibres enter the spinal nerves through the grey communicans and reach the skin incorporated in the peripheral nerves.

The effects of epinephrine, also secreted by the adrenal medulla, and norepinephrine can be widespread because these chemical substances, which result from excitation of the sympathetic postganglionic fibres, are carried by the bloodstream. Adrenergic transmitters stimulate the viscera controlled by the sympathetic division of the autonomic nervous system.

Cholinergic Fibres

Parasympathetic fibres also produce a chemical substance, acetylcholine, which is promptly converted to choline and acetic acid by the action of the enzyme cholinesterase. Acetylcholine is a depolarising substance that aids synaptic transmission at the preganglionic terminal in both sympathetic and parasympathetic ganglia. At the postganglionic terminals of the parasympathetic or craniosacral division, secretion of acetylcholine acts to inhibit the organ. The ability of acetylcholine to excite at the first synapse and inhibit at the second synapse is due to differences in the biochemistry of the target cells. In the heart, for example, parasympathetic stimulation is followed by hyperpolarisation of the cardiac cells and inhibition of the heartbeat. The enzyme cholinesterase quickly destroys acetylcholine, which therefore has effects only locally, where it is secreted. Unlike norepinephrine (noradrenaline), it probably is not carried by the bloodstream.

Test Items

A. 1. d, 2. b, 3. a, 4. c, 5. c, 6. b, 7. a, 8. d, 9. b, 10. c, 11. b, 12. d, 13. c, 14. a, 15. a, 16. c, 17. a, 18. a, 19. a, 20. b.

B. 1. j, 2. g, 3. i, 4. e, 5. h, 6. a, 7. c, 8. b, 9. k, 10. d.
1. a, 2. a, 3. b, 4. d, 5. d, 6. b, 7. c, 8. c, 9. d, 10. b, 11. d, 12. d, 13. d.

C. 1. T, 2. F, 3. T, 4. T, 5. T, 6. T, 7. F, 8. T, 9. T, 10. T, 11. T, 12. T, 13. F, 14. F, 15. T.

10

The Endocrine System

I. CHAPTER SYNOPSIS

The student is introduced to the principal organs of the endocrine system in terms of location, structure, hormones secreted and their physiological effects, and the disorders that result from abnormal secretions. Emphasis throughout is placed on the regulation of hormone secretions by negative feedback systems. There is also a detailed discussion of the general stress syndrome and the stages of the stress response.

The endocrine and nervous systems are the major communications systems within the body. A hormone is a chemical substance synthesised by a specific organ (the endocrine gland) and secreted into the blood, which carries it to other sites where action is exerted. The change in target tissue function resulting from the hormone's action is usually part of a negative feedback loop leading to the maintenance of the internal environment. Although each hormone circulates to all cells of the body, only certain cells are affected; this specificity depends on receptor sites to which the hormone attaches. The quantities of a hormone in the blood are determined by its rate of secretion, destruction, and excretion.

Most hormones cause changes in membrane transport or enzyme activity in the target cells; these primary effects can produce numerous secondary effects. The target cells for some hormones are themselves endocrine glands.

II. OBJECTIVES

After reading the chapter, the student should be able to:

- Explain the different mechanisms of hormone action.
- Explain the relationship between the central nervous system and endocrine glands.
- Explain the action of a hormone on a cell.
- Describe the different feedback mechanisms
- Identify the endocrine glands and list their major hormone secretions and their functions.
- Expain the key differences between peptide and steroid hormones.

III. IMPORTANT TERMS

Using your textbook, define the following terms:

adenyl cyclase (ad′e-nil sy′klace) ______________________________

____

adrenal (a-dree′nul) ______________________________

____

catecholamine (kat-i-kol′uh-meen) ______________________________

____

endocrine (en′do-krine) ______________________________

____

epinephrine (epi-nef′rin) ______________________________

____

feedback (feed′bak) ______________________________

____

glycoprotein (gly-ko-pro′teen) ______________________________

____

homeostasis (ho-mee-os′tah-sis) ______________________________

____

hormone (hor′mone) ______________________________

____

hypophysis (hy-pof′i-sis) ______________________________

____

hypothalamus (hy-po-thal′uh-mus) ______________________________

____

insulin (in′suh-lin) ______________________________

____

loop (loop) ______________________________

____

messenger (mes′an-jur) ______________________________

____

neurosecretory (new-ro-se-kree′-tuh-ree) ______________________________

____

ovaries (o′vur-ees) ______________________________

____

pancreas (pan′kree-us) ______________________________

____

parathyroid (par-uh-thy′royd) ______________________________

____

pituitary (pih-tew′i-ter-ee) ______________________________

____

prostaglandin (pros-tuh-glan′din) ______________________________

____

receptor (re-sep′tur) ______________________________

____

releasing factor (re-lees′-ing fak′tur) ______________________________

____

steroid (ster′oyd) ______________________________

____

target (tahr′gut) ______________________________

____

testes (tes′teez) ______________________________

____

thymus (thy′mus) ______________________________

____

thyroid (thy′royd) ______________________________

____

thyroxine (thy-rok′sin) ______________________________

____

IV. EXERCISES

Complete the following exercises in the order given. A precise set of diagrams and terms has been chosen to describe the endocrine system.

Exercise 10.1

Labelling Write the name of the gland on the space provided below. Colour each gland differently.

Key:
adrenal
hypophysis
ovaries
pancreas
parathyroid
testes
thymus
thyroid

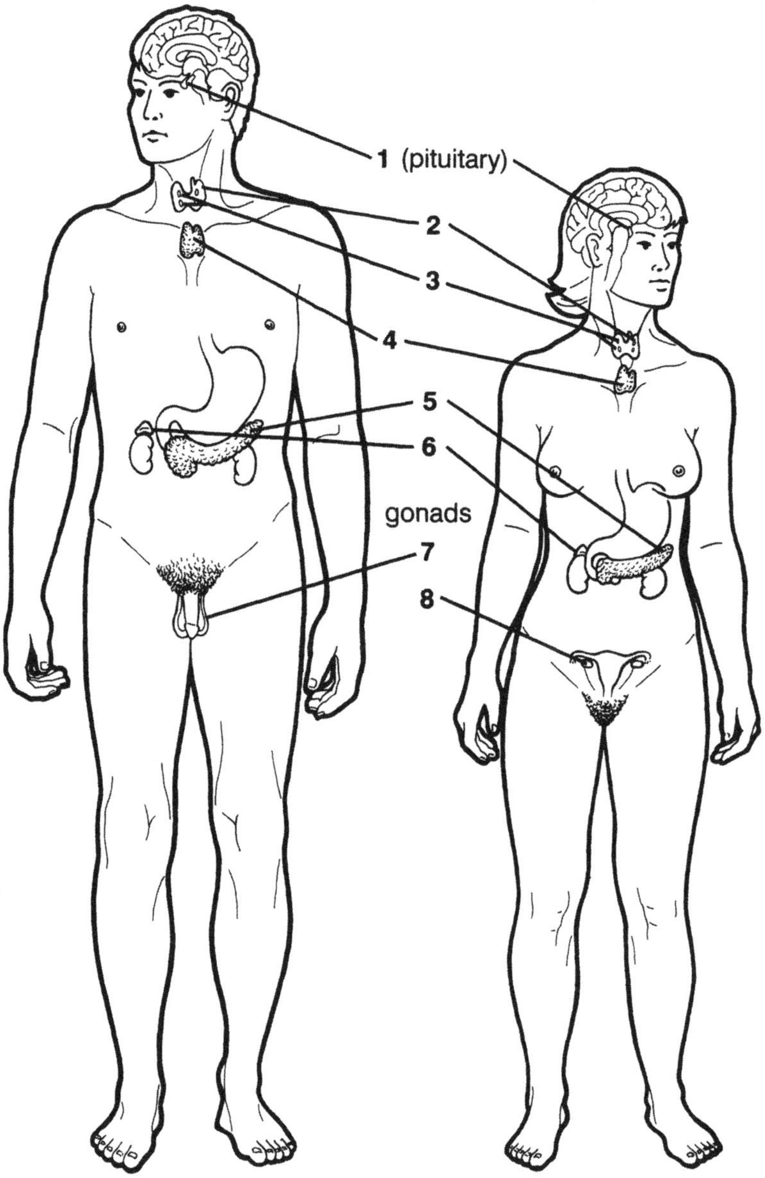

Figure 10.1 General location of the major endocrine glands of the body.

1. ______________________
2. ______________________
3. ______________________
4. ______________________
5. ______________________
6. ______________________
7. ______________________
8. ______________________

Exercise 10.2

Fill in the Blanks. Write the term from the key list in the appropriate spaces provided in the text on the right.

Key:
activities
blood
carried
effects
glycoproteins
homeostasis
hormones
inhibit
maintaining
messengers
organic
proteins
steroids
stimulate
target

HORMONES

Chemical Nature of Hormones

________________ are ________________ compounds of varying structural complexity that are ______________________ by the ________________ to other parts of the body, where they exert their specific _______________________. In simple terms, hormones are chemical ____________ that pass via the bloodstream to the _____________ organ or tissue. They may either ______________ or _____________ a function, but in general they do not initiate a process. Hormones are either _______________, _______________ (combination of a protein and a sugar), or _________________ (fat soluble hormones derived from cholesterol). The one thing that all hormones have in common, whether protein, glycoprotein, or steroid, is the function of _____________ ___________ by modifying the physiological ______________ of cells.

Key:
activates
adenyl cyclase
AMP
ATP
beat
binds
catecholamine
effect
few
increase
influence
interacting
life
metabolism
prostaglandins
receptors
regulate
responses
secondary
sites
small
stimulation
target

Actions of Hormones

Hormones are effective in remarkably ______________ quantities. For example, the injection of a ______________ micrograms of epinephrine (adrenaline) causes a definite ______________ in the rate of heart ______________. There is little doubt that each hormone has some ______________ on the fundamental ______________ of its target cells or tissues. Hormones, therefore, have a marked ______________ on such basic ______________ processes as growth, development, reproduction, energy utilisation, and cell permeability.

Much is known about the way hormones work on their target tissues or cells. Proteins and ______________ (fight or flight) hormones act by first ______________ with receptor ______________ on the cell membrane. The cell membrane contains the ______________ system. The hormone ______________ to specific ______________ in the cell membrane and subsequently ______________ adenyl cyclase. This enzyme converts adenosine triphosphate (__________) into 3,5-cycle ______________, which acts as the second messenger. Cyclic AMP, the ______________ messenger, then moves to other structures.

Although it is not known how the group of locally acting hormones called ______________ directly acts upon cells, it is postulated that they somehow ______________ the formation of cyclic AMP and may be involved in the ______________ of ______________ tissues to hormonal ______________.

Exercise 10.3

Labelling. Write the name of the term or structure on the space provided below. Colour the separate messengers a different colour.

Key:
adenyl
AMP
ATP
endocrine
first
messenger
neurosecretory
receptor
second
specialised

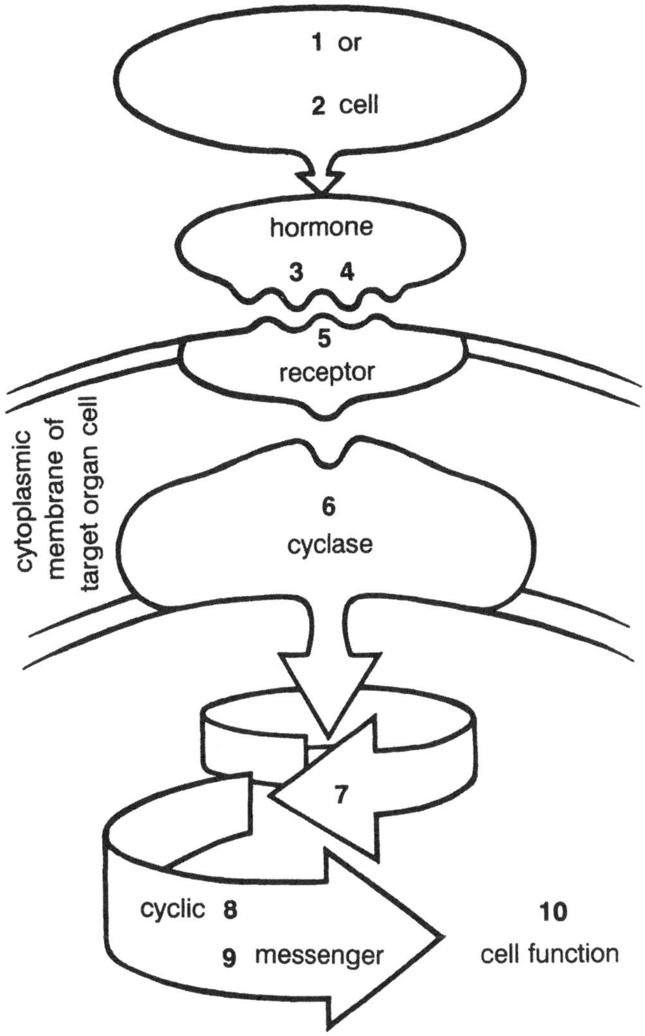

Figure 10.3 Mechanism of hormone action. Hormones act as messengers delivering their message to a membrane receptor in the target cell. Cyclic AMP serves as the second messenger for specialised cell functions.

1. ______________________
2. ______________________
3. ______________________
4. ______________________
5. ______________________
6. ______________________
7. ______________________
8. ______________________
9. ______________________
10. ______________________

Exercise 10.4

Fill in the Blanks. Write the terms from the key list in the appropriate spaces provided in the text on the right.

Key:

common	regulate
continually	regulated
directly	release
hypothalamus	releasing
indirectly	role
minimal	specific
needs	stored
nervous	

Feedback Control Systems

Hormones are secreted __________, and their rate of secretion is __________ by the body's __________. The __________ system controls the endocrine system either __________ or __________. The direct influence is __________ and best illustrated by the effects of the sympathetic nervous system on the secretion of the adrenal medulla. Indirect control is most __________ and is centred around the __________ of the __________. The hypothalamus secretes certain hormones and transfers these hormones to the posterior pituitary where they are __________ Also, the hypothalamus secretes chemical substances, known as __________ factors, which are released into the vascular bed between the hypothalamus and the anterior pituitary. These releasing factors are __________ and __________ the __________ of the anterior hormones.

Key:

effect	negative
feed back	positive
hormone	releasing
inhibit	stimulate
inhibiting	target

The __________ released by the __________ endocrine gland may __________ and influence release of the __________ or __________ substance of the hypothalamus or the pituitary hormone. If the __________ of the feedback is to __________ the overall response of the system, it is termed __________ feedback. If the effect of the feedback is to __________ further hormone release, it is __________ feedback.

Key:

back
direct
high
influence
inhibit
inhibits
long feedback
mechanisms
regulate
release
secretion
short feedback
thyroxine

In many cases the __________ of a hormone is regulated by both positive and negative feedback __________. __________, which is released by the thyroid gland, can __________ the release of thyroid-stimulating hormone in two ways. First, __________ levels __________ the release of thyrotropin- releasing hormone by the hypothalamus, which reduces TSH release by the anterior pituitary. Second, thyroxine __________ the __________ of TSH by __________ effect on the cells of the anterior pituitary. This particular type of feedback pathway (from target gland to pituitary) is called a __________ loop. Additionally, the pituitary hormones may feed __________ to the brain to __________ the releasing or inhibiting substances; this pathway is called a __________ loop.

Exercise 10.5

Labelling. Write the name of the term or structure on the space provided. Colour the feedback loops differently than the anatomy.

Key:
central
feedback
hormone
hypophyseal
long
loop
neurosecretory
releasing
short
stimuli
target

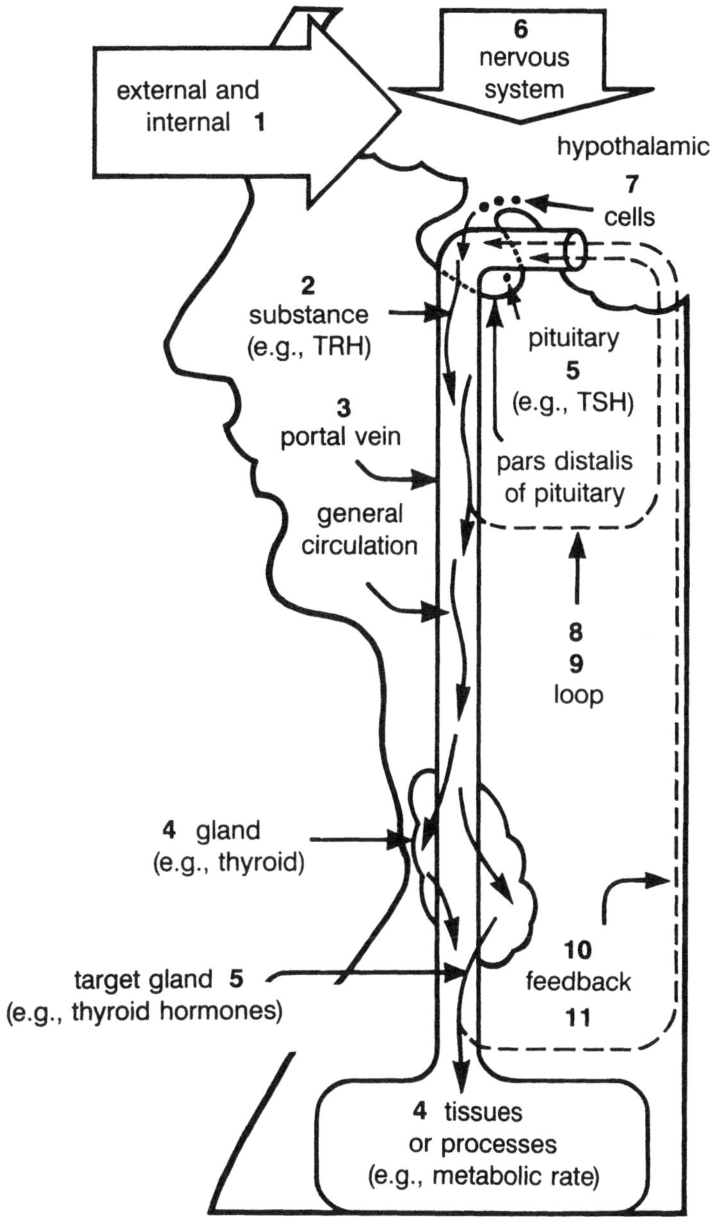

Figure 10.5 Feedback control of endocrine gland activity. External or internal stimuli influence the release of releasing factors from the hypothalamus, which in turn trigger the release of hormones from glands that control important vital functions of the body.

1. ______________________
2. ______________________
3. ______________________
4. ______________________
5. ______________________
6. ______________________
7. ______________________
8. ______________________
9. ______________________
10. ______________________
11. ______________________

V. TEST ITEMS

A. *Multiple Choice.* There is only one answer that is either correct or most appropriate. Circle the best answer for each question.

1. A hormone is a chemical that
a. is produced by living cells
b. regulates metabolic activities
c. is distributed by the blood or lymph
d. all of the above

2. Most hormones are chemically classified as
a. nucleic acids or amino acid based
b. amino acid based or carbohydrates
c. steroid or peptide based
d. carbohydrates or nucleic acids

3. Insulin is secreted by the pancreas when
a. blood sugar level is high
b. blood sugar level is low
c. glucagon is secreted
d. the gallbladder secretes bile

4. In a feedback system,
a. input is fed back into the system
b. input serves no useful purpose
c. output is fed back into the system
d. output is never an important factor

5. Hormones
a. are produced by exocrine glands
b. are carried in the blood to virtually all parts of the body
c. remain at constant concentration in the blood
d. are none of the above

6. Which of the following statements describes steroid hormones?
a. They bind to receptors on the target cell plasma membrane
b. They activate membrane-associated enzymes
c. They activate specific target cell genes
d. They lead to the production of second messengers

7. Which endocrine gland is not under the control of the anterior pituitary gland?
a. the thyroid
b. the parathyroids
c. adrenal cortex
d. the gonads

8. During a general stress syndrome, the alarm reaction is initiated by
a. neurohumor of the hypothalamus
b. hormones of the adrenal cortex
c. hypothalamic stimulation of the sympathetic nervous system and adrenal medulla
d. hormones of the anterior pituitary

9. A child who exhibits dwarfism, mental retardation, yellowish skin colour, and fat pads in the face and abdomen is probably suffering from
a. cretinism
b. pituitary dwarfism
c. acromegaly
d. a goiter

10. An individual with spasms, twitches, and convulsions probably has a defective
    a. thyroid
    b. parathyroid
    c. adrenal medulla
    d. pineal gland

11. The fight-or-flight responses that are brought about by sympathetic stimulation are duplicated by the action of which endocrine gland?
    a. anterior pituitary
    b. adrenal medulla
    c. thyroid
    d. posterior pituitary

12. In a strict sense, the posterior pituitary is not an endocrine gland because it
    a. has a rich blood supply
    b. does not make hormones
    c. is not near the brain
    d. contains ducts

13. Which gland is primarily concerned with sodium and potassium salt balance?
    a. parathyroids
    b. thyroid
    c. adrenal cortex
    d. anterior pituitary

14. Hyperglycemia, increased urine production, thirst, and ketosis are all symptoms of
    a. hyperthyroidism
    b. diabetes mellitus
    c. diabetes insipidus
    d. hyperinsulinism

15. If a person is diagnosed as having a high metabolic rate, which endocrine gland is probably malfunctioning?
    a. parathyroids
    b. thymus
    c. posterior pituitary
    d. thyroid

16. Which of the following hormones is naturally antagonistic to insulin?
    a. aldosterone
    b. parathyroid hormone
    c. calcitonin
    d. glucagon

17. The hormone somatotropin does which of the following?
    a. regulates the growth of the skeleton
    b. helps to regulate the activities of the adrenal glands
    c. causes lymphocytes to be produced
    d. causes decreased activity of the exocrine portion of the pancreas

18. Parathormone (parathyroid hormone) does which of the following?
    a. It aids in the maintenance of normal blood levels of calcium and phosphorous
    b. It aids in the maintenance of normal blood levels of sodium and potassium
    c. It influences the production of prolactin
    d. It responds to the stimulus of the thyrotropic hormone

19. The function of calcitonin is to
a. prevent calculi from forming
b. increase blood sodium levels
c. lower blood calcium levels
d. cause calcification of the pineal gland at the time of puberty

20. Proper carbohydrate metabolism is dependent on the production of insulin by the
a. parathyroids
b. adrenals
c. liver
d. pancreas

B. *Matching.* Each of the terms in Column B refers to a word or phrase in Column A. Insert the letter of the term from Column B that best describes each word or phrase in Column A. Some terms may be used more than once or not at all.

	Column A		*Column B*
1. ____	adrenal medulla	**a.**	iodine
2. ____	stimulates the ovary	**b.**	aldosterone
3. ____	regulates Na^+ and K^+	**c.**	calcitonin
4. ____	contraction of smooth muscle in blood vessels	**d.**	antidiuretic hormone (vasopressin)
5. ____	controls body growth	**e.**	follicle stimulating hormone (FSH)
6. ____	development of male sex characteristics	**f.**	testosterone
7. ____	another form of oestrogen	**g.**	oestradiol
8. ____	involved in calcium homeostasis	**h.**	parathyroid hormone (parathormone)
9. ____	inhibits ovarian function	**i.**	insulin
10. ____	long term steroid stress hormone	**j.**	norepinephrine (noradrenaline)
11. ____	decreases blood sugar	**k.**	glucagon
12. ____	required for thyroxine synthesis	**l.**	growth hormone (somatotropin)
13. ____	alpha cells of the pancreas	**m.**	prolactin
14. ____	stimulates uterine muscle	**n.**	oxytocin
15. ____	acts antagonistically to parathyroid hormone	**o.**	cortisol
		p.	melatonin

C. *True or False.* Write a *T* or an *F* in the space provided to indicate true or false.

___ **1.** People with kidney or liver disease may suffer from hormone excesses due to a decreased rate of destruction of the hormones by these organs.

___ **2.** One of the ways hormones work is to alter the transport of certain molecules across cell membranes.

___ **3.** Some reflexes are mediated by hormones.

___ **4.** Hormones are secreted by exocrine glands into ducts leading to the body cavities.

___ **5.** Hormones must be present in high concentrations in the blood in order to have any physiological effect on the organism.

___ **6.** In general, the end result of most hormone action is a change in the metabolic activity in the target-organ cells.

___ **7.** Hormones may be released from the terminals of neurons.

___ **8.** The hypothalamic releasing factors are not true hormones because they do not reach their target tissue by way of the circulatory system.

___ **9.** The release of a hormone into the blood may be initiated in some cases by stimulating the nerves into the gland.

___ **10.** Hormones cannot cause their target cells to perform new activities, but only accelerate or modify the existing capabilities of the cell.

___ **11.** Hormones are necessary for the regulation of the internal environment under the varying conditions imposed on the organism by a changing external environment.

___ **12.** Endocrine glands use ducts, whereas exocrine glands are ductless.

___ **13.** Long-distance communication between cells is accomplished by nerves and/or hormones.

___ **14.** A type of feedback in which an increase in the output of a system results in a decrease in the input is known as positive feedback.

___ **15.** Releasing factors of the hypothalamus stimulate the release by the adenohypophysis of TSH, ACTH, LH, and growth hormone.

___ **16.** That portion of the adrenal gland essential for life is the cortex.

___ **17.** Negative feedback results in an increase in the production of hormones by the hypophysis.

___ **18.** The pancreas is both an exocrine and endocrine gland.

___ **19.** Thyroid-stimulating hormone is a trophic hormone.

___ **20.** Hormones are secreted by their ducts to their target organ(s).

Answer Sheet—Chapter 10

Exercise 10.1

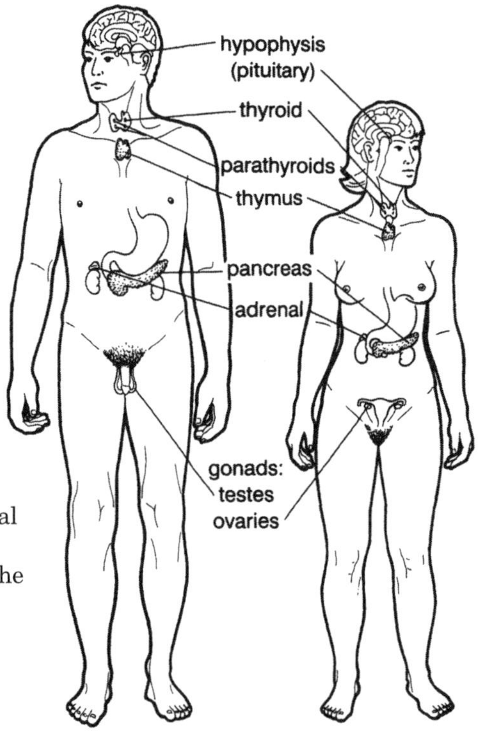

Figure 10.1 General location of the major endocrine glands of the body.

Exercise 10.2

HORMONES

Chemical Nature of Hormones

Hormones are organic compounds of varying structural complexity that are carried by the blood to other parts of the body where they exert their specific effects. In simple terms, hormones are chemical messengers that pass via the bloodstream to the target organ or tissue. They may either stimulate or inhibit a function, but in general they do not initiate a process. Hormones are either proteins, glycoproteins (combination of a protein and a sugar), or steroids (fat soluble hormones derived from cholesterol). The one thing that all hormones have in common, whether protein, glycoprotein, or steroid, is the function of maintaining homeostasis by modifying the physiological activities of cells.

Actions of Hormones

Hormones are effective in remarkably small quantities. For example, the injection of a few micrograms of epinephrine (adrenaline) causes a definite increase in the rate of the heart beat. There is little doubt that each hormone has some effect on the fundamental metabolism of its target cells or tissues. Hormones, therefore, have a marked influence on such basic life processes as growth, development, reproduction, energy utilisation, and cell permeability.

Much is known about the way hormones work on their target tissues or cells. Protein and catecholamine (fight or flight) hormones act by first interacting with receptor sites on the cell membrane. The cell membrane contains the adenyl cyclase system. The hormone binds to specific receptors in the cell membrane and subsequently activates adenyl cyclase. This enzyme converts adenosine triphosphate (ATP) into 3,5-cyclic AMP, which acts as the second messenger. Cyclic AMP, the secondary messenger, then moves to the other structures.

Although it is not known how the group of locally acting hormones called prostaglandins directly acts upon cells, it is postulated that they somehow regulate the formation of cyclic AMP and may be involved in the responses of target tissues to hormonal stimulation.

Exercise 10.3

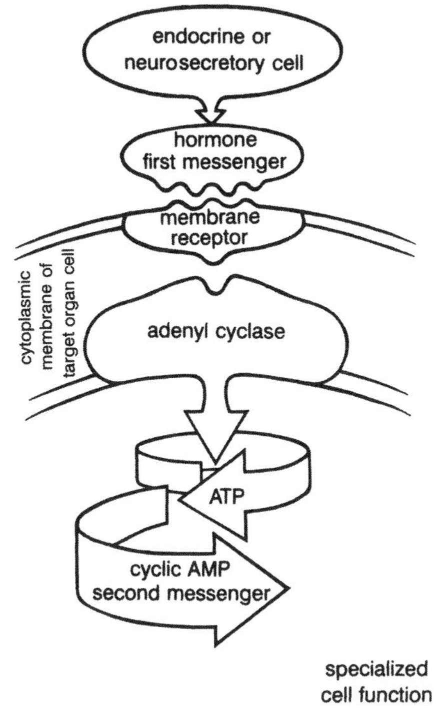

Figure 10.3 Mechanism of hormone action. Hormones act as messengers delivering their message to a membrane receptor in the target cell. Prostaglandins appear to regulate hormonal activity influencing adenyl cyclase and cyclic AMP activity within the cell. Cyclic AMP serves as the second messenger for specialised cell functions.

Exercise 10.4

Feedback Control Systems

Hormones are secreted continually, and their rate of secretion is regulated by the body's needs. The nervous system controls the endocrine system either directly or indirectly. The direct influence is minimal and best illustrated by the effects of the sympathetic nervous system on the secretion of the adrenal medulla. Indirect control is most common and is centred around the role of the hypothalamus. The hypothalamus secretes certain hormones and transfers these hormones to the posterior pituitary where they are stored. Also, the hypothalamus secretes chemical substances, known as releasing factors, that are released into the vascular bed between the hypothalamus and the anterior pituitary. These releasing factors are specific and regulate the release of the anterior pituitary hormones.

The hormone released by the target endocrine gland may feed back and influence release of the releasing or inhibiting substance of the hypothalamus or pituitary hormone. If the effect of the feedback is to inhibit the overall response of the system, it is termed negative feedback. If the effect of the feedback is to stimulate further hormone release, it is positive feedback.

In many cases the secretion of a hormone is regulated by both positive and negative feedback mechanisms. Thyroxine, which is released by the thyroid gland, can regulate the release of thyroid-stimulating hormone in two ways. First, high levels inhibit the release of thyrotropin-releasing hormone by the hypothalamus, which reduces TSH release by the anterior pituitary. Second, thyroxine inhibits the release of TSH by direct effect on the cells of the anterior pituitary. This particular type of feedback pathway (from target gland to pituitary) is called a long feedback loop. Additionally, the pituitary hormones may feed back to the brain to influence the releasing or inhibiting substances; this pathway is called a short feedback loop.

Exercise 10.5

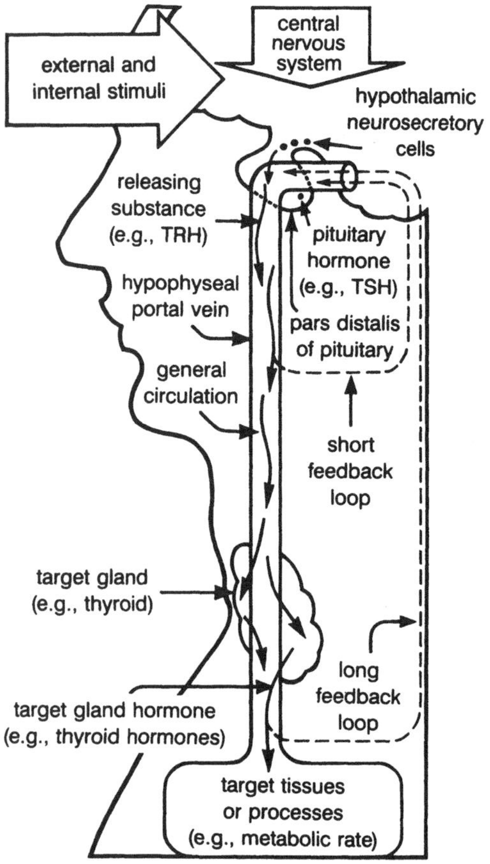

Figure 10.5 Feedback control of endocrine gland activity. External or internal stimuli influence the release of releasing factors from the hypothalamus, which in turn trigger the release of hormones from glands that control important vital functions of the body.

Test Items

A. 1. d, 2. c, 3. a, 4. c, 5. b, 6. c, 7. b, 8. c, 9. a, 10. b, 11. b, 12. b, 13. c, 14. b, 15. d, 16. d, 17. a, 18. a, 19. c, 20. d.

B. 1. j, 2. e, 3. b, 4. d, 5. l, 6. f, 7. g, 8. h, 9. p, 10. o, 11. i, 12. a, 13. k, 14. n, 15. c.

C. 1. T, 2. T, 3. T, 4. F, 5. F, 6. T, 7. T, 8. F, 9. T, 10. T, 11. T, 12. F, 13. T, 14. F, 15. T, 16. T, 17. F, 18. T, 19. F, 20. F.

11

The Special Senses

I. CHAPTER SYNOPSIS

Our perception of the external world is determined by the physiological mechanisms involved in the processing of sensory information transmitted by nerve fibres to the brain from various receptors located throughout the body.

Sensations may be classified as cutaneous, visceral, olfactory, gustatory, visual, auditory, and position sense. The three components of a sensory mechanism are a sense organ or receptor, a pathway to the brain, and a sensory area in the cerebral cortex. In a sense organ or receptor the property of excitability is most highly developed, and each is specialised to respond to a specific type of stimulus. The process of projection, the sensation of afterimages, adaptation, and variability of intensity are all characteristics of sensations. Touch, pressure, heat, cold, and pain comprise the cutaneous senses. There are two types of pain: visceral and somatic. Somatic pain has been subdivided into superficial or cutaneous pain and deep pain. Muscle sense, also called proprioceptive or kinesthetic sense, provides nonvisual information on position of body parts. Adequate stimuli for visceral receptors are of three types, and the impulses from these receptors may follow one of three basic pathways. Organic sensation and visceral pain impulses are initiated by visceral receptors. The olfactory epithelium of the nasal cavity and the taste buds in the papillae of the tongue are the location of receptors for the senses of smell and taste. Receptors for vision lie in the retina of the eyeball and are discussed with associated structures of the eye that make vision possible. Hearing, the sense by which sounds are appreciated, involves the function of structures of the external ear, middle ear, and cochlear portions of the inner ear. Position sense involves the orientation of the head in space, the movement of the body through space, and the sense of balance and equilibrium of the body. The vestibule and semicircular canals of the inner ear are used in position sense. Position sense involves the orientation of the head in space, the movement of the body through space, and the sense of balance and equilibrium of the body. The vestibule and semicircular canals of the inner ear are used in position sense.

II. OBJECTIVES

After reading the chapter, the student should be able to:

- Describe the sensory mechanisms.
- Differentiate among interceptors, proprioceptors, and exteroceptors and give examples of each.
- Define chemoreceptor, pressoreceptor, and photoreceptor and relate their significance.
- Describe referred pain.
- Describe the anatomy of the eyeball and its protective structures.
- Explain the physical phenomenon of refraction and how it operates in focusing.
- Explain depth perception and relate binocular vision with diplopia and hemianopia.
- Describe the anatomy of the ear.
- Follow the transmission of sound from the tympanic membrane to the basilar membrane.
- Explain the Place theory of hearing.
- Differentiate between static and dynamic equilibrium.

III. IMPORTANT TERMS

Using your textbook, define the following terms:

accommodation (a-kom-uh-day′shun) ______________________________

____

adaptation (ad-ap-tay′shun) ______________________________

____

astigmatism (a-stig′muh-tiz-em) ______________________________

____

auditory (aw′di-tor-ee) ____________________

auricle (aw′ri-kul) ____________________

cataract (kat′uh-ract) ____________________

chemoreceptor (keem′o-re-sep-tur) ____________________

choroid (kor′oyd) ____________________

cochlea (kok′lee-uh) ____________________

concave (kon′kave) ____________________

conjunctivitis (kun-junk-ti-vy′tis) ____________________

convex (kon′veks) ____________________

cornea (kor′nee-uh) ____________________

Corti (kor′ti) ____________________

diplopia (di-plo′pee-uh) ____________________

eustachian (yoo-stay′shun) ____________________

exteroceptors (ek-stur-o-sep′turs) ____________________

fovea (fo′vee-uh) ____________________

glaucoma (glaw-ko′muh) ____________________

hyperopia (hy-pur-o′pee-uh) ____________________

incus (ing′kus) ______________________________

____

interoceptor (in-tur-o-sep′tur) ______________________________

____

iris (i′ris) ______________________________

____

malleus (mal′ee-us) ______________________________

____

myopia (my-o′pee-uh) ______________________________

____

nystagmus (nis-tag′mus) ______________________________

____

optic (op′tik) ______________________________

____

photoreceptor (foto-re-sep′tur) ______________________________

____

pupil (pew′pil) ______________________________

____

refraction (ree-frak′shun) ______________________________

____

retina (ret-i′-nuh) ______________________________

____

rhodopsin (ro-dop′sin) ______________________________

____

sclera (skler′uh) ______________________________

____

stapes (stay′peez) ______________________________

____

tympanic (tim-pan′ik) ______________________________

____

vestibular (ves-tib′yoo-lur) ______________________________

____

IV. EXERCISES

Complete the following exercises in the order given. A precise set of terms and diagrams has been chosen to describe the special senses.

Exercise 11.1

Fill in the Blanks. Write the terms from the key list in the appropriate spaces provided in the text on the right.

Key:
alike
brain
change
CNS
composition
conscious
decodes
dendrites
environments
impulses
information
intensity
interpret
interpreted
interprets
odor
other
pathways
peripheral
photoreceptors
pigments
receptor
receptors
sensation
sensory
specialised
stimuli
structure
tissue
unconscious

SENSORY MECHANISMS

A ____________ organ, or ____________, is a ____________ nervous ____________ situated at the ____________ endings of the ____________ of afferent neurons. The receptor's primary function is to ____________ the body with ____________, both ____________ and ____________, about degrees of ____________ in the organism's external and internal ____________.

Three important features of sense organs should be emphasised:

1. Specific ____________ are particularly sensitive to specific ____________. However they can also respond to ____________ stimuli of sufficient ____________. For example, pressure on the eyeball causes a sensation of light.

2. Specific sensitivity to certain stimuli is due to the ____________ and ____________ of the receptor. For example, light-absorbing ____________ are found in the ____________ of the eye.

3. The type of ____________ elicited by a receptor depends on which nerve ____________ are activated, not on how they are activated. All nerve ____________ are essentially ____________, regardless of the stimulus that initiates them. The impulse is transmitted to the ____________, where it is ____________. For example, the region of the cerebrum receiving impulses from an olfactory receptor ____________ and ____________ them as a specific odor or aroma. If an olfactory receptor is artificially stimulated, the same nerve pathways to the ____________ will be activated, and the brain will ____________ the arriving impulses as a specific ____________.

Exercise 11.2

Labelling. Write the name of the structure on the space provided.
Colour the three layers of the eye a different colour.

Key:

capsule	conjunctiva	iris	optic	rectus	superior
choroid	cornea	lens	posterior	retina	vision
ciliary	fovea	ligaments	pupil	sclera	

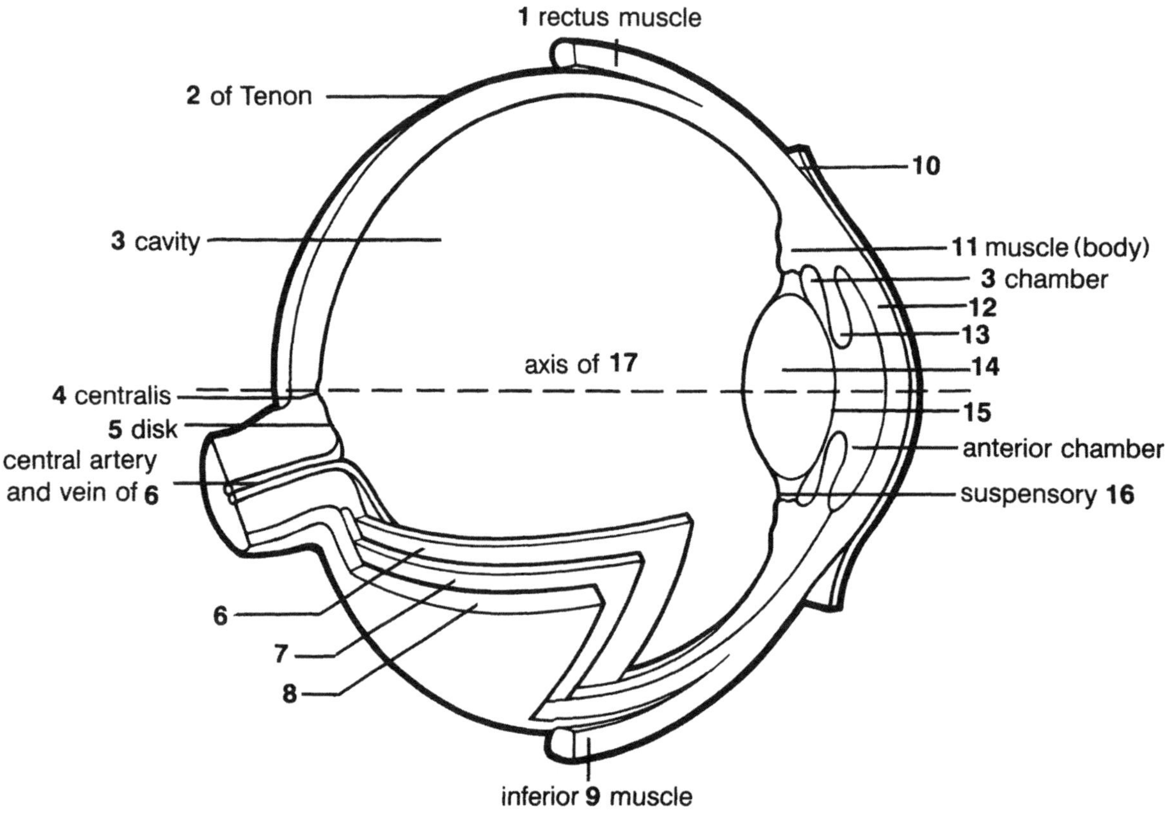

Figure 11.2 Structure of the eye, transverse section.

1. ______________________
2. ______________________
3. ______________________
4. ______________________
5. ______________________
6. ______________________
7. ______________________
8. ______________________
9. ______________________
10. ______________________
11. ______________________
12. ______________________
13. ______________________
14. ______________________
15. ______________________
16. ______________________
17. ______________________

Exercise 11.3

Labelling. Write the name of the structure on the space provided. Colour the temporal bone different from the ear mechanism.

Key:

auditory	Corti	inner	middle	stapes (stirrup)
auricle	eustachian	jugular	oval	temporal
cochlea	external	malleus (hammer)	round	tympanic
cochlear	incus (anvil)	meatus	semicircular canals	vestibular

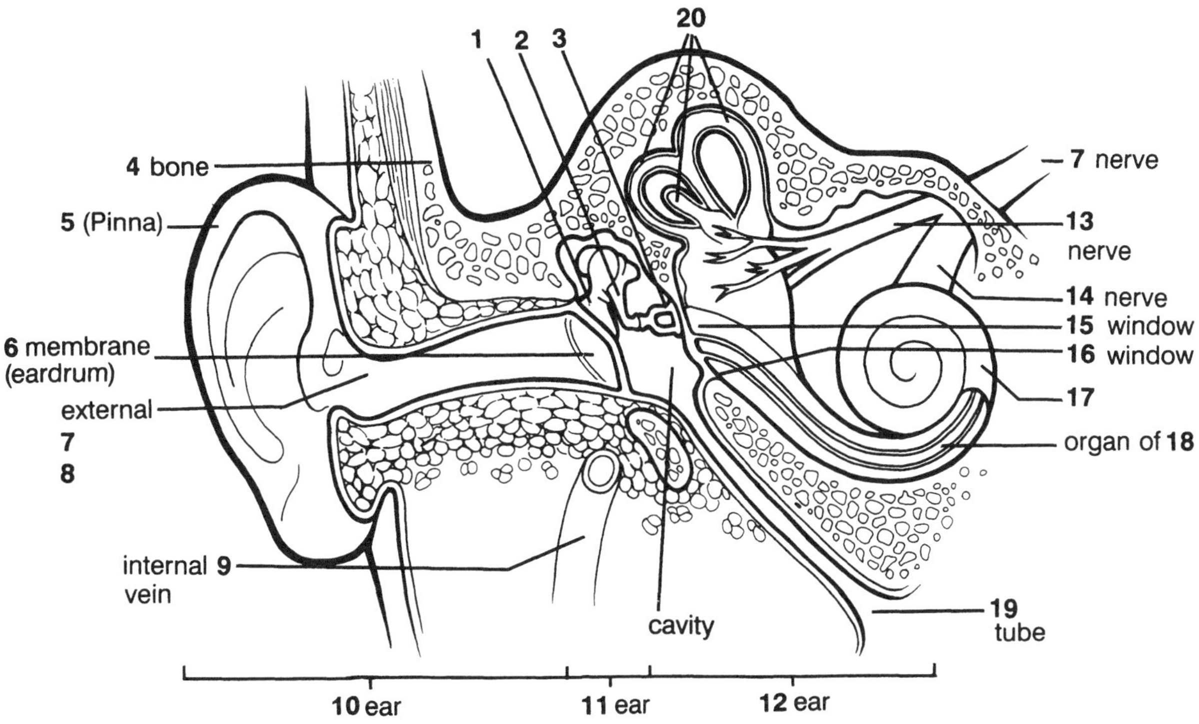

Figure 11.3 Frontal view of the outer ear, middle ear, and internal ear. A section of the cochlear duct has been cut away to show the position of the organ of Corti.

1. ______________________
2. ______________________
3. ______________________
4. ______________________
5. ______________________
6. ______________________
7. ______________________
8. ______________________
9. ______________________
10. ______________________
11. ______________________
12. ______________________
13. ______________________
14. ______________________
15. ______________________
16. ______________________
17. ______________________
18. ______________________
19. ______________________
20. ______________________

V. TEST ITEMS

A. *Multiple Choice.* There is only one answer that is either correct or most appropriate. Circle the best answer for each question.

1. While focusing on a close object, accommodation occurs due to
   a. the ability of the lens to change shape
   b. the muscles of the eyeball coordinating the position of each eye
   c. a change in the shape of the eyeball
   d. a change in the thickness of the cornea

2. As a result of nerve damage, an injured person cannot see at all with the left eye but has no trouble seeing with the right eye. The site of injury is probably in the
   a. optic chiasma
   b. left occipital lobe
   c. left optic tract
   d. left optic nerve

3. A physician who specialises in disorders of the eye is a/an
   a. optician
   b. optometrist
   c. ophthalmologist
   d. neurologist

4. A blockage of the canal of Schlemm might result in
   a. a sty
   b. glaucoma
   c. conjunctivitis
   d. a cataract

5. Otitis media may follow throat infections because the
   a. auditory canal connects the middle ear with the tympanic membrane
   b. eustachian tube opens into the inner ear
   c. mucosa of the nasopharynx is continuous with that of the middle ear
   d. mastoid sinus opens into the middle ear

6. The main function of the rods is
   a. depth perception
   b. vision in dim light
   c. colour vision
   d. refraction

7. Which of the following is likely to result in conduction deafness?
   a. stiffness of the joints between the bones of the middle ear
   b. hardening of the perilymph
   c. loss of the organs of Corti
   d. sclerosis of the membranous labyrinth

8. The blind spot is the place where
   a. there are more rods than cones
   b. there are more cones than rods
   c. the optic nerve leaves the eyeball
   d. the iris attaches to the cornea

9. The organs of Corti are receptors for
   a. light rays
   b. equilibrium
   c. taste
   d. hearing

10. Aqueous humour drains from the anterior chamber into the
a. vitreous body
b. lacrimal duct
c. mastoid sinuses
d. canal of Schlemm

11. The most frequent infection of the eye is
a. conjuctivitis
b. retinitis
c. otitis media
d. iritis

12. The fovea centralis is the place where
a. nerve impulses for equilibrium are concentrated
b. visual acuity is greatest
c. high-pitched tones are received
d. the optic nerve leaves the eyeball

13. The cortical region for vision is located in the
a. temporal lobe
b. frontal lobe
c. occipital lobe
d. parietal lobe

14. The chemical reaction associated with vision takes place in the
a. aqueous humour
b. iris
c. vitreous humour
d. retina

15. Which of these is a true statement?
a. Hearing is not dependent on the inner ear
b. All parts of the organ of Corti hear all ranges of sound
c. The loud music young people listen to cannot damage their ears
d. Hearing is dependent on pressure waves

16. Puncturing the eardrum so that it is inoperative would
a. not affect your sense of hearing
b. prevent the normal transmission of sound vibration
c. destroy the sense receptors for hearing
d. account for why some people who hear still cannot sing on tune

17. The cochlea
a. is a coiled structure found in the inner ear
b. contains three fluid-filled canals
c. contains the organ of Corti
d. all of these

18. The bones of the middle ear
a. respond to a change in the position of the head
b. transmit sound waves
c. are sense receptors connected to the auditory nerve
d. all of these

19. A mucous membrane that lines the inner surface of the eyelid and continues as the surface layer of the eyeball is called
a. the conjunctiva
b. the choroid
c. the sclera
d. none of the foregoing

20. The sense of taste and of smell are detected by
  a. thermoreceptors
  b. chemoreceptors
  c. electromagnetic receptors
  d. mechanoreceptor

B. *Matching.* Each of the words or phrases in Column B refers to a term in Column A. Insert the letter of the word or phrase from Column B that best describes each term in Column A. Some words or phrases may be used more than once or not at all.

	Column A		*Column B*
1. ___	sensory unit	**a.**	sensitive to pressure changes
2. ___	interoceptors	**b.**	the distance between two successive wave peaks
3. ___	lacrimal gland	**c.**	associated with temperature sensitivity
4. ___	wavelength	**d.**	opaque (cloudy) lens
5. ___	modalities	**e.**	receptors located in the walls of the viscera
6. ___	cataract	**f.**	nearsighted (shortsighted)
7. ___	free nerve endings	**g.**	change the shape of the lens
8. ___	myopic eye	**h.**	keeps the eyeball moist
9. ___	ciliary muscles (body)	**i.**	a single afferent neuron plus all the receptors it innervates make up a __________
10. ___	mechanoreceptor		
		j.	therapy

	Column A		*Column B*
1. ___	hyperopic	**a.**	a protein
2. ___	opsin	**b.**	anvil
3. ___	optic chiasma	**c.**	optic crossing
4. ___	incus	**d.**	detects changes in both motion and posture
5. ___	cochlea	**e.**	related to the loudness of sound
6. ___	vestibular system	**f.**	inner ear
7. ___	amplitude	**g.**	elevates the eye
8. ___	superior rectus	**h.**	a farsighted (longsighted) eye
9. ___	inferior rectus	**i.**	depresses the eye
10. ___	erythrolabe	**j.**	a photopigment sensitive to red light

C. *True or False.* Write a *T* or an *F* in the space provided to indicate true or false.

___ **1.** The crystalline lens has a fixed refractive index.

___ **2.** Aqueous humour of the eye, like cerebrospinal fluid, is constantly being manufactured and resorbed.

___ **3.** Iris of the eye and ciliary body constitute the extrinsic muscles of the eye.

___ **4.** The near point of vision moves closer with increasing age.

___ **5.** Pain frequently seems to arise at locations other than the area in which a disorder occurs.

___ **6.** Adaptation to odors is a relatively slow process.

___ **7.** The sensory components of cranial nerves conveying impulses from the special receptors have their cell bodies outside the brain.

___ **8.** All taste sensation is dependent upon the integrity of the seventh cranial nerve.

___ **9.** Hair cells in contact with the tectorial membrane are stimulated when the membrane vibrates.

___ **10.** Deafness due to injury to the auditory centre of the brain could be alleviated by the use of a hearing aid.

___ **11.** Otoliths are associated with body equilibrium.

___ **12.** The inner ear is characterised by the presence of auditory ossicles.

___ **13.** Impulses associated with hearing pass from the utricle and saccule to the vestibulocochlear nerve.

___ **14.** Pressure within the ear is relieved by the passage of air through the eustachian (auditory) tube.

___ **15.** The part of the body affected by impacted cerumen is the anterior chamber of the eye.

___ **16.** The macula lutea contains the area of sharpest vision.

___ **17.** The vitreous humour is situated between the lens and retina.

___ **18.** Taste and smell are perceived through stimulation of dissolved substances acting upon chemoreceptors (chemical receptors).

___ **19.** The stapes fits into the fenestra cochlea or round window.

___ **20.** The portion of the basilar membrane involved increases as sound intensity is increased.

Answer Sheet—Chapter 11

Exercise 11.1

SENSORY MECHANISMS

A sensory organ, or receptor, is a specialised nervous tissue situated at the peripheral endings of the dendrites of afferent neurons. The receptor's primary function is to provide the body with information, both conscious and unconscious, about degrees of change in the organism's external and internal environments.

Three important features of sense organs should be emphasised:

1. Specific receptors are particularly sensitive to specific stimuli. However, they can also respond to other stimuli of sufficient intensity. For example, pressure on the eyeball causes a sensation of light.

2. Specific sensitivity to certain stimuli is due to the structure and composition of the receptor. For example, light-absorbing pigments are found in the photoreceptors of the eye.

3. The type of sensation elicited by a receptor depends on which nerve pathways are activated, not on how they are activated. All nerve impulses are essentially alike, regardless of the stimulus that initiates them. The impulse is transmitted to the CNS, where it is interpreted. For example, the region of the cerebrum receiving impulses from an olfactory receptor decodes and interprets them as a specific odor or aroma. If an olfactory receptor is artificially stimulated, the same nerve pathways to the brain will be activated, and the brain will interpret the arriving impulses as a specific odor.

Exercise 11.2

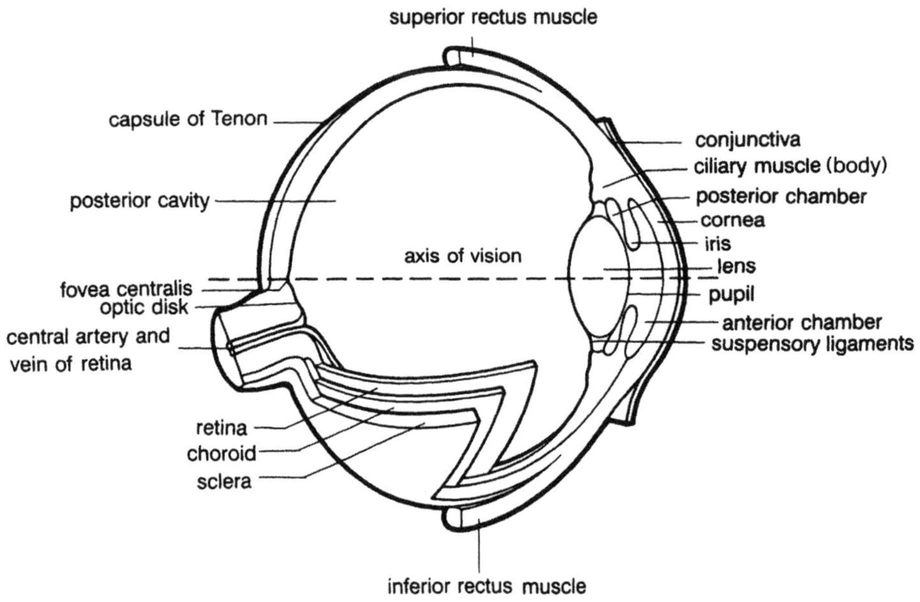

Figure 11.2 Structure of the eye, transverse section.

Exercise 11.3

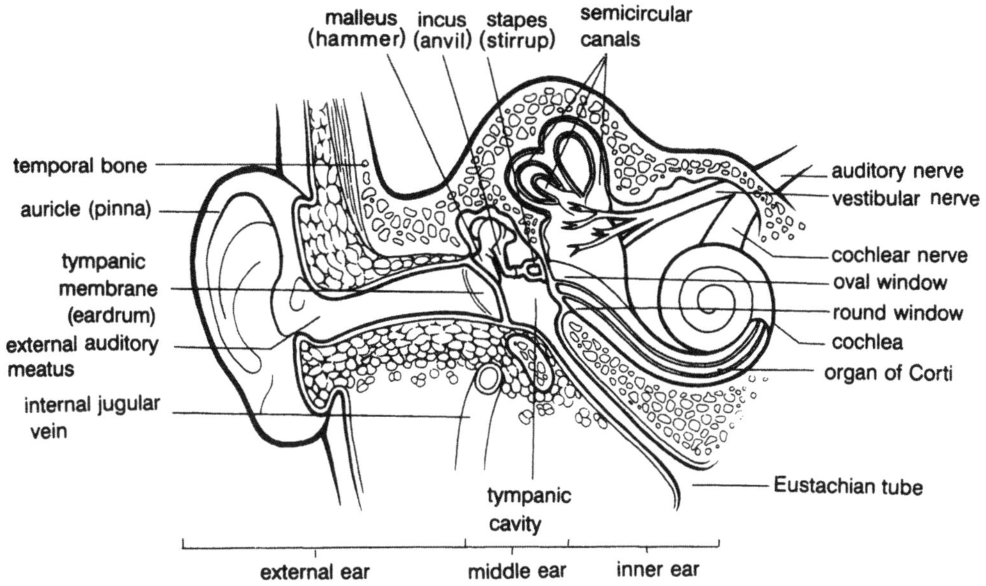

Figure 11.3 Frontal diagram of the outer ear, middle ear, and internal ear. A section of the cochlear duct has been cut away to show the position of the organ of Corti.

Test Items

A. 1. a, 2. d, 3. c, 4. b, 5. c, 6. b, 7. a, 8. c, 9. d, 10. d, 11. a, 12. b, 13. c, 14. d, 15. d, 16. b, 17. d, 18. b, 19. a, 20. b.

B. 1. i, 2. e, 3. h, 4. b, 5. j, 6. d, 7. c, 8. f, 9. g, 10. a.
1. h, 2. a, 3. c, 4. b, 5. f, 6. d, 7. e, 8. g, 9. i, 10. j.

C. 1. T, 2. T, 3. F, 4. F, 5. T, 6. F, 7. T, 8. F, 9. T, 10. F, 11. T, 12. F, 13. F, 14. T, 15. F, 16. T, 17. T, 18. T, 19. F, 20. T.

12

The Blood

I. CHAPTER SYNOPSIS

The central theme of this chapter is that blood maintains the constancy of the internal environment, and, in the process, it too remains constant within limits—blood protein content, pH, pressure, and osmotic pressure are relatively constant, for example.

Blood helps maintain the integrity of the tissues through the exchange of molecules that takes place at the capillaries. This exchange is an important portion of the chapter, and it is considered in detail. The major concern of this chapter is to analyse the structure and function of blood and to note interrelations in maintaining homeostasis. This is developed through a study of the origin and functions of the formed elements in blood and a comparison of the location and composition of plasma and interstitial fluid. The transportation of respiratory gases, the reticulocyte count, the differential count, phagocytosis, the antigen-antibody response, blood clotting, clotting tests, and the ABO and Rh blood grouping systems are considered. Among the blood disorders discussed are several kinds of anaemia, polycythaemia, infectious mononucleosis, and leukaemia.

The human body is continually subjected to stress by invasion of microorganisms (e.g. viruses and bacteria) whose growth, if unchecked, will disrupt the homeostasis and normal functioning of the body through the release of toxic materials and the destruction of cells. The human body has a number of passive (anatomical barriers such as the skin) and active (the immune system and phagocytic activity of the WBCs) defenses against these invaders. The body cells also wear out and must be removed, and abnormal or mutant cell types that arise must be destroyed for they put stress on normal homeostasis. Thus, this chapter deals with the immune system and the physiological mechanisms that allow the body to recognise either material foreign to itself or stressful situations and to neutralise or eliminate them.

II. OBJECTIVES

After reading the chapter, the student should be able to:

- List the functions of blood.
- Describe the characteristics of blood.
- Define haematocrit (packed red cell volume).
- Explain the functions of haemoglobin.
- Describe how an erythrocyte is produced and how older or damaged erythrocytes are removed and destroyed.
- Differentiate between the intrinsic and extrinsic factors.
- Explain the relationship of haemolysis and a high bilirubin level.
- Distinguish among the kinds of leukocytes (leucocytes) and their functions.
- Differentiate between leukopaenia (leucopaenia) and leukocytosis.
- Define diapedesis and relate its role in inflammation.
- Describe a thrombocyte (platelet) and explain its role in the clotting mechanism.
- Define immunity.
- Explain the role of B and T lymphocytes in the immune reaction.

III. IMPORTANT TERMS

Using your textbook, define the following terms:

agglutination (a-gloo-ti-nay′shun) ______________________________

____

allergen (al′ur-jen) ______________________________

____

anaemia (uh-nee′mee-uh) ______________________________

____

antibody (an′tee-bod-ee) ______________________________

____

anticoagulant (ant-ee-ko-ag′yoo-lunt) ______________________________

____

antigen (an′ti-jen) ______________________________

____

bilirubin (bil-i-roo′bin) ______________________________

____

coagulation (ko-ag-yoo-lay′shun) ______________________________

____

diapedesis (dye-uh-pe-dee′sis) ______________________________

____

erythrocyte (e-rith′ro-sight) ______________________________

____

extrinsic (ek-strin′sik) ______________________________

____

haematocrit (hem′ah-to-krit) ______________________________

____

haemoglobin (hee′muh-glo-bin) ______________________________

____

haemopoietic (hee-mo-poy-et′ik) ______________________________

____

heparin (hep′uh-rin) ______________________________

____

histamine (his′tuh-meen) ______________________________

____

intrinsic (in-trin′sik) ______________________________

____

leucocyte (lew′ko-sight) ______________________________

____

lysis (ly′sis) ______________________________

____

platelet (playt′lit) ______________________________

____

thrombocyte (throm′bo-sight) ______________________________

____

thrombus (throm′bus) ______________________________

____

IV. EXERCISES

Complete the following exercises in the order given. A precise set of terms and diagrams have been chosen to describe the blood.

Exercise 12.1

Fill in the Blanks. Write the name of the characteristic of blood (provided in the key list) in the space provided in the text on the right.

Key:
arteries
bright red
dark red
density
flows
less
oxygenated
pH
6 L
slowly
temperature
thicker
veins
viscosity
volume
volume
water
weight

CHARACTERISTICS OF BLOOD

Blood is __________ (indicating that it is well __________) in the __________ and __________ (__________ oxygenated) in the veins. It __________ four to five times more __________ than water because it is four to five times __________ (a property called __________). Its specific gravity (__________ compared with water) varies between 1.045 and 1.065 (__________ is 1.000), and its __________ and __________ values are 38°C (100.4°F) and about 7.38, respectively. The __________ of blood in the body has been measured in many ways but can be expected to vary with the size of the body. A useful estimate is that its __________ is 8% of the body's weight. The blood __________ of a man of average size is approximately __________.

Key:
anticoagulants
cells and cell
clotting
corpuscles
erythrocytes
55%
formed
hematocrit
homogeneous
leucocytes
lower
opaque
percentage
plasma
plasma
thrombocytes
transparent
upper
venipuncture
yellow

Seen with the naked eye, blood appears to be ________ and ________; but, on microscopic examination, it consists of ________ fragments and an intercellular fluid, the ________.

When blood is obtained from a person's vein (by ________) and transferred to a test tube, and ________ is prevented by adding certain chemicals called ________, it separates into two distinct layers. The ________ layer, which is ________ and ________, contains most of the chemical components of the blood in solution; this is the ________. Plasma constitutes about ________ of the blood's volume. The ________ portion of the blood sample consists of ________ elements: the red blood cells (________), the white blood cells (________), and the platelets (________).These are often called ________, meaning little bodies. The ________ of total blood volume contributed by these formed elements is called the ________.

Exercise 12.2

Labelling. Write the name of the formed element in the space provided. Colour each cell differently.

Key:
basophil
eosinophil
erythrocytes
lymphocytes
monocytes
neutrophil
thrombocytes

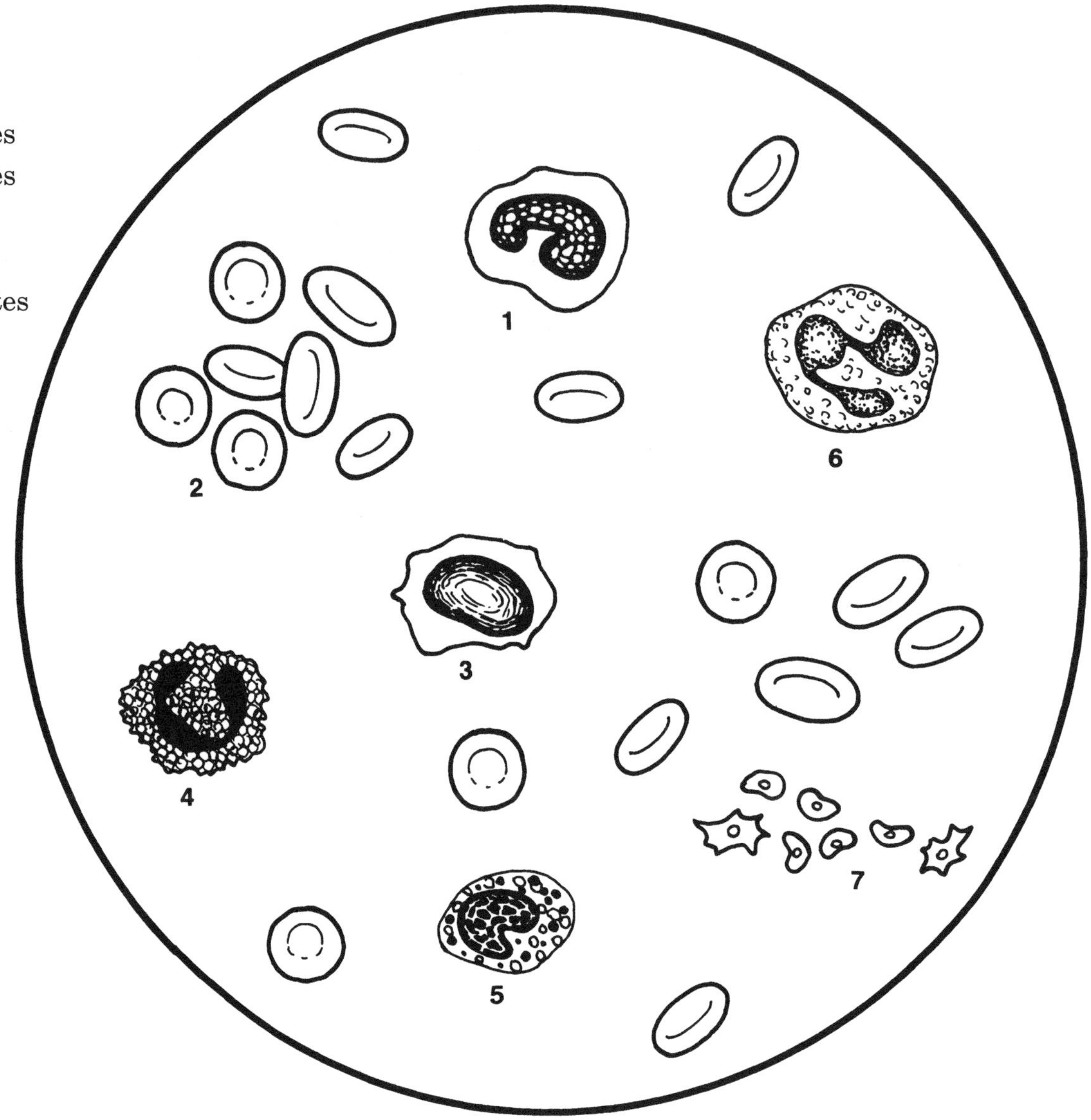

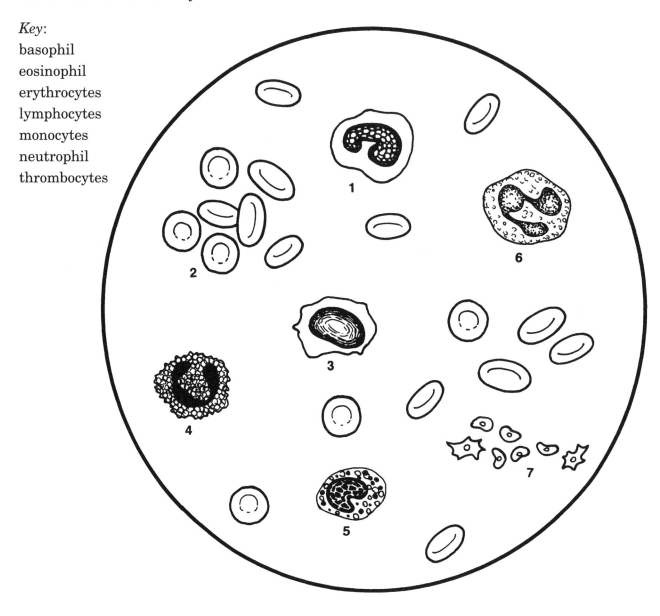

Figure 12.2 Microscopic blood smear.

1. ______________________
2. ______________________
3. ______________________
4. ______________________
5. ______________________
6. ______________________
7. ______________________

Exercise 12.3

Labelling. Write the name of the blood factor on the space provided. Colour each area differently.

Key:
circulation
erythrocyte
excreted
extrinsic
gastric
haemopoietic
intrinsic
RBC
stimulate
WBC

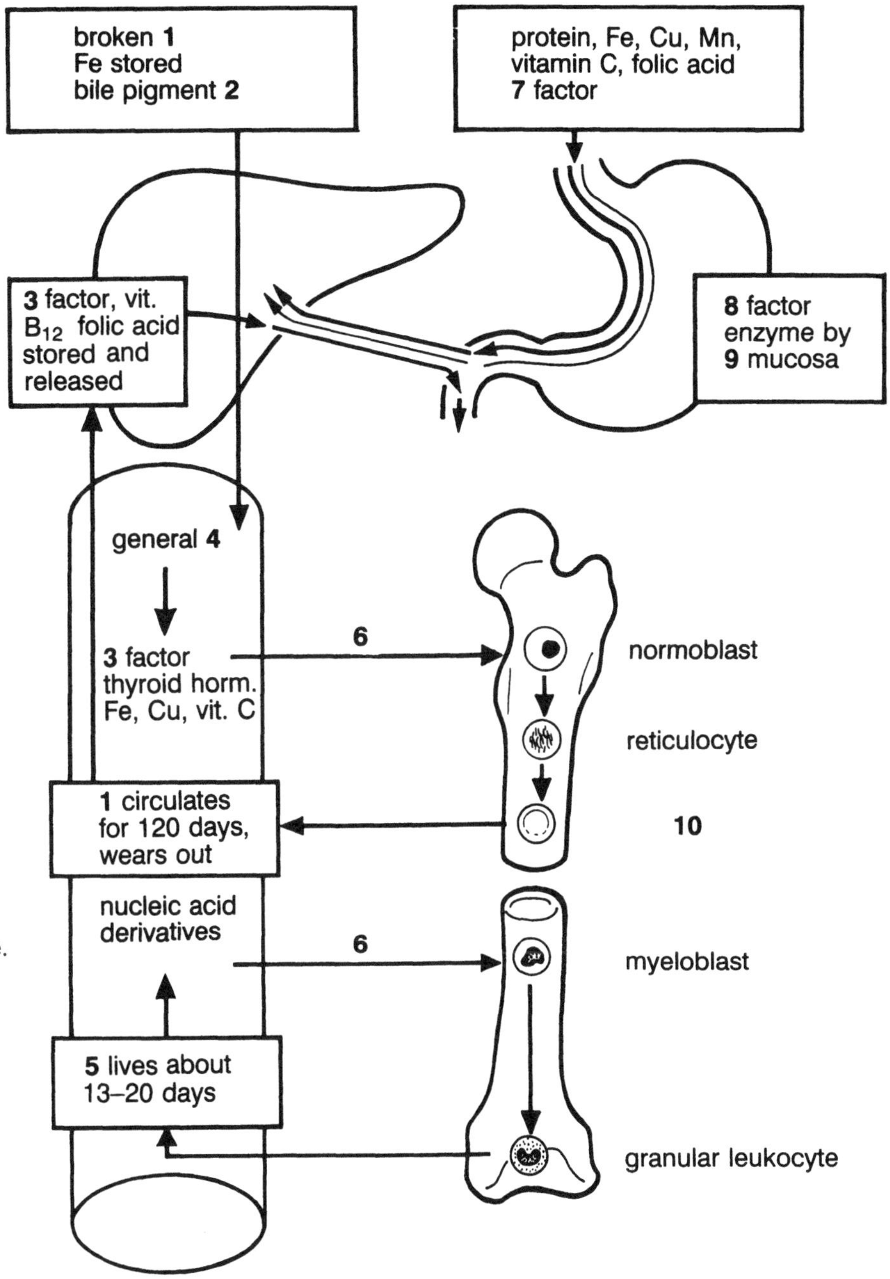

Figure 12.3 Sequence of events in, and elements essential for, normal blood formation. RBC, red blood cell; WBC, white blood cell; vit., vitamin; horm., hormone.

1. ______________________
2. ______________________
3. ______________________
4. ______________________
5. ______________________
6. ______________________
7. ______________________
8. ______________________
9. ______________________
10. ______________________

V. TEST ITEMS

A. *Multiple Choice.* There is only one answer that is either correct or most appropriate. Circle the best answer for each question.

1. Oxygen is carried in the blood in the form of
a. carboxyHb
b. haematocrit
c. oxyHb
d. cyanosis

2. A person with blood type A has antibodies for type
a. B
b. O
c. Rh
d. A

3. Inability of the blood to transport adequate amounts of oxygen may be due to a deficiency of
a. platelets
b. fibrin
c. leucocytes
d. haemoglobin

4. B lymphocytes' prime responsibility is to
a. attack the foreign body
b. produce haemoglobin
c. produce antibodies
d. be a killer cell

5. Haemoglobin is
a. carried in red blood cells
b. an oxygen transporter
c. made of protein and heme
d. all of the above

6. The two enzymes in the clotting processes are
a. fibrin and thromboplastin
b. thromboplastin and thrombin
c. platelets and fibrin
d. prothrombin and calcium

7. A person with normal blood volume and white cell count but low red cell count or low haemoglobin content is suffering from
a. haemophilia
b. anaemia
c. leukaemia
d. mononucleosis

8. In a severe allergic reaction, anaphylactic shock is caused by the prolonged effects of
a. histamine
b. epinephrine (adrenaline)
c. heparin
d. fibrinogen

9. The normal erythrocyte count for an adult is
a. 3–4 million/mm^3
b. 8 million/mm^3
c. 4.5–5 million/mm^3
d. 3 million/mm^3

10. In the healthy adult, erythrocytes are formed in the
    a. liver
    b. red bone marrow
    c. lymphoid tissue
    d. spleen

11. The hematocrit test tells the physician the volume of
    a. white blood cells
    b. blood platelets
    c. lymphocytes
    d. packed red cell volume

12. The most actively phagocytic cells and most amoeboid cells are the
    a. lymphocytes
    b. neutrophils
    c. basophils
    d. eosinophils

13. The blood group composing the smallest percentage in the general white population is blood type
    a. A
    b. B
    c. AB
    d. Rh–

14. Blood type AB is the universal recipient because
    a. it has no antibodies
    b. it has no antigens
    c. it has all antigens
    d. it has all antibodies

15. An antibody is
    a. a protein that reacts with an antigen
    b. a white corpuscle that phagocytises invading bacteria
    c. a carbohydrate
    d. a blood platelet

16. Immunity is
    a. the opposite to allergic
    b. dependent on the proper functioning of the nervous system
    c. dependent on the presence of antibodies
    d. a factor that increases with age

17. A vaccine contains
    a. penicillin
    b. horse serum
    c. treated antigens
    d. antibodies

18. A sample of type O blood will agglutinate with
    a. anti-A serum
    b. both anti-A and -B serum
    c. anti-B serum
    d. neither anti-A nor -B serum

19. Which of these is most specifically responsible for antibody-mediated immunity?
   a. T cell
   b. B cell
   c. platelets
   d. all of the above

20. A key role of T cells is
   a. phagocytosis
   b. production of histamine
   c. rejecting foreign tissue transplants
   d. production of heparin

B. *Matching.* Each of the words or phrases in Column B refers to a term in Column A. Insert the letter of the word or phrase from Column B that best describes each term in Column A. Some words or phrases may be used more than once or not at all.

Column A	*Column B*
1. ___ ADH (vasopressin)	**a.** derived from B lymphocytes
2. ___ Rh incompatibility	**b.** release histamine
3. ___ plasma cells	**c.** phagocytise bacteria
4. ___ transfusion reaction	**d.** a hormone released when dehydrated
5. ___ cortisol	**e.** stimulates gluconeogenesis
6. ___ destroy cance cells	**f.** antibodies against self-tissue
7. ___ autoimmune	**g.** atopic allergy
8. ___ active immunity	**h.** erythroblastosis foetalis (haemolytic disease of the newborn)
9. ___ hay fever	**i.** a special type of tissue rejection
10. ___ basophils	**j.** self-protein molecules that are antigenic
11. ___ passive immunity	**k.** cell-mediated immunity
12. ___ clones	**l.** recipient receives preformed antibody
13. ___ histocompatibility antigens	**m.** different populations of B cells
14. ___ macrophages	**n.** antibodies are built up as a result of actual contact

	Column A		Column B
1. ___	stimulate antibody production	a.	antibody
2. ___	fibrinogen	b.	vitamin K
3. ___	platelets	c.	major protein in a blood clot
4. ___	red bone marrow	d.	anticoagulant
5. ___	erythropoietin	e.	hormone that regulates erythrocyte production
6. ___	spleen and liver	f.	development of white blood cells
7. ___	autoimmune	g.	manufactures red blood cells during foetal life
8. ___	agglutinin	h.	manufactures red blood cells in adults
9. ___	leucopoiesis	i.	thromboplastin
10. ___	prothrombin	j.	antigens

C. *True or False.* Place a *T* or an *F* in the space provided to indicate true or false.

___ **1.** The release of histamine from damaged tissues produces inflammation (reddening) by increasing the permeability of capillaries to red blood cells that accumulate in the extracellular spaces surrounding the damaged tissue.

___ **2.** When a blood vessel is severed or injured, its immediate response is to constrict.

___ **3.** The event transforming blood into a solid clot is the conversion of plasma fibrinogen to fibrin.

___ **4.** Vitamin K is an essential cofactor in the liver's synthesis of prothrombin and the plasma factors.

___ **5.** Bilirubin is a breakdown component of haemoglobin.

___ **6.** About 70% of the total body iron is in haemoglobin.

___ **7.** Vitamin B regulates the rate of erythrocyte production.

___ **8.** Polymorphonuclear granulocytes refers to the three types of blood cells with lobulated nuclei and cytoplasmic granules.

___ **9.** The cells of the body believed to form antibodies are called neutrophils.

___ **10.** Any substance capable of stimulating antibody production is an antigen.

___ **11.** Substances such as heparin and dicumarol that promote fibrinolysis are classified as anticoagulants.

___ **12.** Blood type O is referred to as the universal recipient because it has neither A nor B antibodies in its plasma.

___ **13.** The normal range for clotting time is between 5 and 15 minutes.

___ **14.** In contrast with plasma, both lymph and interstitial fluid lack thrombocytes and erythrocytes.

____ **15.** Excessive loss of red blood cells through bleeding may result in sickle cell anaemia.

____ **16.** An abnormal increase in the number of red blood cells is referred to as haemolysis.

____ **17.** Slight fever, sore throat, stiff neck, cough, malaise, and a high monocyte and leukocyte count are indicative of a disorder of white blood cells called leukemia.

____ **18.** Antibodies are produced by plasma cells.

____ **19.** Antibodies are all composed of polypeptide chains.

____ **20.** The lymphocyte is the largest of the white blood cells.

Answer Sheet—Chapter 12

Exercise 12.1

CHARACTERISTICS OF BLOOD

Blood is bright red (indicating that it is well oxygenated) in the arteries and dark red (less oxygenated) in the veins. It flows four to five times more slowly than water because it is four to five times thicker (a property called viscosity). Its specific gravity (density compared with water) varies between 1.045 and 1.065 (water is 1.000), and its temperature and pH values are 38°C (100.4°F) and about 7.38, respectively. The volume of blood in the body has been measured in many ways but can be expected to vary with the size of the body. A useful estimate is that its weight is 8% of the body's weight. The blood volume of a man of average size is approximately 6 L.

Seen with the naked eye, blood appears to be opaque and homogeneous; but on microscopic examination, it consists of cells and cell fragments and an intercellular fluid, the plasma. When blood is obtained from a person's vein (by venipuncture) and transferred to a test tube, and clotting is prevented by adding certain chemicals called anticoagulants, it separates into two distinct layers. The upper layer, which is yellow and transparent, contains most of the chemical components of the blood in solution; this is the plasma. Plasma constitutes about 55% of the blood's volume. The lower portion of the blood sample consists of the formed elements: the red blood cells (erythrocytes), the white blood cells (leucocytes), and the platelets (thrombocytes). These are often called corpuscles, meaning little bodies. The percentage of total blood volume contributed by these formed elements is called the hematocrit.

Exercise 12.2

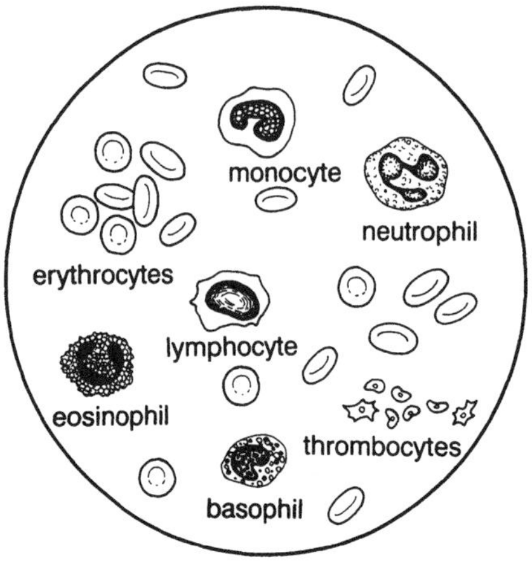

Figure 12.2 Microscopic blood smear.

Exercise 12.3

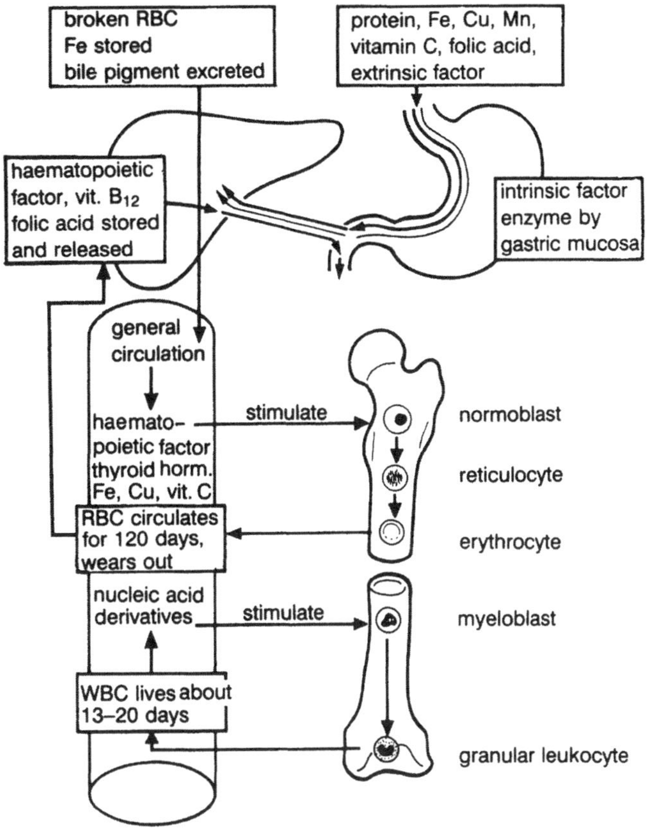

Figure 12.3 Sequence of events in, and elements essential for, normal blood formation. RBC, red blood cell; WBC, white blood cell; vit., vitamin; horm., hormone.

Test Items

A. 1. c, 2. a, 3. d, 4. c, 5. d, 6. b, 7. b, 8. a, 9. c, 10. b, 11. d, 12. b, 13. c, 14. a, 15. a, 16. c, 17. c, 18. d, 19. b, 20. c.

B. 1. d, 2. h, 3. a, 4. i, 5. e, 6. k, 7. f, 8. o, 9. g, 10. b, 11. l, 12. n, 13. j, 14. c.
1. j, 2. c, 3. i, 4. h, 5. e, 6. g, 7. d, 8. a, 9. f, 10. b.

C. 1. F, 2. T, 3. T, 4. T, 5. T, 6. T, 7. F, 8. T, 9. F, 10. T, 11. T, 12. F, 13. T, 14. T, 15. F, 16. F, 17. F, 18. T, 19. T, 20. F.

13

The Heart

I. CHAPTER SYNOPSIS

This chapter presents the major anatomical and physical features of the heart. Among the principal physiological aspects considered are the initiation and conduction of the heartbeat, the electrocardiogram, the heart's blood supply, the major events of the cardiac cycle, heart sounds, cardiac output and stroke volume, regulation of heart rate and circulatory shock, and homeostasis.

In a multicellular organism such as a human being, diffusion from the surface of the body is too slow a process to deliver nutrients and oxygen to the cells of the body and to remove waste products and carbon dioxide. The circulatory system provides the body with a mechanism for rapidly exchanging matter between the external and internal environments. The heart, acting as a pump, provides the force necessary to produce a bulk flow of blood that is channeled to the tissues through blood vessels where the exchange of matter between the blood and interstitial fluid occurs.

II. OBJECTIVES

After reading the chapter, the student should be able to:

- Identify the structures of the heart and trace the cardiac cycle.
- Describe the two sets of heart valves and explain their function in cardiac blood flow.

- Explain why the sinoatrial node is the pacemaker of the heart.
- Define coronary artery disease (CAD).
- List and explain at least two kinds of myocardial infarctions (heart attacks).
- Describe the cardiac reflex in relation to the neurochemical control.
- Explain congenital heart disease and give examples.

III. IMPORTANT TERMS

Using your textbook, define the following terms:

apex (ay′pecks) ______________________________

____

atrium (ay′tree-um) ______________________________

____

bicuspid (bye-kus′pid) ______________________________

____

bradycardia (bra-dee-kahr′dee-uh) ______________________________

____

circumflex (sur′kum-flecks) ______________________________

____

coronary (kor′o-ner-ree) ______________________________

____

diastole (dye-as′tuh-lee) ______________________________

____

endocardium (en-do-kahr′dee-um) ______________________________

____

epicardium (epi-kahr′dee-um) ______________________________

____

foramen (fo-ray′men) ______________________________

____

infarction (in-fahrk′shun) ______________________________

____

ischaemia (is-kee′mee-uh) ______________________________

____

murmur (mur′mur) ______________________________

____

myocardium (migh-o-kahr′dee-um) ______________________________

____

pericardium (per-ri-kahr′dee-um) ______________________________

____

Purkinje (pur-kin′je) ______________________________

____

septum (sep′tum) ______________________________

____

sinoatrial (sigh-no-ay′tree-ul) ______________________________

____

stenosis (ste-no′sis) ______________________________

____

systole (sis′tuh-lee) ______________________________

____

tachycardia (ta-ki-kahr′dee-uh) ______________________________

____

tricuspid (trye-kus′pid) ______________________________

____

umbilical (um-bil′i-kul) ______________________________

____

valve (valv) ______________________________

____

ventricle (ven′tri-kul) ______________________________

____

IV. EXERCISES

Complete the following exercises in the order given. A precise set of terms and diagrams has been chosen to describe the heart.

Exercise 13.1

Labelling. Write the name of the structure on the space provided. Colour the right and left sides of the heart blue and red, respectively.

Key:

aorta	atrium	pulmonary	superior	veins
aortic	bicuspid	semilunar	tricuspid	ventricle
apex	inferior	septum	valve	

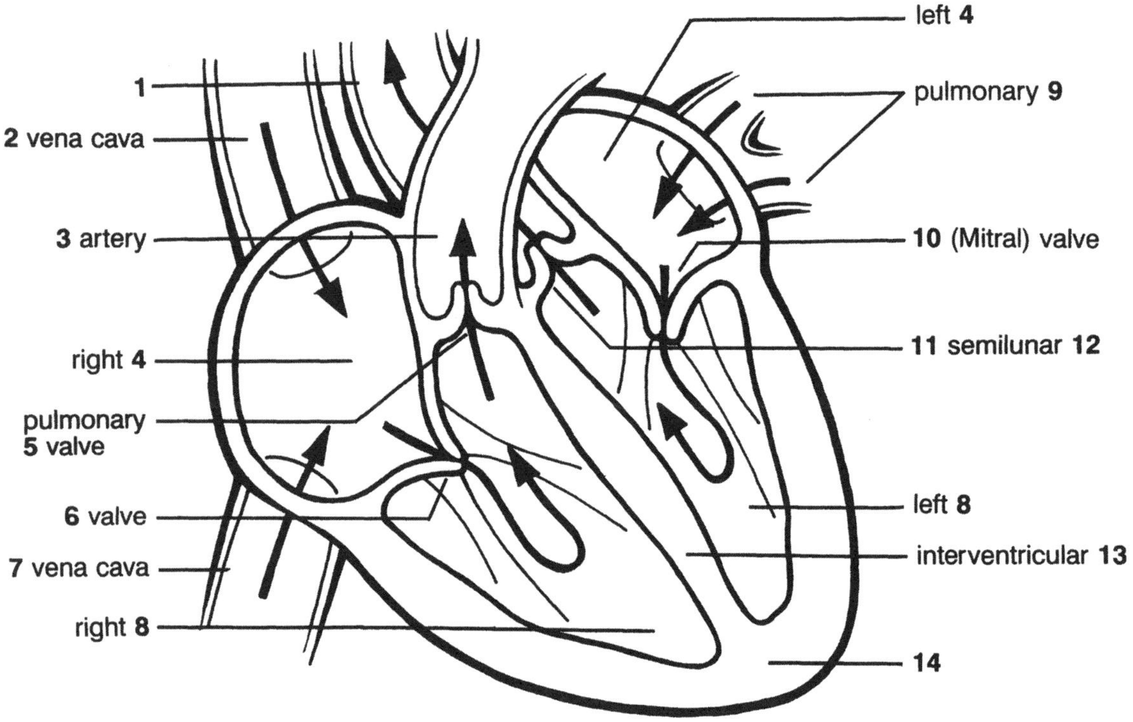

Figure 13.1 The heart. Arrows indicate direction of blood flow.

1. ______	8. ______
2. ______	9. ______
3. ______	10. ______
4. ______	11. ______
5. ______	12. ______
6. ______	13. ______
7. ______	14. ______

Exercise 13.2

Labelling. Write the name of the structure on the space provided. Colour the excitation system black and the heart tissue light red.

Key:

atrioventricular	interventricular	sinoatrial
atrium	myocardium	ventricle
His	Purkinje	

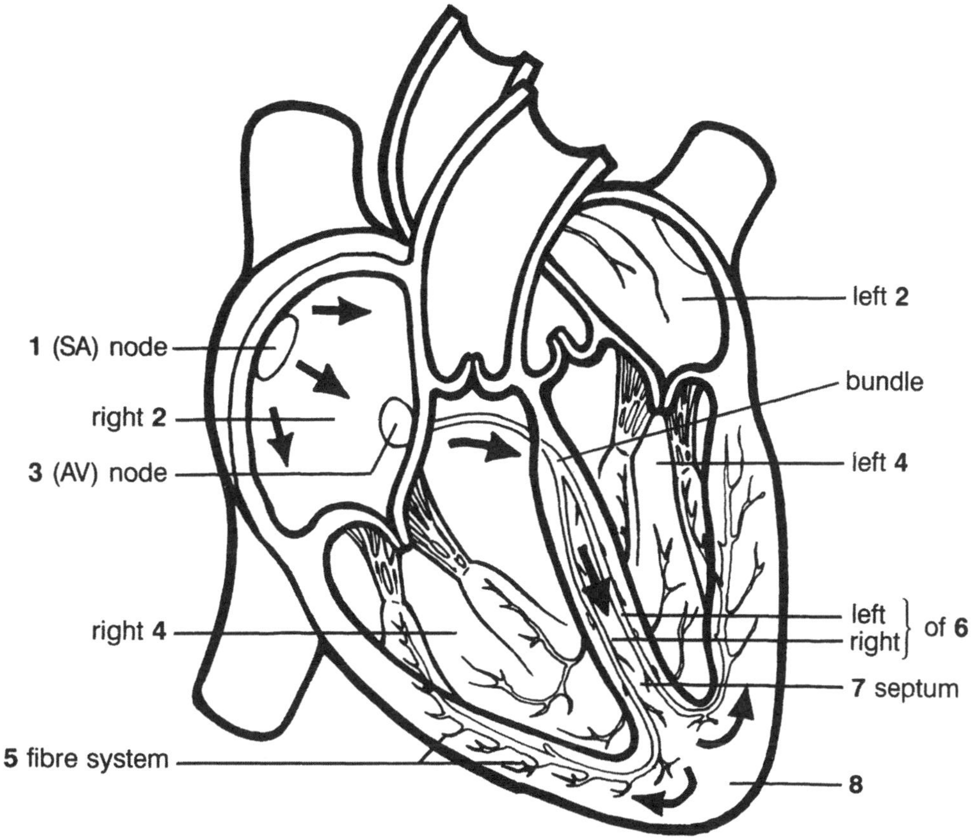

Figure 13.2 Excitation-conduction system. An impulse is conducted from its point of origin, the right atrium, to its destination, the myocardium.

1. ______________________
2. ______________________
3. ______________________
4. ______________________
5. ______________________
6. ______________________
7. ______________________
8. ______________________

Exercise 13.3

Labelling. Write the name of the structure on the space provided. Colour the arteries, veins, pericardium, and fat.

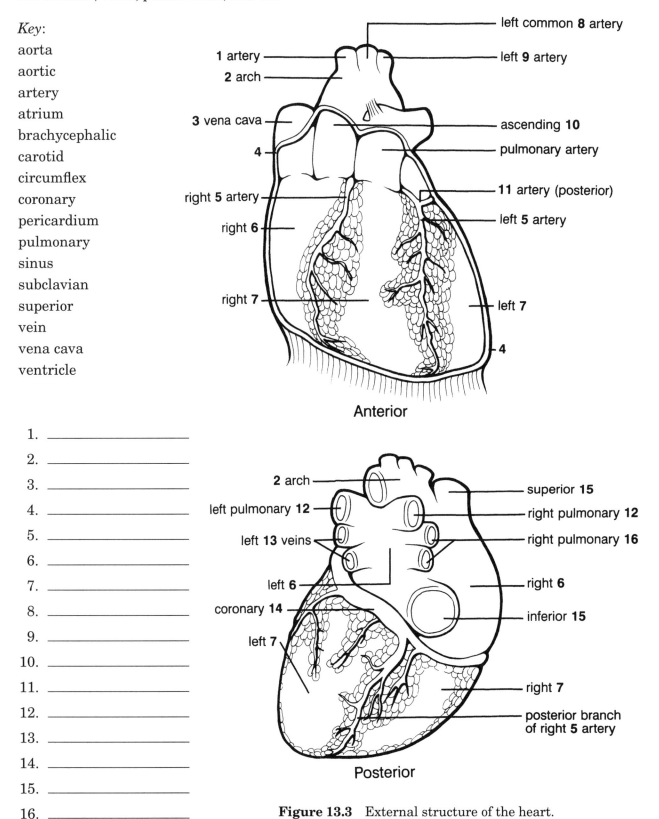

Key:
aorta
aortic
artery
atrium
brachycephalic
carotid
circumflex
coronary
pericardium
pulmonary
sinus
subclavian
superior
vein
vena cava
ventricle

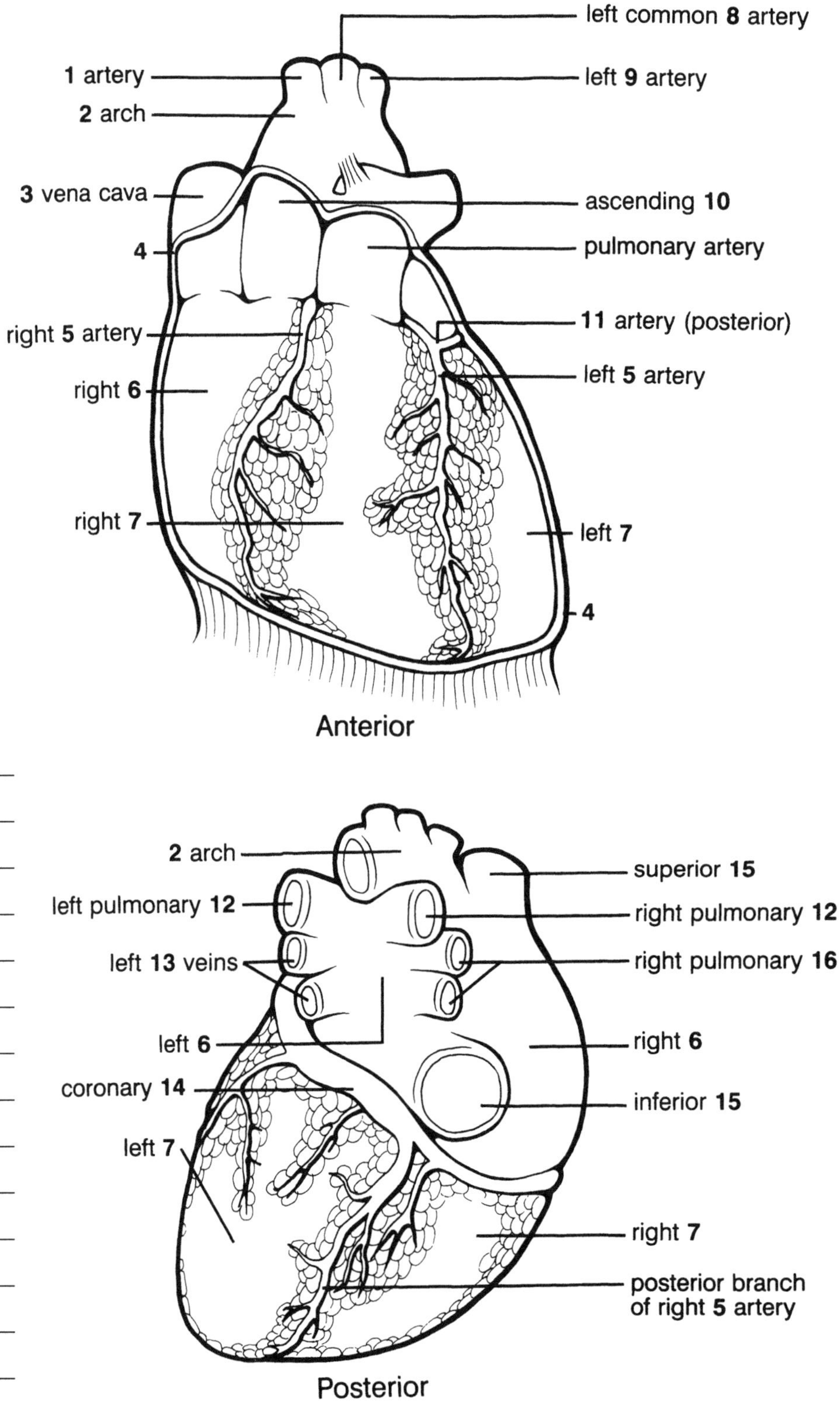

1. ____________
2. ____________
3. ____________
4. ____________
5. ____________
6. ____________
7. ____________
8. ____________
9. ____________
10. ____________
11. ____________
12. ____________
13. ____________
14. ____________
15. ____________
16. ____________

Figure 13.3 External structure of the heart.

Exercise 13.4

Labelling. Write the name of the structure on the space provided. Colour the different vessels and organs.

Key:
aorta
arch
arteriosus
atrium
foramen
iliac
liver
lung
placenta
pulmonary
umbilical
vena cava
ventricle

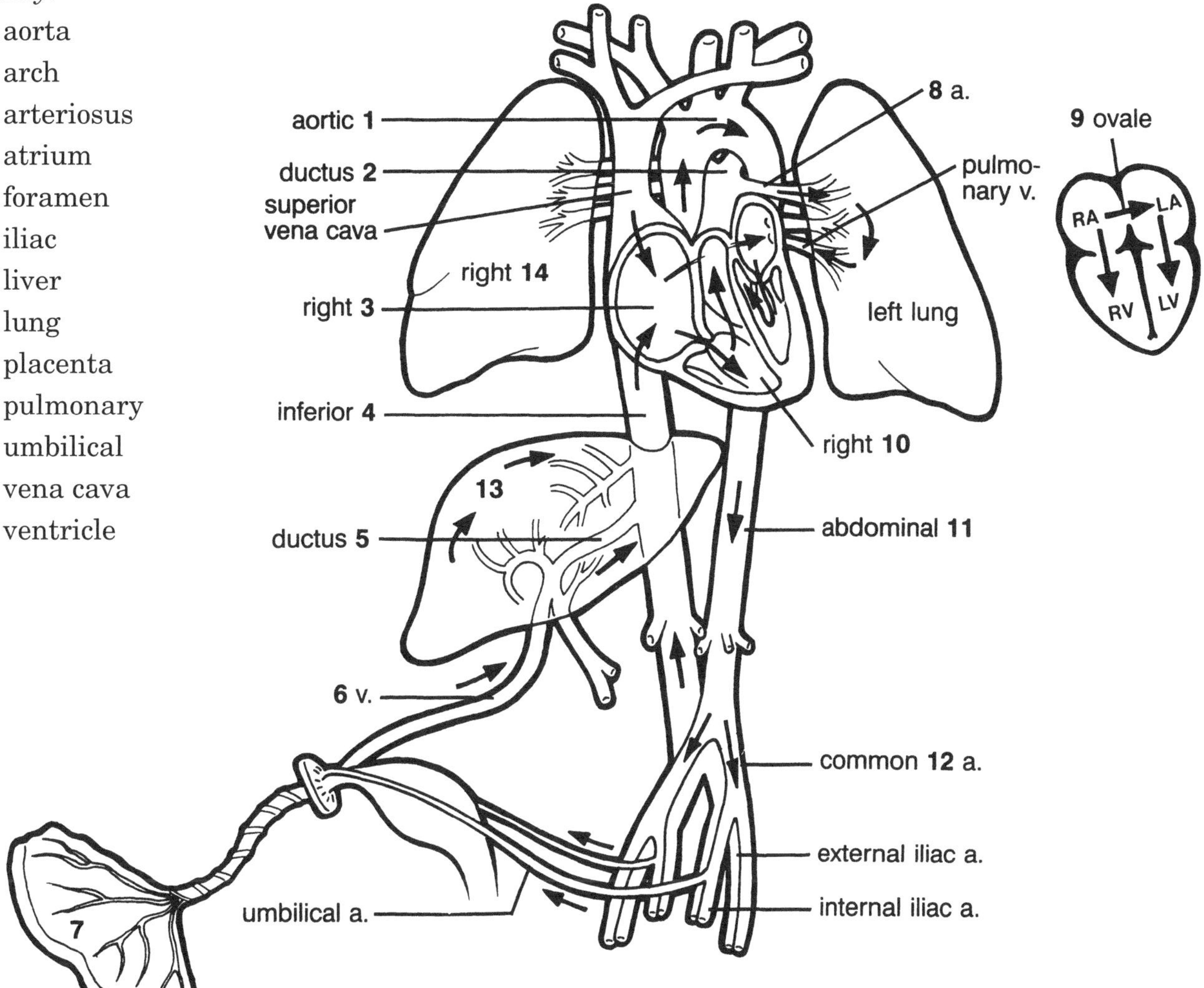

Figure 13.4 Plan of circulation in a mature foetus. Arrows indicate the direction of blood flow. The inset shows the blood flow in the fetal heart. Note the blood flow from the right atrium into both the right ventricle and left atrium through the foramen ovale. RA, right atrium; LA, left atrium; RV, right ventricle; LV, left ventricle.

1. ______________________
2. ______________________
3. ______________________
4. ______________________
5. ______________________
6. ______________________
7. ______________________
8. ______________________
9. ______________________
10. ______________________
11. ______________________
12. ______________________
13. ______________________
14. ______________________

V. TEST ITEMS

A. *Multiple Choice.* There is only one answer that is either correct or most appropriate. Circle the best answer for each question.

1. High blood pressure is technically called
   a. hypotension
   b. hypotenicity
   c. hypertenicity
   d. hypertension

2. The tricuspid valve lies between the
   a. left atria and left ventricle
   b. right and left atria
   c. right and left ventricles
   d. right atria and right ventricle

3. When the quantity of adrenaline (epinephrine) is increased
   a. the heart will speed up
   b. the heart will slow down
   c. the blood volume will increase
   d. the blood volume will decrease

4. Which layer of the heart contracts?
   a. epicardium
   b. myocardium
   c. endocardium
   d. pericardium

5. Which of the following acts as the heart's natural pacemaker?
   a. SA node
   b. AV node
   c. bundle of His
   d. Purkinje fibres

6. Normal systolic pressure in the adult is
   a. 70 cc
   b. 120 mm Hg
   c. 30 ml
   d. 80 mm Hg

7. Which of the following chambers pumps blood into the systemic circulatory system?
   a. right atrium
   b. left atrium
   c. right ventricle
   d. left ventricle

8. Freshly oxygenated blood is received by the
   a. right atrium
   b. left atrium
   c. right ventricle
   d. left ventricle

9. The membranous sac surrounding the heart is known as the
   a. pericardium
   b. endocardium
   c. myocardium
   d. epicardium

10. The P wave of the ECG correlates with the
   a. depolarisation of the AV node
   b. atrial depolarisation
   c. ventricular repolarisation
   d. depolarisation of the ventricle

11. Which of the following correctly depicts the functional differences between the left and right sides of the heart?
   a. The right side of the heart works against greater resistance than the left side of the heart
   b. The left side of the heart pumps more blood than the right side of the heart
   c. Starling's law of the heart applies to the left ventricle but not to the right ventricle
   d. The partial pressure of oxygen in the blood of the left ventricle is lower than it is in the right ventricle

12. Which of the following blood vessels carries deoxygenated blood?
   a. pulmonary arteries
   b. pulmonary veins
   c. coronary arteries
   d. aorta

13. The two distinct heart sounds, described phonetically as *lubb* and *dupp*, represent the
   a. contraction of the ventricles and the relaxation of the atria
   b. contraction of the atria and the relaxation of the ventricles
   c. closing of the atrioventricular and semilunar valves
   d. surging of blood into the pulmonary artery and aorta

14. During atrial systole, all but which of the following occur?
   a. Deoxygenated blood passes into the right ventricle
   b. Oxygenated blood passes into the left ventricle
   c. The ventricles are in diastole
   d. The semilunar valves are open

15. An operation that attempts to repair an atrial septal defect would be carried out on the
   a. ductus arteriosus
   b. ductus venosus
   c. foramen ovale
   d. interventricular septum

16. A congenital heart disorder that results in cyanosis as a result of the mixing of oxygenated and deoxygenated blood is
   a. patent ductus arteriosus
   b. atrial septal defect
   c. ventricular septal defect
   d. valvular stenosis

17. A myocardial infarction results in
   a. the death of an area of the aorta
   b. an accelerated rate of haematopoiesis
   c. rapid cell division of the layers of the pericardium
   d. death of an area of the heart muscle

18. A "blue" baby is probably
  a. suffering from rheumatic heart disease
  b. suffering from arterial sclerosis
  c. not getting enough oxygenated blood throughout the body
  d. not getting enough liver in the body

19. Systole occurs when
  a. the heart muscle contracts
  b. the heart muscle relaxes
  c. the atrioventricular valve closes
  d. the semilunar valve closes

20. The heartbeat originates in the
  a. AV node
  b. pacemaker
  c. autonomic nervous system
  d. pericardium

B. *Matching.* Each of the phrases in Column B refers to a term in Column A. Insert the letter of the phrase from Column B that best describes each term in Column A. Some words or phrases may be used more than once or not at all.

Column A

1. ____ noradrenaline (norepinephrine)
2. ____ intrinsic control
3. ____ SA node
4. ____ systole
5. ____ T wave
6. ____ ectopic foci
7. ____ adrenaline (epinephrine)
8. ____ intercalated disks
9. ____ murmur
10. ____ fibrillation
11. ____ apex
12. ____ intrathoracic
13. ____ myocardium
14. ____ Starling's law of the heart
15. ____ arteries

Column B

a. increases cardiac output
b. increases ventricular and atrial contractility
c. the external pressure surrounding the heart
d. the direct proportion between the diastolic volume of the heart and the force of the contraction
e. an inherent property of cardiac muscle
f. under constant influence of nerves and hormones
g. a leaky valve
h. ventricular contraction
i. ventricular repolarisation
j. disorganised contractions
k. caffeine may cause
l. "tight junctions"
m. the tip of the left ventricle
n. heart muscle
o. carries blood away from the heart

Column A		Column B
1. ____ tachycardia	a.	mechanical device for applying electrical shock to the heart
2. ____ defibrillator	b.	heart sound produced by blood passing through a valve or opening caused by a septal defect
3. ____ cardiac arrest	c.	rapid heart rate
4. ____ cyanosis	d.	slightly bluish skin colouration due to oxygen deficiency in systemic blood
5. ____ bradycardia	e.	complete stoppage of the heartbeat
6. ____ murmur	f.	slow heartbeat

C. *True or False.* Place a *T* or an *F* in the space provided to indicate true or false.

___ **1.** The reflex that controls venous blood pressure is the carotid sinus reflex.

___ **2.** Sympathetic stimulation of the heart brings about an increase in heart rate.

___ **3.** The phenomenon by which the length of the cardiac muscle fibre determines the force of contraction is called Starling's law of the heart.

___ **4.** In an ECG, the QRS complex represents the spread of an electrical impulse through the atria.

___ **5.** The mass of conducting cells located in the right atrium and that serves as the pacemaker is called the sinoatrial node.

___ **6.** During ventricular systole, the ventricles are in a period of relaxation.

___ **7.** Under normal circumstances, the right side of the heart contains only deoxygenated blood.

___ **8.** The condition known as mitral stenosis (narrowing) hinders blood's flow from the right atrium into the right ventricle.

___ **9.** The coronary arteries are the first branches off of the thoracic aorta.

___ **10.** Although anastomoses between coronary arteries are numerous, they are small, hence the many deaths from coronary obstruction.

___ **11.** To catheterise the right side of the heart, the catheter must be introduced through a vein.

___ **12.** Whereas the sinoatrial node serves as the natural pacemaker of the heart, the atrioventricular node functions to coordinate ventricular contractions with atrial contractions.

___ **13.** The left ventricle has to pump more blood than the right ventricle because it has to pump the blood through the whole body, not just through the pulmonary system.

___ **14.** The cardiovascular integrating centre is located in the medulla of the brain stem.

___ **15.** The force of contraction of the left ventricle is greater than that of the right ventricle.

Answer Sheet—Chapter 13

Exercise 13.1

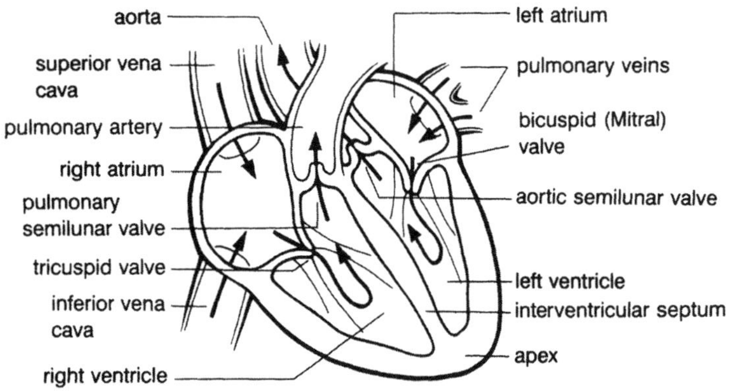

Figure 13.1 The heart. Arrows indicate direction of blood flow.

Exercise 13.2

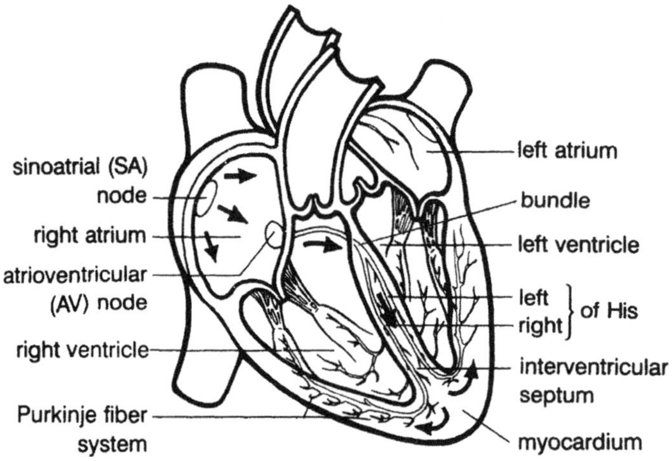

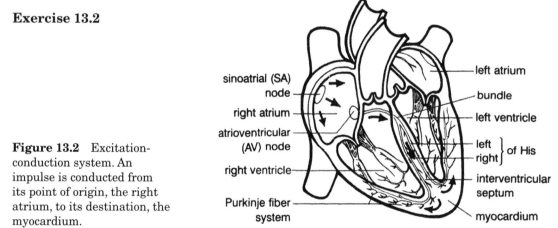

Figure 13.2 Excitation-conduction system. An impulse is conducted from its point of origin, the right atrium, to its destination, the myocardium.

Exercise 13.3

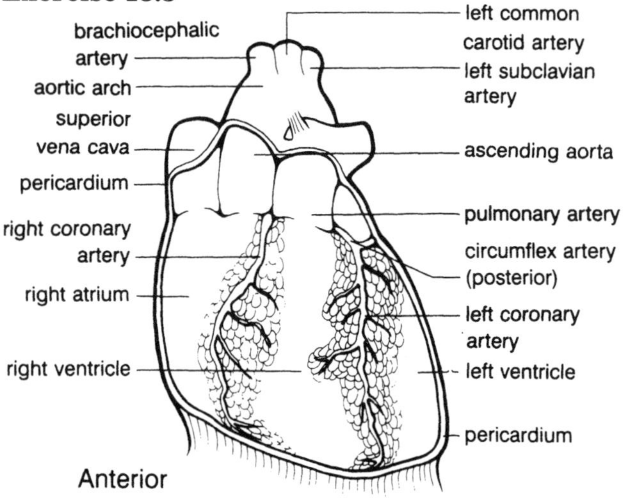

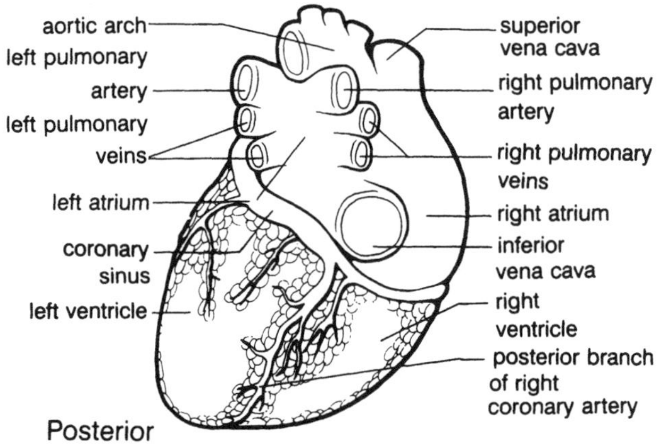

Figure 13.3 External structure of the heart.

Exercise 13.4

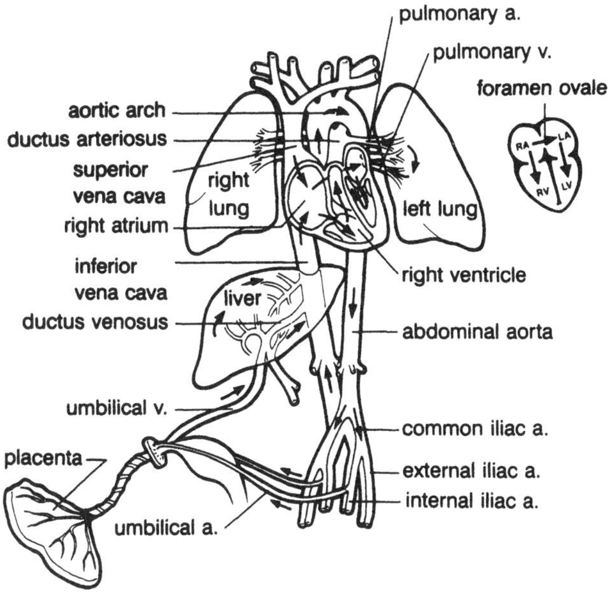

Figure 13.4 Plan of circulation in a mature foetus. Arrows indicate the direction of blood flow. The inset shows the blood flow in the fetal heart. Note the blood flow from the right atrium into both the right ventricle and left atrium through the foramen ovale. RA, right atrium; LA, left atrium; RV, right ventricle; LV, left ventricle.

Test Items

A. 1. d, 2. d, 3. a, 4. b, 5. a, 6. b, 7. d ,8. b, 9. a, 10. b, 11. a, 12. a, 13. c, 14. d, 15. c, 16. b, 17. d, 18. c, 19. a, 20. b.

B. 1. b, 2. e, 3. f, 4. h, 5. i, 6. k, 7. a, 8. l, 9. g, 10. j, 11. m, 12. c, 13. n, 14. d, 15. o.
1. c, 2. a, 3. e, 4. d, 5. f, 6. b.

C. 1. F, 2. T, 3. T, 4. F, 5. T, 6. F, 7. T, 8. F, 9. F, 10. F, 11. T, 12. T, 13. F, 14. T, 15. T.

14

Circulation

I. CHAPTER SYNOPSIS

In the previous chapter, the control of the heart was emphasised. After blood leaves the heart, a variety of control systems and pathways regulate the distribution of blood to the tissues in proportion to the varying metabolic demands of the organs and systems of the body. These control mechanisms are integrated into the overall design of the circulatory system. The overall design, outside of the heart, consists of the arteries, arterioles, capillaries, veins, and the integrated lymphatic system. Thus, this chapter concerns itself with the basic anatomical and physiological modalities of the vascular system in maintaining overall circulatory homeostasis.

II. OBJECTIVES

After reading the chapter, the student should be able to:

- Identify the structural differences between an artery, vein, and capillary.
- Identify the major arteries and veins of the systemic circulation.
- Identify the major pressure and pulse points of the body.
- Differentiate between pulmonary and systemic circulation.
- Describe the anatomical differences between the hepatic portal and foetal circulatory systems.

III. IMPORTANT TERMS

Using your textbook, define the following terms:

alveolar (al-vee-o-lar) ______________________________

____

aneurysm (an′yoo-riz-m) ______________________________

____

apoplexy (ap′o-plek-see) ______________________________

____

arteriole (ahr-teer′-ee-ole) ______________________________

____

arteriosclerosis (ahr-teer-ee-o-skle-ro′sis) ______________________________

____

artery (ahr′tur-ee) ______________________________

____

brachial (bray′kee-ul) ______________________________

____

capillary (kap′i-lair-ee) ______________________________

____

cerebrovascular (ser-re-bro-vas′kew-lur) ______________________________

____

haemorrhage (hem′uh-ridj) ______________________________

____

hepatic (he-pat′ik) ______________________________

____

hypertension (hy-pur-ten′shun) ______________________________

____

oncotic (ong-kot′ik) ______________________________

____

oxygenated (ok′si-ji-nated) ______________________________

____

portal (por′-tul) ____________________

pulmonary (pul′-muh-ner-ee) ____________________

pulse (puls) ____________________

saphenous (sa-fee′-nus) ____________________

shock (shok) ____________________

sphygmomanometer (sfig-mo-mah-nom′-et-ur) ____________________

stethoscope (steth′-ah-skope) ____________________

varicose (var′i-kos) ____________________

vascular (vas′-kew-lur) ____________________

vein (vain) ____________________

venule (ven′-yool) ____________________

vessel (ves-′ul) ____________________

IV. EXERCISES

Complete the following exercises in the order given. A precise set of terms and diagrams has been chosen to describe the circulatory system.

Exercise 14.1

Labelling. Write the name of the artery on the space provided. Colour the arteries red.

Key:
aortic
axillary
brachial
carotid
femoral
iliac
mesenteric
pedis
peroneal
popliteal
radial
renal
subclavian
temporal
tibial
ulnar

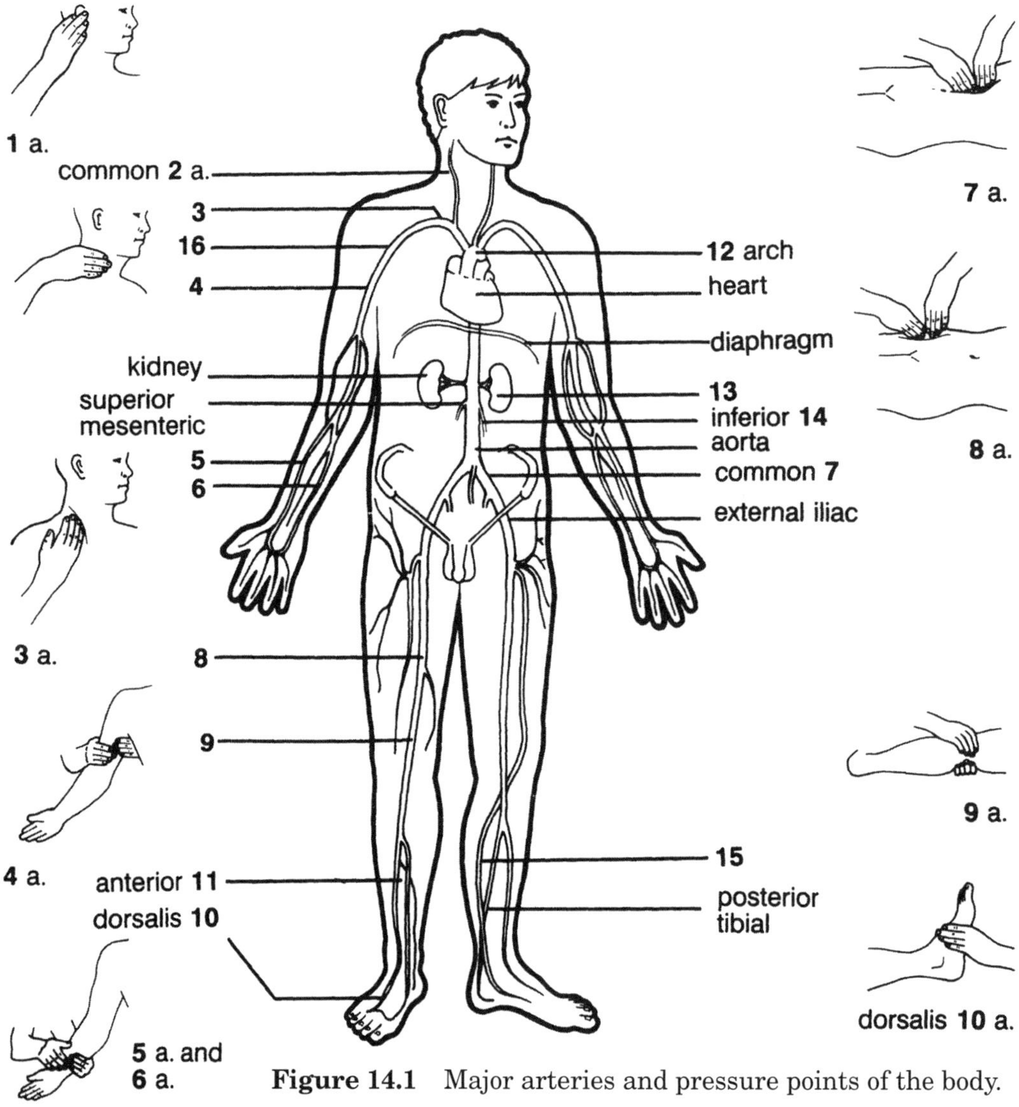

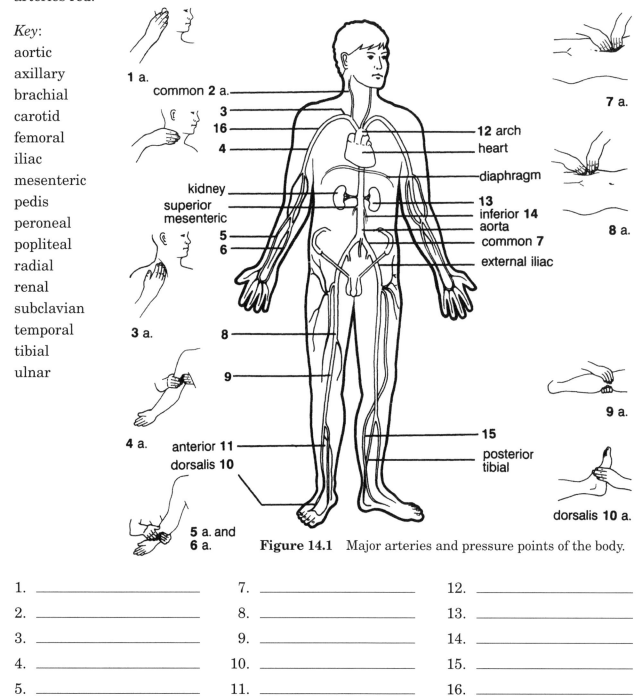

Figure 14.1 Major arteries and pressure points of the body.

1. ____________ 7. ____________ 12. ____________
2. ____________ 8. ____________ 13. ____________
3. ____________ 9. ____________ 14. ____________
4. ____________ 10. ____________ 15. ____________
5. ____________ 11. ____________ 16. ____________

Exercise 14.2

Labelling. Write the name of the vein on the space provided. Colour the veins blue.

Key:
axillary
basilic
brachial
femoral
iliac
innominate
jugular
popliteal
radial
renal
saphenous
subclavian
tibial
ulnar
vena cava

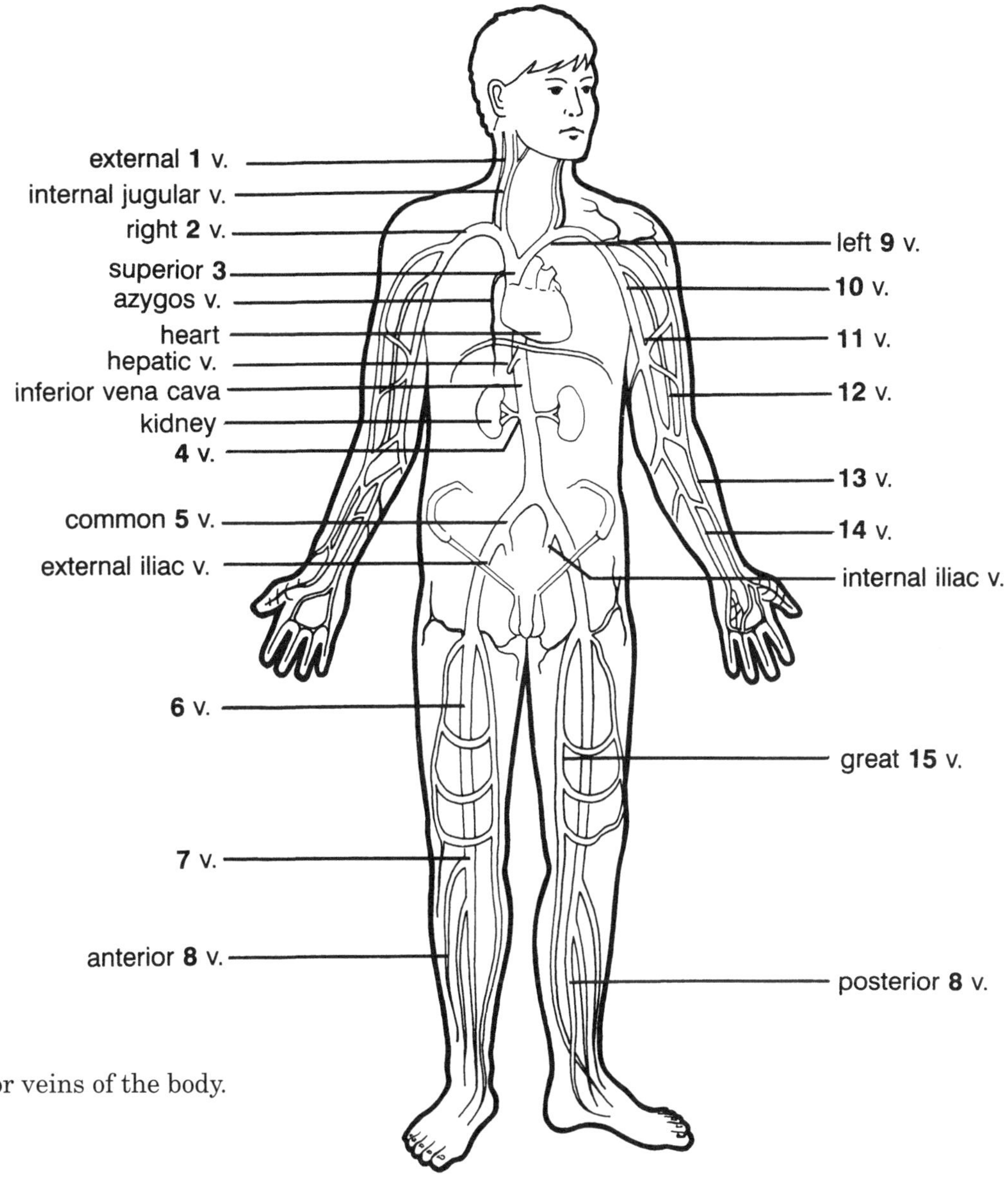

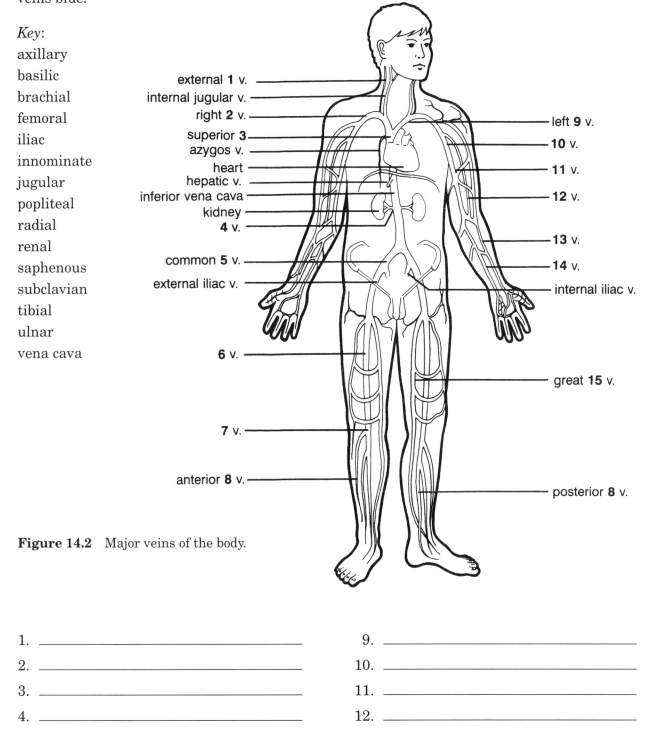

Figure 14.2 Major veins of the body.

1. ______________________
2. ______________________
3. ______________________
4. ______________________
5. ______________________
6. ______________________
7. ______________________
8. ______________________
9. ______________________
10. ______________________
11. ______________________
12. ______________________
13. ______________________
14. ______________________
15. ______________________

Exercise 14.3

Labelling. Write the name of the vein in the space provided. Colour the veins blue and the organs various colours.

Key:
hepatic
iliac
mesenteric
portal
splenic
vena cava

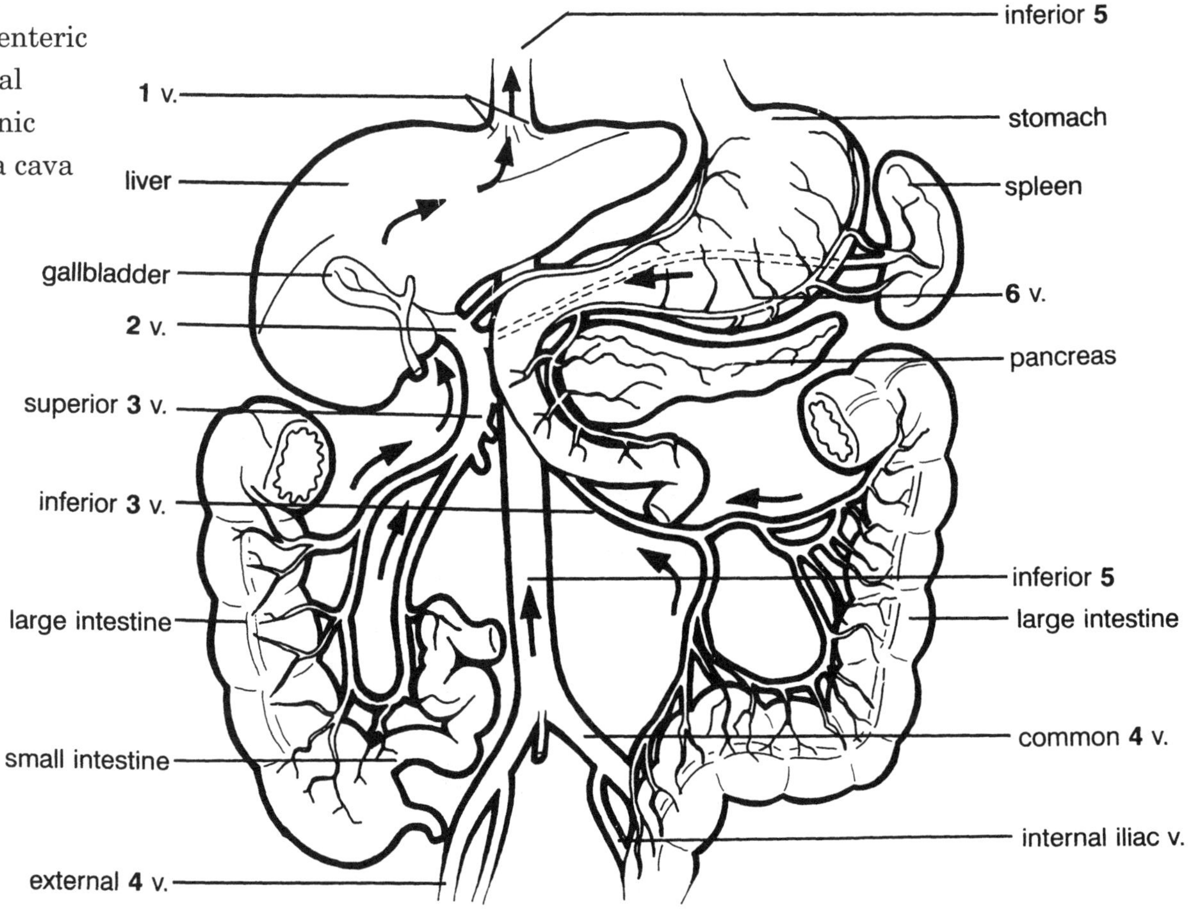

Figure 14.3 The hepatic portal system. Arrows indicate the direction of flow in all abdominal organs, through the liver, to the superior vena cava.

1. ______________________
2. ______________________
3. ______________________
4. ______________________
5. ______________________
6. ______________________

Exercise 14.4

Fill in the Blanks. Write the missing terms from the key list on the left in the appropriate spaces provided in the text on the right.

Key:

alveolar
arterioles
artery
artery
blood
branches
bronchi
capillary
capillary
divides
follows
heart
leaves
left
lungs
lungs
pulmonary
returns
right
right
veins

PULMONARY CIRCULATION

The ______ circulation carries ______ from the ______ to the ______ and back to the heart. The blood ______ the heart by way of the large pulmonary ______ and ______ through the pulmonary ______.

Originating in the ______ ventricle, the pulmonary ______ passes upward and backward for a short distance and then ______ into ______ and ______ branches that enter the ______. Within each lung the artery ______ widely, and each branch closely ______ the subdivisions of the ______. The terminal ______ open into the ______ networks that surround the ______ sacs.

Key:

artery
artery
away
carbon dioxide
carbon dioxide
capillary
carry
condition
direction
left
lung
named
oxygenated
oxygenated
returning
to
two
veins
veins
venules
vessels

The pulmonary ______ entering the ______ atrium have ______ branches from each ______. Their smallest tributaries arise as ______ from the ______ networks of the alveolar air sacs.

Of paramount importance here is the ______ of the blood in these vessels. As we have seen, blood ______ are ______ according to the ______ of flow to or from the heart—not in terms of what they ______. Generally, a vessel leaving the heart is called an ______ and carries ______ blood (red); a vessel ______ to the heart is called a vein and carries ______-laden blood (blue). However, in the pulmonary circulation only, the pulmonary ______ carries ______-laden blood ______ from the heart (to the lungs), and the pulmonary ______ carry ______ blood ______ the heart (from the lungs).

V. TEST ITEMS

A. *Multiple Choice.* There is only one answer that is either correct or most appropriate. Circle the best answer for each question.

1. Blood is pumped to the lungs by the
a. left atrium c. right atrium
b. left ventricle d. right ventricle

2. A resting pulse of 100 or more per minute indicates
a. bradycardia c. tachycardia
b. myocardia d. endocardia

3. In foetal circulation, the blood containing the highest amount of oxygen is found in the
a. umbilical arteries c. aorta
b. ductus venosus d. umbilical veins

4. An abnormal accumulation of fluid in the tissues is called
a. oedema c. diuresis
b. bursitis d. dehydration

5. A rate of blood flow of 0.5 mm per second would indicate that the blood is flowing through a
a. large artery c. arteriole
b. vein d. capillary

6. The opening between the two atria in the foetus is called the
a. foramen ovale c. ductus arteriosus
b. ductus venosus d. umbilical artery

7. In taking blood pressure, the artery most commonly used is the
a. radial c. femoral
b. brachial d. carotid

8. Arterial pressure increases if
a. peripheral resistance fails
b. peripheral resistance increases
c. viscosity decreases
d. vasodilation results

9. The circle of Willis (cerebral arterial circle)
a. is the circle around the stomach made by the celiac and gastric arteries
b. is the circle formed by the arch of the aorta
c. refers to the return of blood through the portal system
d. is at the base of the brain

10. The longest vein in the body, a superficial vein of the leg and thigh, is subject to enlargement called varicose veins. It is the
a. femoral vein c. saphenous vein
b. popliteal vein d. tibial vein

11. In the foetus, the left atrium receives most of its blood from the
a. ductus arteriosus c. foramen ovale
b. fossa ovalis d. pulmonary artery

12. The principal effect of reducing the elasticity of the large arteries is to
a. increase systolic and decrease diastolic pressure
b. decrease systolic pressure
c. increase diastolic pressure
d. do none of the foregoing

13. The circumflex artery is a branch of the
a. right coronary artery
b. common carotid artery
c. pulmonary trunk
d. left coronary artery

14. A reduction in oxygen concentration in the blood brings about vasoconstriction by acting principally on
a. chemoreceptors in the aorta and carotid arteries
b. chemoreceptors in the medulla
c. arterial baroreceptors
d. none of the foregoing

15. Reduction in blood volume often produces
a. hypertension
b. shock
c. vasodilation
d. purpura

16. The stretch receptors termed baroreceptors that are present in the carotid artery and aorta are sensitive to
a. decrease in CO_2
b. decrease in oxygen
c. changes in arterial pressure
d. vasoconstriction

17. Which statement best describes arteries?
a. All carry oxygenated blood to the heart
b. All contain valves to prevent the backflow of blood
c. All carry blood away from the heart
d. Only large arteries are lined with endothelium

18. Which statement is *not* true of veins?
a. They have less elastic tissue and smooth muscle than arteries
b. They contain more fibrous tissue than arteries
c. Most veins in the extremities have valves
d. They always carry deoxygenated blood

19. All arteries of systemic circulation branch from the
a. aorta
b. pulmonary artery
c. superior vena cava
d. circle of Willis

20. A thrombus in the first branch of the aortic arch would affect the flow of blood to the
a. left side of the head and neck
b. myocardium of the heart
c. right side of the head and neck and right upper extremity
d. left upper extremity

B. *Matching.* Each of the words or phrases in Column B refers to a term in Column A. Insert the letter of the word or phrase from Column B that best describes each term in Column A. Some words or phrases may be used more than once or not at all.

	Column A		*Column B*
1. ___	testes	**a.**	spermatic
2. ___	thigh	**b.**	splenic
3. ___	kidney	**c.**	phrenic
4. ___	spleen	**d.**	renal
5. ___	stomach	**e.**	gastric
6. ___	face	**f.**	posterior cerebral
7. ___	occipital lobe of cerebrum	**g.**	plantar
		h.	lumbar
8. ___	diaphragm	**i.**	internal maxillary
9. ___	sole of foot	**j.**	femoral
10. ___	abdominal wall		

	Column A		*Column B*
1. ___	abdominal aorta	**a.**	ulnar artery
2. ___	celiac artery	**b.**	posterior interventricular artery
3. ___	left coronary artery	**c.**	transverse sinuses
		d.	anterior tibial artery
4. ___	coronary sinus	**e.**	inferior mesenteric artery
5. ___	internal jugular veins	**f.**	hepatic artery
		g.	median cubital vein
6. ___	right coronary artery	**h.**	anterior interventricular artery
7. ___	brachial artery	**i.**	great and small cardiac veins
8. ___	popliteal artery	**j.**	superior mesenteric vein
9. ___	basilic vein		
10. ___	portal vein		

C. *True or False.* Place a *T* or an *F* in the space provided to indicate true or false.

___ **1.** Veins tend to have thick walls of elastic fibres and smooth muscle.

___ **2.** The highest velocity blood flow occurs in the capillaries.

___ **3.** Varicosities in the veins that lie in the wall of the rectum are called haemorrhoids.

___ **4.** Blood pressure is increased if either the flow or resistance is increased.

___ **5.** The blood vessels through which blood flows slowest are the veins.

___ **6.** If a blood vessel is stimulated by a vasoconstrictor nerve, the peripheral resistance increases.

___ **7.** The middle layer (tunica media) of arterioles contains large amounts of elastic fibres.

___ **8.** The right side of the heart is concerned with pulmonary circulation.

___ **9.** Blood entering the left atrium of the heart comes directly from the inferior vena cava and the superior vena cava.

___ **10.** The two circulatory paths in the body are called the pulmonary circulation (lesser circulation) and the systemic circulation (greater circulation).

___ **11.** The epithelial linings of the great vessels are continuous with the endocardium.

___ **12.** When vessels communicate with one another, they are said to be anastomose; an anastomosis is a passageway or connection between two vessels.

___ **13.** The spermatic and ovarian arteries are branches of the renal artery.

___ **14.** The unique feature of the portal system is that blood from the digestive tract is detoured through the liver instead of being returned to the inferior vena cava.

___ **15.** Umbilical veins carry oxygenated blood.

Answer Sheet—Chapter 14

Exercise 14.1

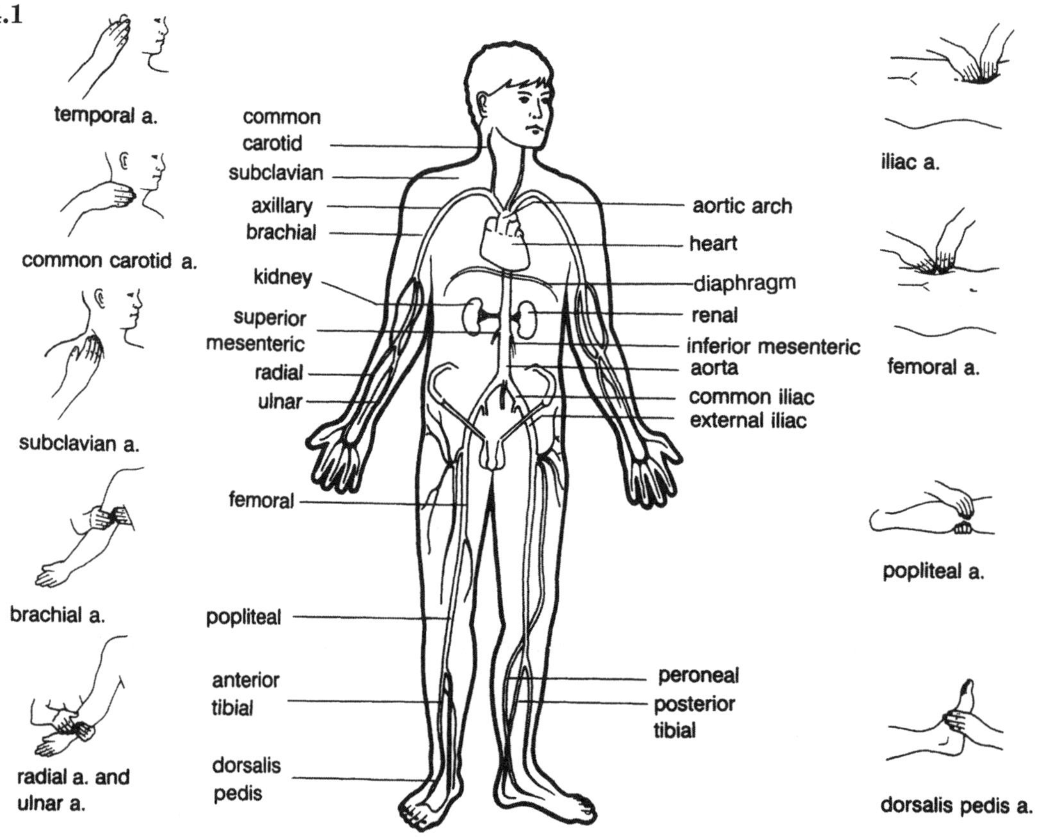

Figure 14.1 Major arteries and pressure points of the body.

Exercise 14.2

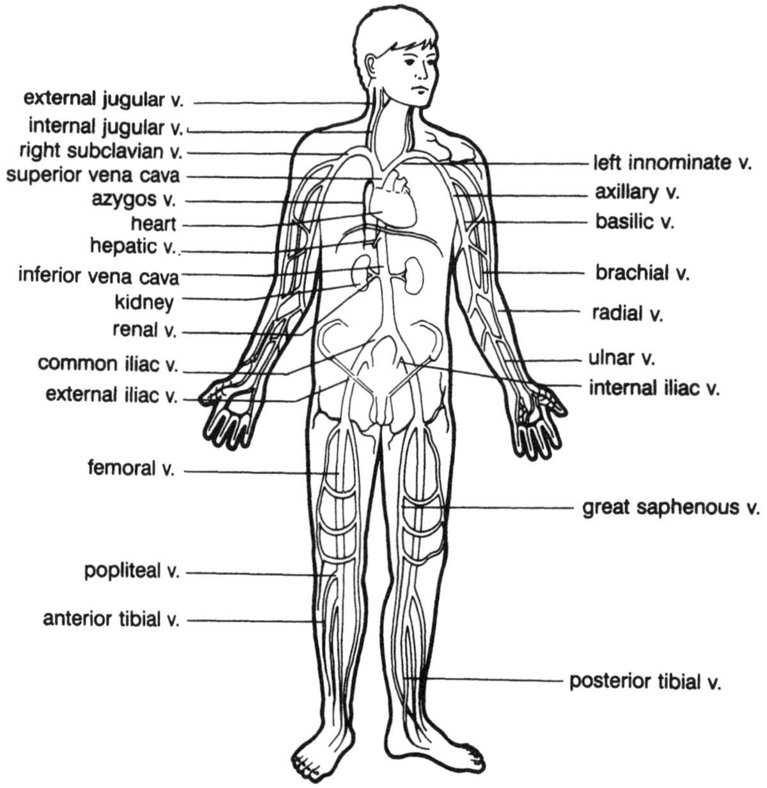

Figure 14.2 Major veins of the body.

Exercise 14.3

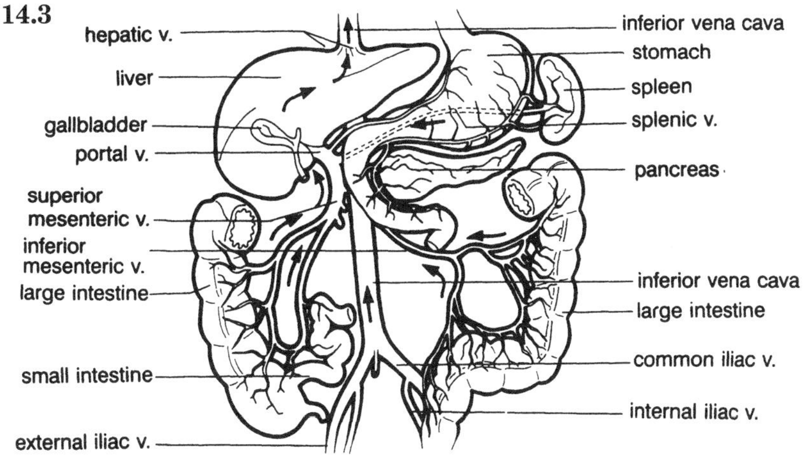

Figure 14.3 The hepatic portal system. Arrows indicate the direction of flow in all abdominal organs, through the liver, to the superior vena cava.

Exercise 14.4

PULMONARY CIRCULATION

The pulmonary circulation carries blood from the heart to the lungs and back to the heart. The blood leaves the heart by way of the large pulmonary artery and returns through the pulmonary veins.

Originating in the right ventricle, the pulmonary artery passes upward and backward for a short distance and then divides into right and left branches that enter the lungs. Within each lung the artery branches widely, and each branch closely follows the subdivisions of the bronchi. The terminal arterioles open into the capillary networks that surround the alveolar sacs.

The pulmonary veins entering the left atrium have two branches from each lung. Their smallest tributaries arise as venules from the capillary networks of the alveolar air sacs.

Of paramount importance here is the condition of the blood in these vessels. As we have seen, blood vessels are named according to the direction of flow to or from the heart—not in terms of what they carry. Generally, a vessel leaving the heart is called an artery and carries oxygenated blood (red); a vessel returning to the heart is called a vein and carries carbon dioxide-laden blood (blue). However, in the pulmonary circulation only, the pulmonary artery carries carbon dioxide-laden blood away from the heart (to the lungs), and the pulmonary veins carry oxygenated blood to the heart (from the lungs).

Test Items

A. 1. d, 2. c, 3. d, 4. a, 5. d, 6. a, 7. b, 8. b, 9. d, 10. c, 11. c, 12. a, 13. d, 14. a, 15. b, 16. c, 17. c, 18. d, 19. a, 20. c.

B. 1. a, 2. j, 3. d, 4. b, 5. e, 6. i, 7. f, 8. c, 9. g, 10. h.
1. e, 2. f, 3. h, 4. i, 5. c, 6. b, 7. a, 8. d, 9. g, 10. j.

C. 1. F, 2. F, 3. T, 4. T, 5. F, 6. F, 7. T, 8. T, 9. F, 10. T, 11. T, 12. T, 13. F, 14. T, 15. T.

15

The Lymphatic System

I. CHAPTER SYNOPSIS

The lymphatic system is composed of lymph, lymph vessels, a series of small masses of lymphoid tissue called lymph nodes, and three organs—tonsils, thymus, and spleen. Other principal areas of study include the role of lymphatic organs in antibody production, the immune response, allergic reactions, the basis for rejection of transplants, immunosuppressive techniques, implantation, and autoimmune diseases.

The lymphatic system is a one-way collecting system that gathers and drains filtered fluid and cellular constituents that accumulate in the spaces between the cells. The larger lymphatic vessels drain into veins, which return the lymph to the blood circulation.

Lymphatic capillaries resemble blood capillaries in structure. Both consist of a single layer of endothelial tissue. The major difference is that the lymphatic capillary has a closed terminal end; lymph fluid is absorbed from the tissue spaces through the endothelial membrane. Most of the tissues of the body, with notable exception of the central nervous system, are drained by lymphatic capillaries.

Larger lymphatic vessels drain the capillary network. The walls of these vessels resemble the walls of veins in structure. The muscle fibres in both the middle and outer layers are longitudinal and oblique, and therefore these larger vessels are contractile; lymphatic capillaries are not.

Lymphatic tissue filters and removes bacteria. Along the course of the lymphatic vessels are small bodies of lymphatic tissue called lymph nodes.

The immune system consists of a variety of chemical and cellular defenses and is heavily reliant on the leukocyte (white blood cell) populations. The sole function of this specialised defensive system is to protect the body against an incredible array of pathogens in general, these enemies fall into three categories: (1) microorganisms (bacteria, viruses, and fungi) that have gained entry into the body, (2) foreign tissue cells that have been transplanted into the body, and (3) the body's own cells that have become cancerous.

The specific immune responses that target a single pathogen are mediated by lymphocytes that mature in the thymus gland (T cells) or in lymphoid tissue elsewhere in the body (B cells). Sensitised T cells are capable of combining with foreign antigens, producing cell-mediated immunity, which defends against some viruses, some bacteria, cancer cells, and tissue transplants. B cells are triggered by contact with foreign antigens to produce large numbers of plasma cells. These cells manufacture antibodies (immunogobulins) that circulate in the blood, producing humoral immunity.

Lymphocytes are the defense specialists that protect the body from pathogenic microorganisms, foreign tissue cells, and disease or infected cells in the body that pose a threat to the normal cell population.

II. OBJECTIVES

After reading the chapter, the student should be able to:

- Describe and identify the anatomical arrangement of a capillary bed.
- Compare the structure of a vein and lymph vessel.
- Identify the major vessels of the lymphatic system.
- Locate the major clusters of lymph nodes in the body.
- Explain how a superficial lymph node protects the body from infection.
- Explain how swollen tender lymph nodes can be of use in identifying locations of infection.
- Explain tissue drainage.
- Describe oedema and explain a number of ways it can occur.
- Distinguish between cell-mediated and humoral immunity.
- Discuss the different types of T cells and the role played by each in the immune response.

III. IMPORTANT TERMS

Using your textbook, define the following terms:

allergen (al′-er jen) ______________________________

____

antibody (an′tee-bo-dee) ______________________________

____

antigen (an′ti-jen) ______________________________

____

capillary (kap′i-lair-ee) ______________________________

____

chyle (kile) ______________________________

____

cisterna (sis-tur′nuh) ______________________________

____

duct (dukt) ______________________________

____

elephantiasis (el-e-fan-ty′uh-sis) ______________________________

____

endothelial (en-do-theel′ee-ul) ______________________________

____

extracellular (eck-struh-sel′yoo-lur) ______________________________

____

Hodgkin's (hoj′-kins) ______________________________

____

immunity (i-myoo′ne-tee) ______________________________

____

intercellular (in-tur-sel′yoo-lur) ______________________________

____

intercostal (in-tur-kos′tul) ______________________________

____

interferon (in-ter-fer′on) ______________________________

____

lacteal (lak′tee-ul) ______________________________

____

lymph (limf) ________________________________

____

lymphoma (lim-fom′a) ________________________________

____

macrophage (mak′ro-faj) ________________________________

____

mastectomy (mas-tek′tuh-mee) ________________________________

____

node (node) ________________________________

____

oedema (Oh-de'ma) ________________________________

____

splenomegaly (spleen-o-meg′uh-lee) ________________________________

____

thoracic (tho-ras′ik) ________________________________

____

IV. EXERCISES

Complete the following exercises in the order given. A precise set of terms and diagrams has been chosen to describe the lymphatic system.

Exercise 15.1

Labelling. Write the name of the structure in the space provided. Colour the vessels different from the surrounding tissue.

Key:

arterial	endothelial	venous
blind	intercellular	
capillary	tissue	

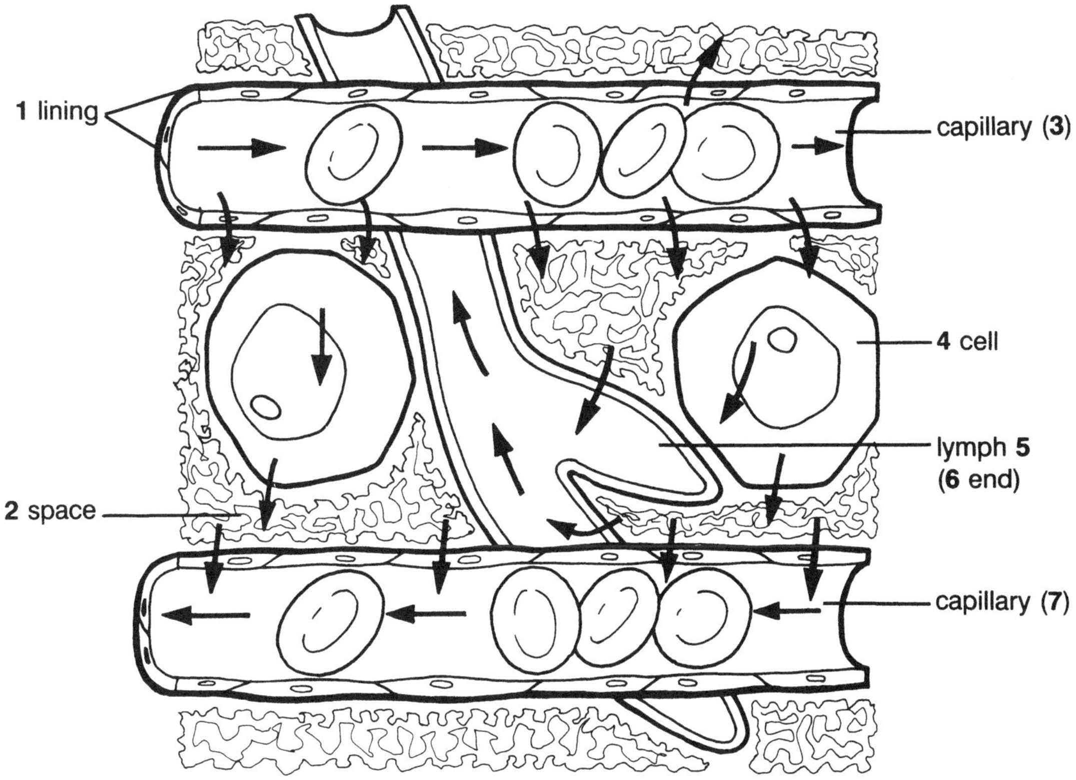

Figure 15.1 Capillary bed, showing how materials diffuse between arterial capillaries and venous capillaries. Materials that are trapped in the intercellular tissue spaces are collected by lymphatic capillaries and returned to the blood system.

1. ______________________
2. ______________________
3. ______________________
4. ______________________
5. ______________________
6. ______________________
7. ______________________

Exercise 15.2

Labelling. Write the name of the structure on the space provided. Colour the organs and vessels differently.

Key:
axillary
capillaries
cisterna
cubital
duct
heart
inguinal
lymph
palmar
parotid
plantar
popliteal
thoracic

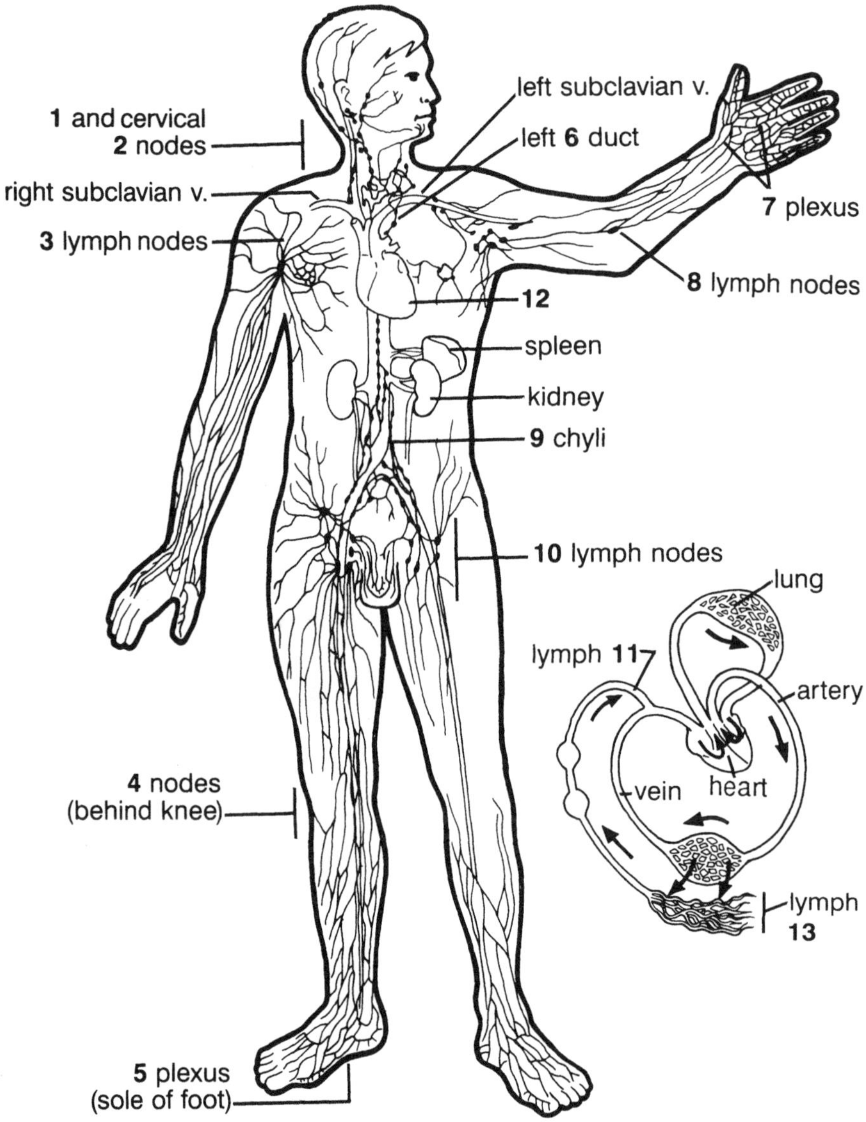

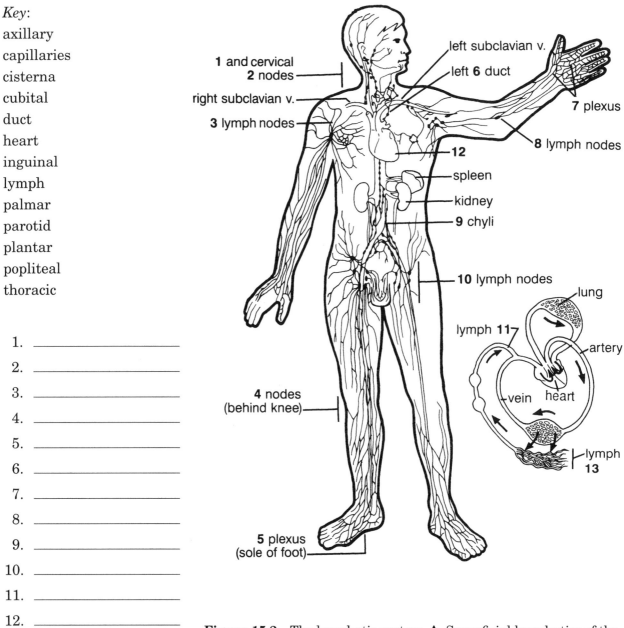

1. ______________________
2. ______________________
3. ______________________
4. ______________________
5. ______________________
6. ______________________
7. ______________________
8. ______________________
9. ______________________
10. ______________________
11. ______________________
12. ______________________
13. ______________________

Figure 15.2 The lymphatic system. **A.** Superficial lymphatics of the body. Locations of the major lymph nodes and organs are also shown. Shaded area indicates the segment of the upper right quadrant of the body that drains into the right lymphatic duct. The remaining area of the body is drained by the left lymphatic (thoracic) duct. **B.** Diagrammatic representation of the lymphatic system, showing its connection with the general circulatory system.

Exercise 15.3

Labelling. Write the name of the structure in the space provided. Colour the organs and vessels differently as in Figure 15.2.

Key:
brachiocephalic
cisterna
heart
intercostals
intestine
jugular
kidney
liver
nodes
pulmonary
spleen
subclavian
thoracic
vena cava
vessels

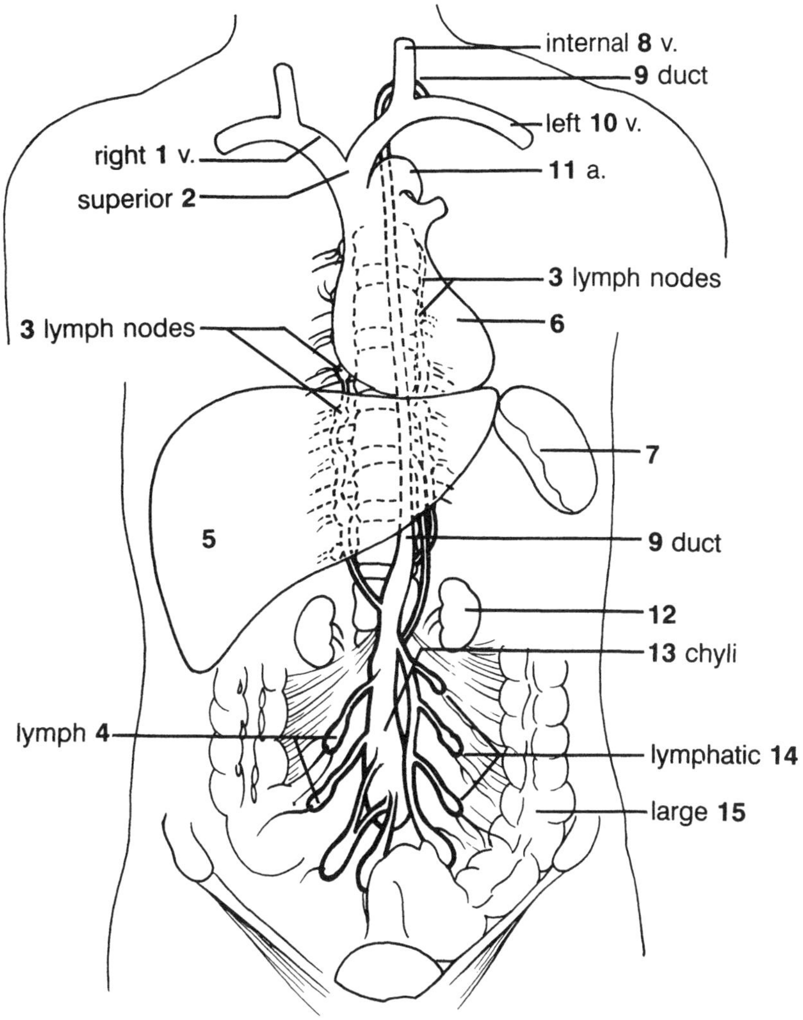

Figure 15.3 Lymphatic drainage to the cisterna chyli and thoracic duct.

1. ______________________
2. ______________________
3. ______________________
4. ______________________
5. ______________________
6. ______________________
7. ______________________
8. ______________________
9. ______________________
10. ______________________
11. ______________________
12. ______________________
13. ______________________
14. ______________________
15. ______________________

Exercise 15.4

Fill in the Blanks. Fill in the blanks in the text on the right with the appropriate terms from the key list.

Key:
antigen
blood
cellular immunity
humoral immunity
lymph
lymphocyte
lymph nodes
macrophages

CELLS OF THE IMMUNE SYSTEM

Immunity is resistance to disease resulting from the presence of foreign substances or ____________ in the body. When this resistance is provided by antibodies released to body fluids, the immunity is called ____________. When living cells provide the protection, the immunity is referred to as ____________. The major cell types on the specific immune responses are two ____________________ populations. Phagocytic cells that act as accessory cells in the immune response are the ____________. Because pathogens are likely to use both ____________ and ____________ as a means of getting around the body, ____________ and other lymphatic tissues (which house the immune cells) are in an excellent position to detect their presence.

V. TEST ITEMS

A. *Multiple Choice.* There is only one answer that is either correct or most appropriate. Circle the best answer for each question.

1. Lymph flow is aided by all the following factors except
  a. breathing
  b. muscular contraction
  c. protein osmotic pressure
  d. valves in lymph vessels

2. Lymph
  a. does not always reach the bloodstream
  b. contains large amounts of protein
  c. carries a lower waste content than the blood
  d. flows against gravity in the lymphatics

3. The lymphatic system returns interstitial fluid to the
  a. liver
  b. blood
  c. cerebrospinal fluid (CSF)
  d. intestinal lumen

4. Which one of the following would not be considered part of the lymphatic system?
  a. thymus
  b. lymph node
  c. tonsil
  d. heart

5. The thoracic duct receives lymph from a dilated vessel called the
  a. cisterna chyli
  b. lacteal
  c. lymph capillary
  d. right lymphatic duct

6. The thoracic duct delivers lymph into the
  a. large lymphatics
  b. lymph capillaries
  c. right lymphatic duct
  d. left subclavian vein

7. A large organ structurally similar to a lymph node but designed to filter blood is the
a. thymus
b. spleen
c. Peyer's patch
d. pharyngeal tonsil

8. Lymphatics and veins are similar in that both
a. contain valves
b. carry oxygenated blood
c. carry deoxygenated blood
d. carry blood away from the heart

9. Lymph
a. flows at approximately the same rate as blood in the veins
b. has the same composition as blood plasma
c. is tissue fluid that enters the lymph capillaries
d. normally contains large numbers of red blood cells

10. Lymph nodes
a. have only one afferent vessel
b. filter lymph
c. produce large numbers of lymphocytes
d. in the extremities are located primarily in the hands and feet

11. The spleen
a. is the primary reservoir for lymph
b. produces large numbers of granulocytes during adulthood
c. destroys worn out red blood cells
d. is necessary for life

12. The lymphatic system and the venous system have which of the following properties in common?
a. They move fluid toward the heart
b. The flow of fluid in the vessels is aided by skeletal muscle contractions
c. They contain red blood cells
d. The walls of the vessels are impermeable to proteins

13. Why should lymph in the thoracic duct have a much higher lymphocyte count than lymph in peripheral lymph spaces?
a. The lymphocytes have just circulated through the tissues and are carrying waste material
b. The lymphocytes have multiplied by mitotic division in the lymph stream
c. The lymphocytes have increased in numbers because this lymph has just passed through numerous lymph nodes
d. The lymphocytes have not as yet been filtered out by passage through the lymph nodes

14. Lymphatic tissue is present in organs other than lymph nodes. Which one of the following is *not* a lymphatic organ?
a. lymphoid nodules and tonsils
b. spleen
c. liver
d. thymus

15. The function of the lymphatic capillaries in the villi of the intestine is to absorb what?
a. sugars
b. fats
c. proteins
d. water

16. An abnormal accumulation of fluid in tissue spaces is called
a. diuresis
b. bursitis
c. oedema
d. anaemia

17. What do we call the lymph that is carrying absorbed fat and has a milk-white appearance?
a. lacteal
b. bile
c. chyle
d. synovial fluid

18. The lymph capillary within the villus of the intestine is called a
a. thoracic duct
b. lacteal
c. chyle duct
d. milk duct

19. Which of the following tonsils are found around the opening of the digestive and respiratory systems?
a. palatine
b. pharyngeal
c. lingual
d. all of the above

20. The major lymph vessel in the body is
a. the thoracic duct
b. the right lymphatic duct
c. the intestinal trunk
d. none of the foregoing

B. *Matching.* Each of the words or phrases in Column B refers to a word or phrase in Column A. Insert the letter of the word or phrase from Column B that best describes each word or phrase in Column A. Some words or phrases may be used more than once or not at all.

Column A		*Column B*
1. ___	oedema	**a.** substance produced in response to an antigen
2. ___	adenitis	**b.** skin eruption
3. ___	antigen	**c.** enlargement of a gland
4. ___	immune	**d.** a benign lymph tumour
5. ___	effusion	**e.** disease caused by a filaria worm
6. ___	lymphosarcoma	**f.** escape of fluid from lymphatics
7. ___	adenopathy	**g.** resistance to a disease
8. ___	antibody	**h.** swelling of tissues
9. ___	hives	**i.** inflammation of adenoids
10. ___	elephantiasis	**j.** a malignant lymphatic tumour
		k. interacts with antibodies

Column A		Column B
1. ___	phagocytic cell	a. stem cell
2. ___	cell-mediated immunity	b. B lymphocyte
3. ___	produces plasma cells	c. lymphangitis
4. ___	excessive tissue fluid	d. infectious mononucleosis
5. ___	produces blood cells	e. macrophage
6. ___	inflamed lymph vessels	f. lymphoma
7. ___	benign or malignant tumour of lymphatic tissue	g. Hodgkin's disease
8. ___	inflammation of lymph nodes	h. T lymphocytes
9. ___	viral infection of lymph nodes	i. lymphosarcoma
10. ___	chronic malignant disorder of lymph nodes	j. oedema

C. *True or False.* Place a *T* or an *F* in the space provided to indicate true or false.

___ **1.** The excessive accumulation of lymph in tissue spaces is referred to as edema.

___ **2.** The combination of antibodies with antigens on a bacterial cell wall kills the bacterium.

___ **3.** The initial interaction of antigens with the body's defense system leading to the formation of antibodies occurs in cells located in the lymph nodes.

___ **4.** The body produces larger quantities of antigens the first time it encounters a foreign antigen than upon subsequent encounters with the same antigen.

___ **5.** The phagocytosis of bacteria by white blood cells is increased when the bacterial surface antigens have combined with antibodies.

___ **6.** The increased blood flow accompanying inflammation ensures an adequate supply of leukocytes, which play a crucial role in the immune response.

___ **7.** Interferon is particularly effective against bacterial invasions.

____ **8.** Specific interferon molecules attack only those foreign substances that fit their protein structure.

____ **9.** The interferon system reacts rapidly, with increased synthesis beginning within hours of the onset of the infection.

____ **10.** Antibodies cannot enter intact human cells, but interferon can.

____ **11.** In general, the B cells and the T cells serve identical functions.

____ **12.** Antigens are identical proteins except for a relatively small number of amino acids occupying the first positions in the chain.

____ **13.** The transfer of actively formed antibodies from one person (or animal) to another confers a resistance known as active immunity.

____ **14.** Persons with type AB blood have neither anti-A nor anti-B antibodies.

____ **15.** Lymphatic vessels have valves.

____ **16.** The main thoracic duct empties into the left brachiocephalic vein.

____ **17.** Lymphatic tissue is present only in lymph nodes and nodules, which are present only in certain special regions of the body, such as the axillary region.

____ **18.** Mast cells and basophils are the main sources of histamine—a vasodilatory substance.

____ **19.** Any organic molecule, usually large, that has been recognised as foreign by the body's defense system, can function as an antigen.

____ **20.** Lymph is returned to the heart by a system of vessels structured like arteries.

Answer Sheet—Chapter 15

Exercise 15.1

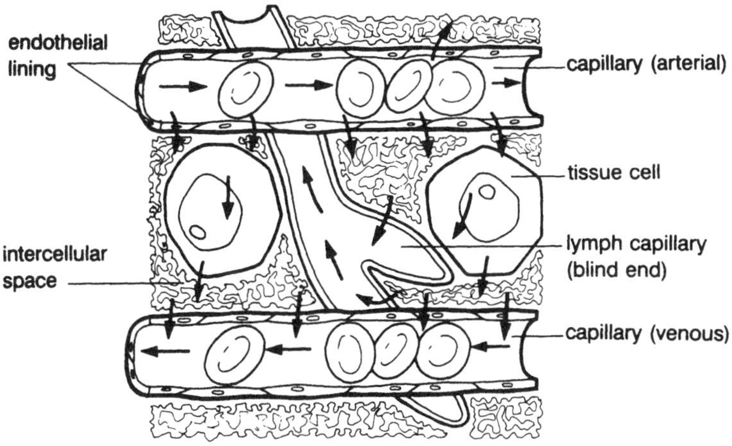

Figure 15.1 A capillary bed, showing how materials diffuse between arterial capillaries and venous capillaries. Materials that are trapped in the intercellular tissue spaces are collected by lymphatic capillaries and returned to the blood system.

Exercise 15.2

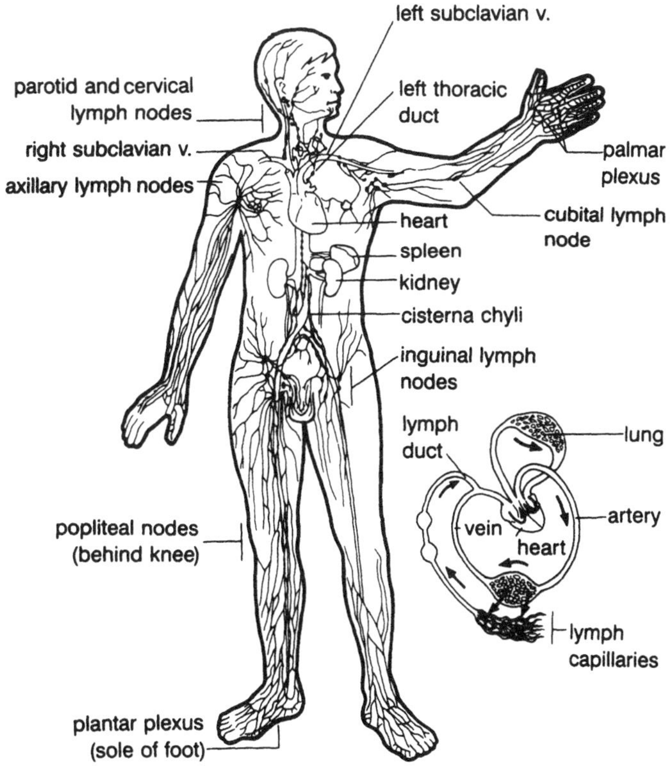

Figure 15.2 The lymphatic system. **A.** Superficial lymphatics of the body. Locations of the major lymph nodes and organs are also shown. Shaded area indicates the segment of the upper right quadrant of the body that drains into the right lymphatic duct. The remaining area of the body is drained by the left lymphatic (thoracic) duct. **B.** Diagrammatic representation of the lymphatic system, showing its connection with the general circulatory system.

Exercise 15.3

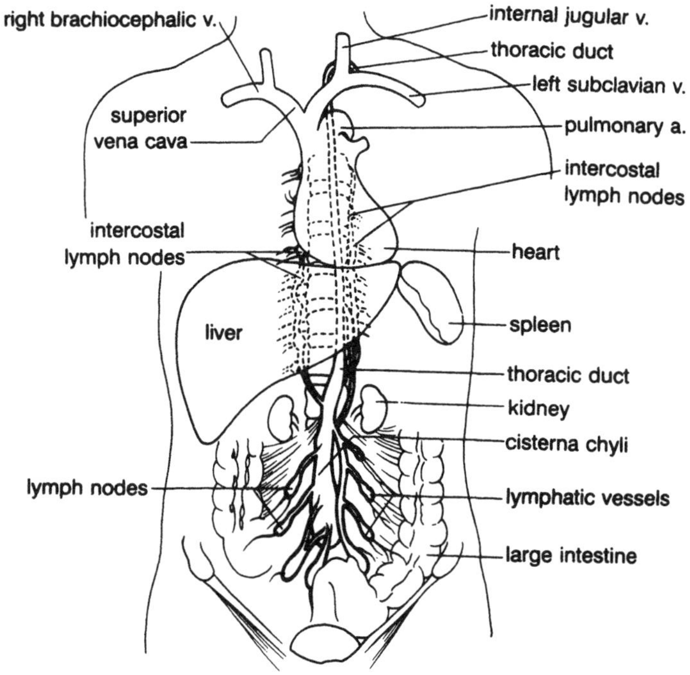

Figure 15.3 Lymphatic drainage to the cisterna chyli and thoracic duct.

Exercise 15.4

CELLS OF THE IMMUNE SYSTEM

Immunity is resistance to disease resulting from the presence of foreign substances or <u>antigens</u> in the body. When this resistance is provided by antibodies released to body fluids, the immunity is called <u>humoral immunity</u>. When living cells provide the protection, the immunity is referred to as <u>cellular immunity</u>. The major cell types on the specific immune responses are two <u>lymphocyte</u> populations. Phagocytic cells that act as accessory cells in the immune response are the <u>macrophages</u>. Because pathogens are likely to use both <u>blood</u> and <u>lymph</u> as a means of getting around the body, <u>lymph nodes</u> and other lymphatic tissues (which house the immune cells) are in an excellent position to detect their presence.

Test Items

A. 1. c, 2. d, 3. b, 4. d, 5. a, 6. d, 7. b, 8. a, 9. c, 10. c, 11. c, 12. a, 13. c, 14. c, 15. b, 16. c, 17. c, 18. b, 19. d, 20. a.

B. 1. h, 2. i, 3. k, 4. g, 5. f, 6. j, 7. c, 8. a, 9. b, 10. e.
1. e, 2. h, 3. b, 4. j, 5. a, 6. c, 7. f, 8. g, 9. d, 10. i.

C. 1. T, 2. F, 3. T, 4. F, 5. T, 6. T, 7. F, 8. F, 9. T, 10. F, 11. F, 12. F, 13. F, 14. T, 15. T, 16. T, 17. F, 18. T, 19. T, 20. F.

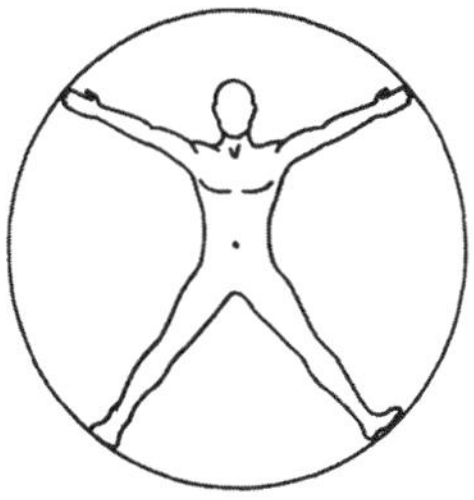

16

The Respiratory System

I. CHAPTER SYNOPSIS

The utilisation of oxygen by the mitochondria during the process of oxidative phosphorylation provides the major mechanism for the synthesis of adenosine triphosphate (ATP) by the cells of the body. The mitochondria are also the site of carbon dioxide production, the major metabolic waste product. The lungs and circulatory system provide the mechanisms for delivering oxygen to the cells and removing the carbon dioxide. During the course of evolution, specialised proteins (haemoglobin) evolved, which increase the oxygen-carrying capacity of the blood. The conversion of carbon dioxide to carbonic acid in the red blood cells and its dissociation into bicarbonate and hydrogen ions provide a mechanism for regulating the acidity of body fluids by controlling the volume of expired carbon dioxide. The levels of carbon dioxide and oxygen in the blood are powerful regulatory agents for controlling the activity of both the respiratory and cardiovascular systems. Thus, this chapter examines the organisation of the respiratory system, the steps involved in respiration, ventilation, and exchange and transport of gases in the body.

II. OBJECTIVES

After reading the chapter, the student should be able to:

- Label the structures of the respiratory system.
- Identify two functions of the cilia and mucous cells.

- Define respiration, ventilation, inspiration, and expiration.
- Describe the Hering-Breuer control of breathing.
- Explain the oxygen-associated chemoreceptor mechanism for the control of ventilation.
- Explain the process of gaseous exchange in the alveoli and in the tissue.

III. IMPORTANT TERMS

Using your textbook, define the following terms:

alveolar (al-vee′uh-lur) ____________________

____

aspiration (as-pi-ray′shun) ____________________

____

atrium (ay′tree-um) ____________________

____

bronchiole (bronk′ee-ole) ____________________

____

bronchus (bron′k-us) ____________________

____

concha (kong′kuh) ____________________

____

cortex (kor′teks) ____________________

____

dyspnea (disp-nee′uh) ____________________

____

emphysema (em′fi-see-muh) ____________________

____

epiglottis (epi-glot′is) ____________________

____

expiration (ek-spi-ray′shun) ____________________

____

glottis (glot′is) ____________________

____

hyaline (hy′uh-lin) ______________________________

____

inspiration (in-spi-ray′shun) ______________________________

____

intrapulmonary (in-truh-pool′muh-nerr-ee) ______________________________

____

intrathoracic (in-truh-tho-ras′ik) ______________________________

____

larynx (lar′inks) ______________________________

____

lingual (ling′gwul) ______________________________

____

nasopharynx (nay-zo-far′inks) ______________________________

____

oropharynx (or-o-far′inks) ______________________________

____

phrenic (fren′ik) ______________________________

____

pneumotaxic (new-mo-taks′ik) ______________________________

____

respiration (res-pi-ray′shun) ______________________________

____

tonsil (ton′sil) ______________________________

____

vagus (vay′gus) ______________________________

____

ventilation (ven-ti-lay′shun) ______________________________

____

IV. EXERCISES

Complete the following exercises in the order given. A precise set of terms and diagrams has been chosen to describe the respiratory system.

Exercise 16.1

Labelling. Write the name of the structure on the space provided. Colour the nasal and oral passages differently.

Key:
concha
epiglottis
glottis
larynx
lingual
mandible
nasopharynx
oesophagus
oral
oropharynx
thyroid
tongue
tonsil
trachea

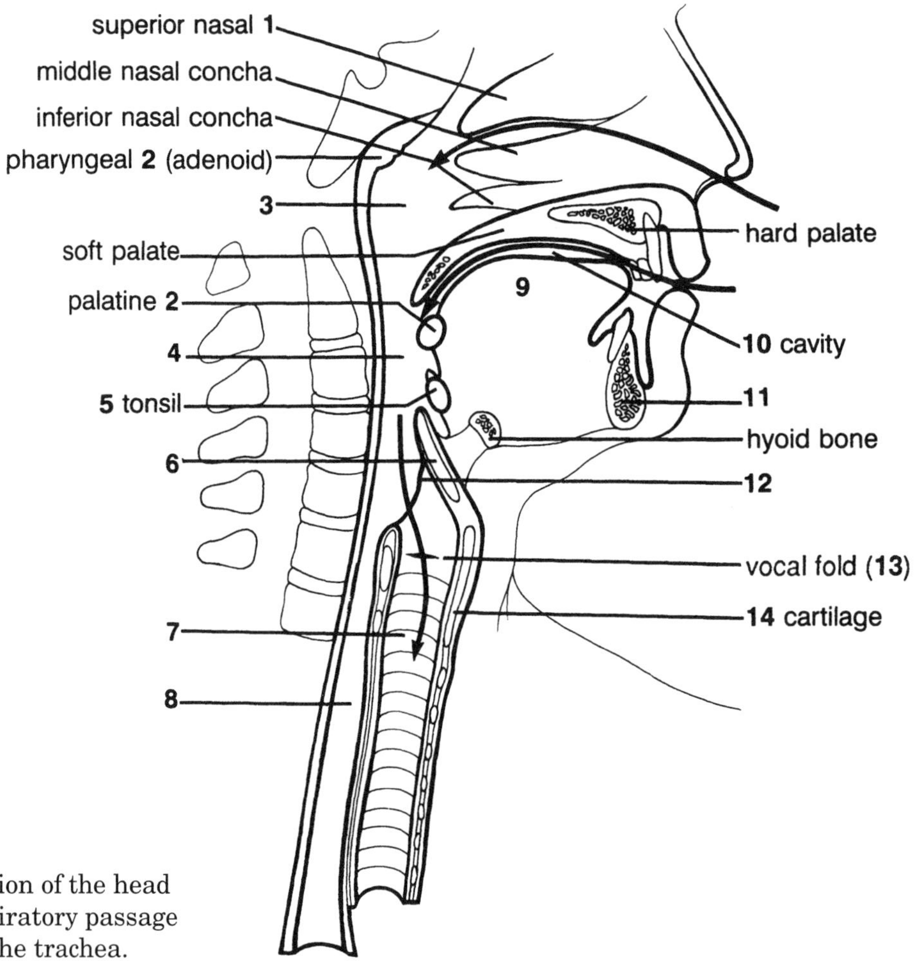

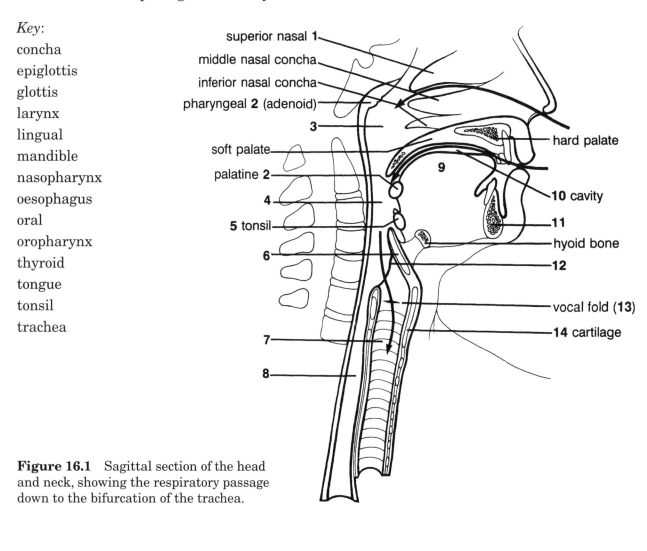

Figure 16.1 Sagittal section of the head and neck, showing the respiratory passage down to the bifurcation of the trachea.

1. ______________________
2. ______________________
3. ______________________
4. ______________________
5. ______________________
6. ______________________
7. ______________________
8. ______________________
9. ______________________
10. ______________________
11. ______________________
12. ______________________
13. ______________________
14. ______________________

Exercise 16.2

Labelling. Write the name of the structure on the space provided. Colour the respiratory tract different from the lung mass.

Key:
alveolar
alveoli
atrium
bronchiole
bronchioles
bronchus
capillary
duct
glottis
respiratory
sacs
trachea

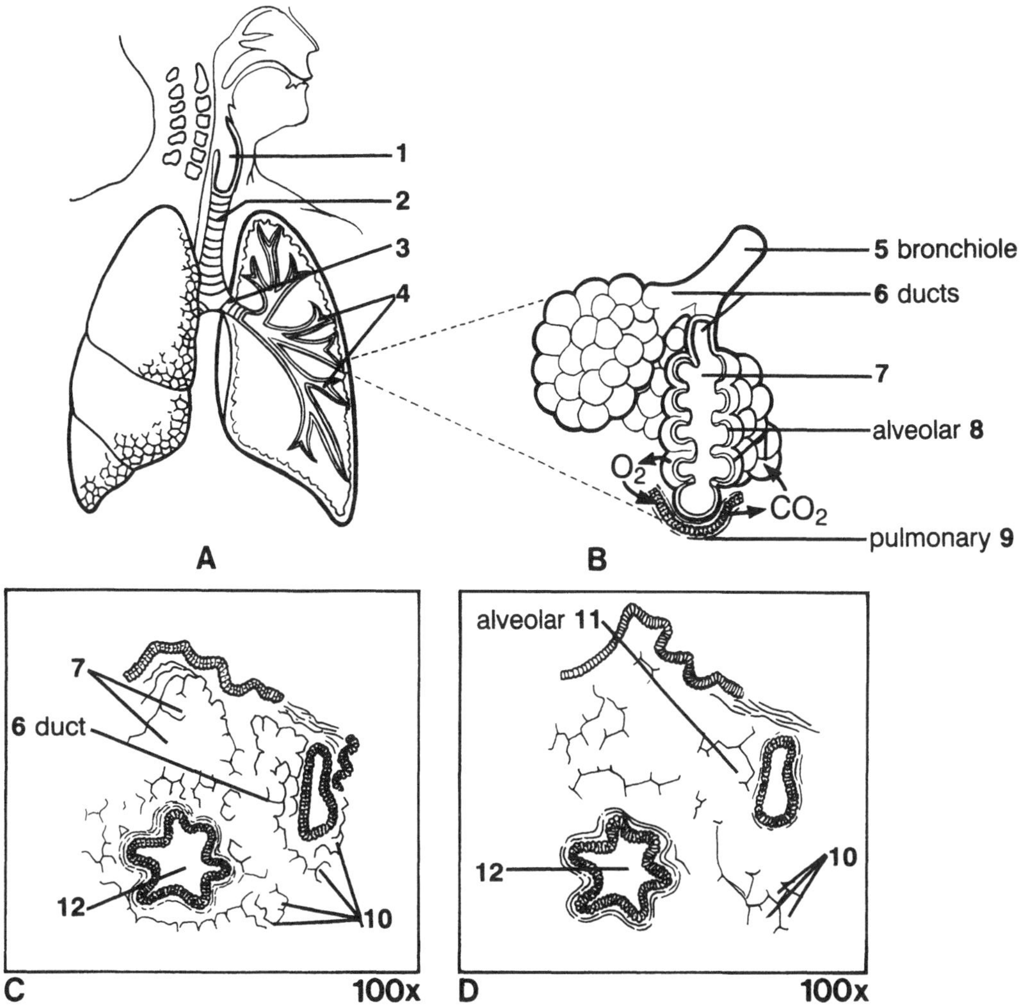

Figure 16.2 Internal structure of the lungs. **A.** Relationship of the lungs to the head and neck. **B.** External and internal appearance of a lung lobule, showing the atrium and alveolar space. **C.** Section of a lung, magnified 100 times. **D.** Section of a similar lung with emphysema. Note the decreased number of alveolar spaces and consequent diminishing of the surface area available for gaseous exchange.

1. ______________________
2. ______________________
3. ______________________
4. ______________________
5. ______________________
6. ______________________
7. ______________________
8. ______________________
9. ______________________
10. ______________________
11. ______________________
12. ______________________

Exercise 16.3

Labelling. Write the name of the structure on the space provided. Colour the various organs and tissues differently.

Key:
aortic
carotid
cerebrum
cortex
CO_2
diaphragm
expiratory
glossopharyngeal
inspiratory
intercostal
medulla
phrenic
pneumotaxic
stretch
vagus
voluntary

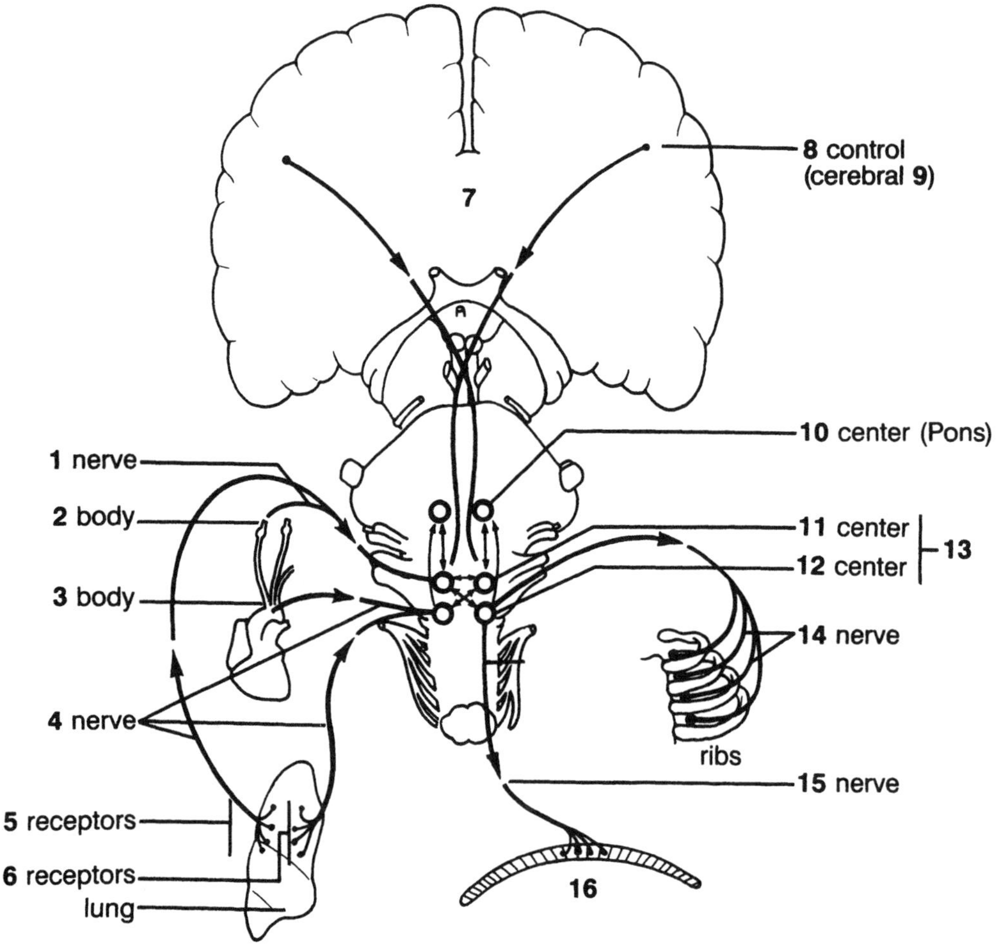

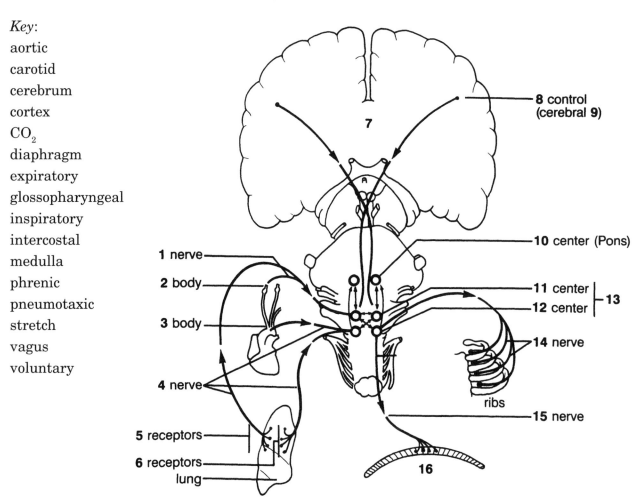

Figure 16.3 Chemical and nervous control of respiration. Arrows indicate direction of nerve impulses.

1. ______________________
2. ______________________
3. ______________________
4. ______________________
5. ______________________
6. ______________________
7. ______________________
8. ______________________
9. ______________________
10. ______________________
11. ______________________
12. ______________________
13. ______________________
14. ______________________
15. ______________________
16. ______________________

Exercise 16.4

Fill in the Blanks. Write the correct term from the key list in the space provided in the text on the right.

Key:
alveoli
aorta
arterial
arteries
blood
carbon dioxide
carbon dioxide
cellular
lungs
oxygen
oxygen
returned
returns
tissues
veins
vena cava
venous

GASEOUS EXCHANGE

____________ gas exchange takes place in all body ____________; cells take up ____________ from the ____________ and add ____________ to it. When this occurs, blood becomes ____________. As we have seen, this carbon dioxide-rich blood then ____________ to the heart, entering through the ____________. From the heart, venous blood is pumped through the short, paired pulmonary ____________ to the ____________, where these arteries branch into extensive capillary networks spread over the ____________. Pulmonary gas exchange takes place here; ____________ leaves the blood and ____________ enters. Thus blood becomes ____________. This oxygen-rich blood is ____________ to the heart by the pulmonary ____________, and this blood in turn is redistributed throughout the body by the ____________.

Key:
air
capillary
cell
determined
direction
greater
into
pressure
saturated
venous
vessel

The ____________ in which the gases move is ____________ by the prevailing ____________ gradients, or tension gradients, between blood ____________ and organ ____________. Specifically, atmospheric ____________ in the alveoli contains only a little carbon dioxide, but the ____________ blood that flows into the lungs from the body is virtually ____________ with the gas. The pressure gradient of carbon dioxide is ____________ in the ____________; therefore, carbon dioxide diffuses ____________ the alveolus.

Key:
blood
capillary
from
high
into
into
low
low
oxygen
oxygen
oxygen
pressure
respiratory
reverse
tension
tissue
waste

Predictably, the pressure pattern is the ________________ for oxygen. Blood flowing into the body is ________________ poor. The air in the alveoli contains a maximal content of oxygen; therefore oxygen diffuses ________________ the ________________ from the alveolus to satisfy the increased alveolar ________________ gradient.

Just as in the lungs, cellular gas exchange in the other body tissues is governed by ________________ gradients. Cells continuously use up ________________ in internal respiration, and the tension of this gas in cells is therefore ________________. The arterial tension is high, however, and the ________________ diffuses ________________ the blood ________________ the tissue cells. At the same time, since ________________ carbon dioxide is produced as a ________________ product of cellular metabolism, the carbon dioxide tension within the tissue cells is ________________. Arterial blood has a ________________ carbon dioxide tension, and the gas therefore diffuses from the ________________ cells into the ________________.

V. TEST ITEMS

A. *Multiple Choice.* There is only one answer that is either correct or most appropriate. Circle the best answer for each question.

1. Which of the following is considered to be the functional unit of the lungs?
a. bronchus
b. alveolus
c. trachea
d. bronchioles

2. The term used to describe a lack of oxygen in a person is
a. hyperoxia
b. hypercapnia
c. hypoxia
d. hyperventilation

3. Emphysema is a chronic obstructive pulmonary disease (COPD) that is related to
a. a high blood count
b. anaemia
c. air pollution
d. polycythemia

4. The walls of the alveoli are composed of
a. columnar epithelium
b. stratified squamous epithelium
c. simple squamous epithelium
d. loose connective tissue

5. Oxygen and carbon dioxide are exchanged in the lungs by
a. anoxia
b. filtration
c. active transport
d. simple diffusion

6. Damage to which of the following would stop breathing?
a. pneumotaxic centre
b. stretch receptors
c. the medulla
d. the cerebrum

7. The space between the pleura of the lungs that extends from the breastbone to the backbone is the
a. cranium
b. mediastinum
c. hypogastric region
d. epigastric region

8. A rise in the carbonic acid content of the blood has what effect on respiration?
a. The respiratory rate increases and the breathing becomes stronger and deeper
b. The respiratory rate decreases and the breathing becomes shallow and weaker
c. The chemoreceptors become depressed
d. The pressoreceptors become depressed

9. Which of the following is true of the foetal lungs prior to birth?
a. They are completely filled with mucus
b. They totally fill the thoracic cavity
c. Amniotic fluid is breathed in and out of the lungs
d. Intrapleural pressure is greater than atmospheric pressure

10. Which portion of the pharynx serves solely as a respiratory passageway?
a. nasopharynx
b. oral pharynx
c. laryngeal pharynx
d. oesophagus

11. Too rapid decompression after exposure to high atmospheric pressure may cause gas bubbles to form in the blood and tissues, a dangerous condition called the bends. What is the gas that causes the bends?
a. carbon dioxide
b. oxygen
c. ammonia
d. nitrogen

12. Why is the inhalation of carbon monoxide so dangerous?
a. It causes an increase in the respiratory rate
b. It causes a rise in blood pressure
c. Because haemoglobin has a much greater affinity for carbon monoxide (CO) than it does for oxygen
d. It causes a breakdown of the surface active agent in the alveoli

13. Upon opening the chest, which structure would you see first?
a. parietal pleura
b. secondary bronchi
c. visceral pleura
d. pleural cavity

14. The heart lies in what cavity between the lungs, with the diaphragm forming the floor?
a. abdominal cavity
b. pleural cavity
c. pericardial cavity
d. peritoneal cavity

15. Where are the inspiratory and expiratory centres located?
a. lungs
b. intercostal muscles
c. cerebellum
d. medulla

16. It is in what structures that the oxygen of the air and carbon dioxide of the blood can be exchanged?
a. lacteals of the villi
b. pleura
c. bronchioles
d. alveoli

17. Name the cartilaginous structure that contains the vocal folds.
a. pharynx
b. larynx
c. epiglottis
d. bronchus

18. The greatest amount of carbon dioxide in the blood is carried by
a. bicarbonate ions, HCO_3
b. haemoglobin
c. blood plasma
d. carbonic anhydrase

19. The reaction of carbon dioxide with water is a relatively slow process, yet this reaction occurs within the red cells in a fraction of a second. What is responsible for speeding up this reaction?
a. cytochrome oxidase
b. ATP
c. phosphorylase
d. carbonic anhydrase

20. If a person inhales the maximum amount of air and then exhales as much as possible, the total exchange represents his
a. tidal air flow
b. residual air volume
c. inspiratory reserve
d. vital capacity

B. *Matching.* Each of the phrases in Column B refers to a term in Column A. Insert the letter of the word or phrase from Column B that best describes each term in Column A. Some words may be used more than once or not at all.

Column A		Column B	
1. ___	alveoli	**a.**	an air space under a concha
2. ___	ethmoid	**b.**	a bone of the nasal cavity
3. ___	adenoids	**c.**	a large cavity within a maxillary bone
4. ___	mediastinum	**d.**	a common passage for air and food
5. ___	pharynx	**e.**	the sites of gas exchange within the lungs
6. ___	tonsils	**f.**	the slight dilation of each nasal cavity just inside the nostril
7. ___	hilum	**g.**	hypertrophied pharyngeal tonsils
8. ___	pseudostratified epithelium	**h.**	lymphoid tissue
9. ___	meatus	**i.**	produces sounds
10. ___	larynx	**j.**	the largest cartilage in the larynx
11. ___	mucus	**k.**	separates each lung
12. ___	paranasal sinus	**l.**	the main surface depression of the lung
13. ___	diaphragm	**m.**	contains cilia
14. ___	thyroid	**n.**	is constantly moved by cilia to the pharynx
15. ___	vestibule	**o.**	the principal muscle of respiration

Column A		Column B
1. ___ apnea	a.	sounds heard in the lungs that resemble bubbling
2. ___ diphtheria	b.	irregular breathing beginning with shallow breaths that increase in depth and rapidity then decrease and cease altogether
3. ___ hypoxia	c.	a temporary absence of respirations
4. ___ orthopnea	d.	oxygen starvation
5. ___ pneumothorax	e.	bacterial infection that causes the membranes of the pharynx and larynx to become enlarged and leathery
6. ___ bronchitis	f.	presence of clot in a pulmonary arterial vessel that stops circulation to a part of the lungs
7. ___ pulmonary embolism	g.	reduction in oxygen supply to cells
8. ___ rales	h.	normal quiet breathing
9. ___ respirator	i.	viral infection that causes inflammation of respiratory mucous membranes and fever
10. ___ influenza	j.	presence of more than normal air in the pleural cavity
11. ___ dyspnea	k.	a collapsed lung or portion of a lung
12. ___ eupnea	l.	inability to breathe in a horizontal position
13. ___ asphyxia	m.	labored or difficult breathing
14. ___ Cheyne-Stokes respiration	n.	metal chamber that encloses the chest to induce inspiration and expiration
15. ___ atelectasis	o.	inflammation of the bronchi and bronchioles

C. *True or False.* Place a *T* or an *F* in the space provided to indicate true or false.

___ **1.** The palatine tonsils are located on the posterior wall of the nasopharynx.

___ **2.** During inspiration, contraction of the diaphragm and external intercostal muscles increases the size of the thoracic cavity.

___ **3.** Tidal volume is usually about 500 cc.

___ **4.** During expiration, the intrathoracic (intrapleural) pressure becomes positive.

___ **5.** During quiet breathing, expiration is brought about by the contraction of the external intercostal muscles.

___ **6.** Vital capacity may be measured as the maximum amount of air expired after a maximum inspiration.

___ **7.** Most of the CO_2 in the blood is carried by haemoglobin.

___ **8.** Irritation of the vagus nerve will result in deep, slow breathing.

___ **9.** An increase in the concentration of carbon dioxide in the blood increases ventilation by chemical stimulation of the respiratory centre in the medulla.

___ **10.** Enlarged chest, degeneration of alveolar sacs, high levels of carbon dioxide in the blood, and development of fibrous connective tissue are all symptoms of pneumonia.

___ **11.** Gases move between the blood and lungs by the process of filtration.

___ **12.** Inflammation of the membrane around the lung is referred to as bronchitis.

___ **13.** Any sudden increase in arterial blood pressure will decrease the rate of respiration.

___ **14.** The top portion of the nose communicates with the pharynx through the internal nares.

___ **15.** The major portion of carbon dioxide is carried in the blood as the bicarbonate ion.

___ **16.** The pneumotaxic centre is located in the medulla and assumes a role in the control of respirations.

___ **17.** If a person undergoes continued hypoventilation, the pCO_2 will increase.

___ **18.** A spasmodic contraction of the expiratory muscles that forcefully expels air through the nose and mouth is called cough.

___ **19.** The combination of external cardiac communication and exhaled air ventilation constitutes heart-lung resuscitation.

___ **20.** The term *eupnea* refers to cessation of breathing at the end of a normal expiration.

Answer Sheet—Chapter 16

Exercise 16.1

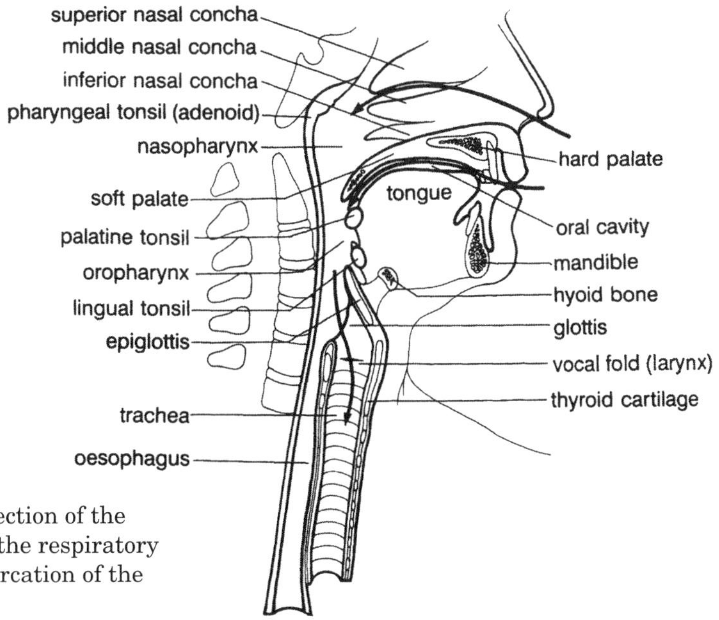

Figure 16.1 Sagittal section of the head and neck, showing the respiratory passage down to the bifurcation of the trachea.

Exercise 16.2

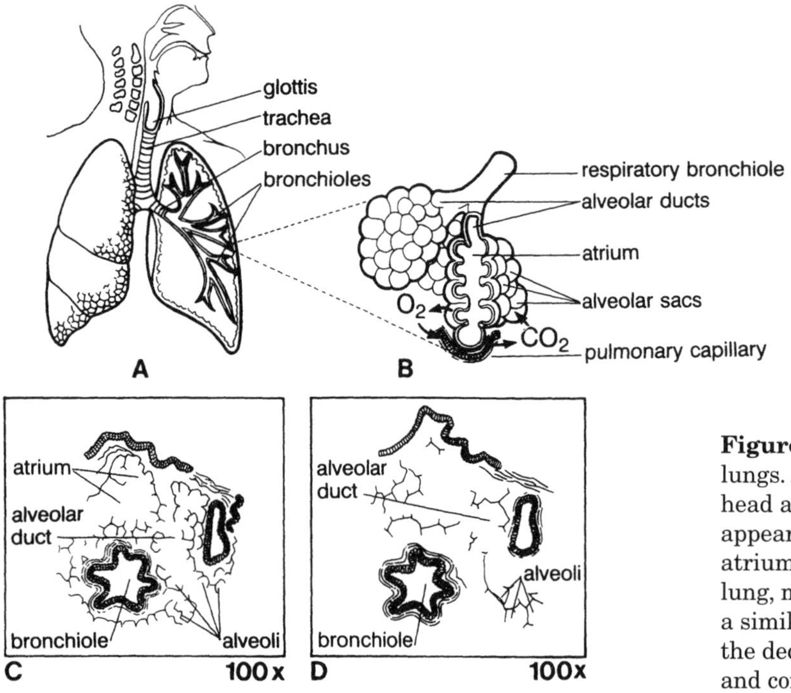

Figure 16.2 Internal structure of the lungs. **A.** Relationship of the lungs to the head and neck. **B.** External and internal appearance of a lung lobule, showing the atrium and alveolar space. **C.** Section of a lung, magnified 100 times. **D.** Section of a similar lung with emphysema. Note the decreased number of alveolar spaces and consequent diminishing of the surface area available for gaseous exchange.

Exercise 16.3

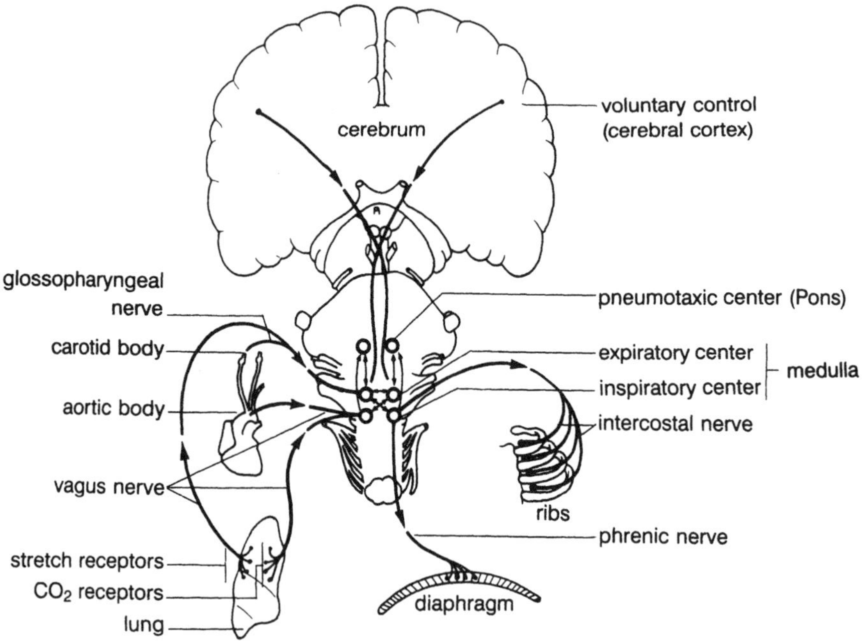

Figure 16.3 Chemical and nervous control of respiration. Arrows indicate direction of nerve impulses.

Exercise 16.4

GASEOUS EXCHANGE

Cellular gas exchange takes place in all body tissues; cells take up oxygen from the blood and add carbon dioxide to it. When this occurs, blood becomes venous. As we have seen, this carbon dioxide-rich blood then returns to the heart, entering through the vena cava. From the heart, venous blood is pumped through the short, pulmonary arteries to the lungs, where these arteries branch into extensive capillary networks spread over the alveoli. Pulmonary gas exchange takes place here; carbon dioxide leaves the blood and oxygen enters. Thus blood becomes arterial. This oxygen-rich blood is returned to the heart by the pulmonary veins, and this blood in turn is redistributed throughout the body by the aorta.

The direction in which the gases move is determined by the prevailing pressure gradients, or tension gradients, between blood vessel and organ cell. Specifically, atmospheric air in the alveoli contains only a little carbon dioxide, but the venous blood that flows into the lungs from the body is virtually saturated with the gas. The pressure gradient of carbon dioxide is greater in the capillary; therefore, carbon dioxide diffuses into the alveolus.

Predictably, the pressure pattern is the reverse for oxygen. Blood flowing into the lungs from the body is oxygen poor. The air in the alveoli contains a maximal content of oxygen; therefore oxygen diffuses into the capillary from the alveolus to satisfy the increased alveolar pressure gradient.

Just as in the lungs, cellular gas exchange in the other body tissues is governed by tension gradients. Cells continuously use up oxygen in internal respiration, and the tension of this gas in cells is therefore low. The arterial tension is high, however, and the oxygen diffuses from the blood into the tissue cells. At the same time, since respiratory carbon dioxide is produced as a waste product of cellular metabolism, the carbon dioxide tension within the tissue cells is high. Arterial blood has a low carbon dioxide tension, and the gas therefore diffuses from the tissue cells into the blood.

Test Items

A. 1. b, 2. c, 3. c, 4. c, 5. d, 6. c, 7. b, 8. a, 9. c, 10. a, 11. d, 12. c, 13. a, 14. c, 15. d, 16. d, 17. b, 18. a, 19. d, 20. d.

B. 1. e, 2. b, 3. g, 4. k, 5. d, 6. h, 7. l, 8. m, 9. a, 10. i, 11. n, 12. c, 13. o, 14. j, 15. f.
1. c, 2. e, 3. g, 4. l, 5. j, 6. o, 7. f, 8. a, 9. n, 10. i, 11. m, 12. h, 13. d, 14. b, 15. k.

C. 1. F, 2. T, 3. T, 4. F, 5. F, 6. T, 7. F, 8. T, 9. T, 10. F, 11. F, 12. F, 13. T, 14. T, 15. T, 16. F, 17. T, 18. F, 19. T, 20. F.

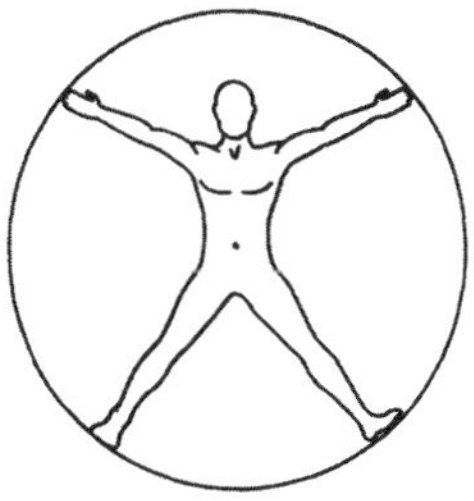

17

The Alimentary Tract

I. CHAPTER SYNOPSIS

Throughout the text the synthesis of molecules, contraction of muscles, transport of molecules or ions across cell membranes, and maintenance of body temperature are discussed. For these activities, the body depends on its ability to extract and use the chemical potential energy locked within the structure of chemical bonds. Without sufficient energy, the cells die. This chapter deals with the concept of energy, the mechanisms of trapping chemical energy in a form that can be used by cells (ATP synthesis), the properties of enzymes, which catalyze the many chemical reactions in cells, and the general metabolic pathways for the breakdown, synthesis, and interconversion of carbohydrates, fats, and proteins. The student is introduced to metabolism and nutrition.

The digestive process is considered by region, in which the anatomy, physiology, physical processes, and chemical processes of each region are discussed together. There is also emphasis on the nervous and hormonal control of digestion.

II. OBJECTIVES

After reading the chapter, the student should be able to:

- Identify the anatomy of the alimentary tract.
- Explain how saliva is produced and its effect on carbohydrates.

- Describe peristalsis and its control mechanism.
- Differentiate between the cardiac and pyloric sphincters in reference to position and function.
- Define peptic ulcer and where it is found.
- Identify the sites and formation of bile.
- Describe the role of bile in digestion.
- Identify the function of hormones in digestion and give examples.
- Explain how the end products of digestion are absorbed by villi.
- Explain how each of the three foodstuffs are metabolised for energy, synthesis, and storage.

III. IMPORTANT TERMS

Using your textbook, define the following terms:

ampulla (am-pul′uh) ______________________________

____

anal (ay′nul) ______________________________

____

appendix (a-pen′diks) ______________________________

____

bile (bile) ______________________________

____

bolus (bo′lus) ______________________________

____

carbohydrate (kahr-bo-high′drate) ______________________________

____

defaecation (def-e-kay′shun) ______________________________

____

diarrhoea (dye-uh-ree′uh) ______________________________

____

diverticulum (dye-vur-tik′yoo-lum) ______________________________

____

enzyme (en′zime) ______________________________

____

fat (fat) ______________________________

jaundice (jawn′dis) ______________________________

parietal (puh-rye′e-tul) ______________________________

protein (pro′teen) ______________________________

pyloric (pye-lo′rik) ______________________________

rugae (roo′guy) ______________________________

sinusoid (sy′nuh-soid) ______________________________

sphincter (sfink′tur) ______________________________

substrate (sub′strayt) ______________________________

ulcer (ul′sur) ______________________________

varices (var′i-seez) ______________________________

vitamin (vy′tuh-min) ______________________________

IV. EXERCISES

Complete the following exercises in the order given. A precise set of terms and diagrams has been chosen to describe the alimentary tract.

Exercise 17.1

Labelling. Write the name of the structure on the space provided. Colour the organs differently.

Key:

anal	mouth
appendix	oesophagus
ascending	parotid
caecum	pharynx
descending	pyloric
diaphragm	rectum
duodenum	sigmoid
gallbladder	spleen
ilium	stomach
jejunum	transverse
liver	valve

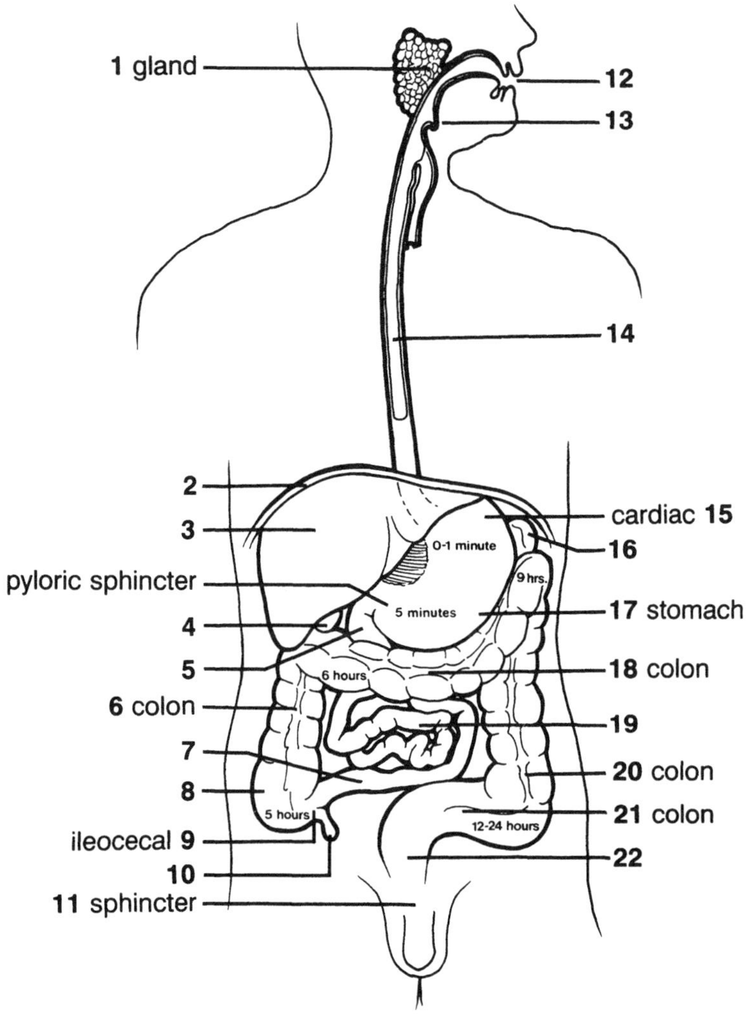

Figure 17.1 Human digestive tract. Times indicated along the tract represent how long it takes food to pass through each area during the process of digestion.

1. ______________ 9. ______________ 17. ______________
2. ______________ 10. ______________ 18. ______________
3. ______________ 11. ______________ 19. ______________
4. ______________ 12. ______________ 20. ______________
5. ______________ 13. ______________ 21. ______________
6. ______________ 14. ______________ 22. ______________
7. ______________ 15. ______________
8. ______________ 16. ______________

Exercise 17.2

Labelling. Write the name of the structure on the space provided. Colour the various layers of the stomach a different colour.

Key:
cardiac
chief
curvature
duodenum
furrow
gastric
mucous
muscle
oesophagus
parietal
pyloric
rugae
smooth
sphincter
submucosa

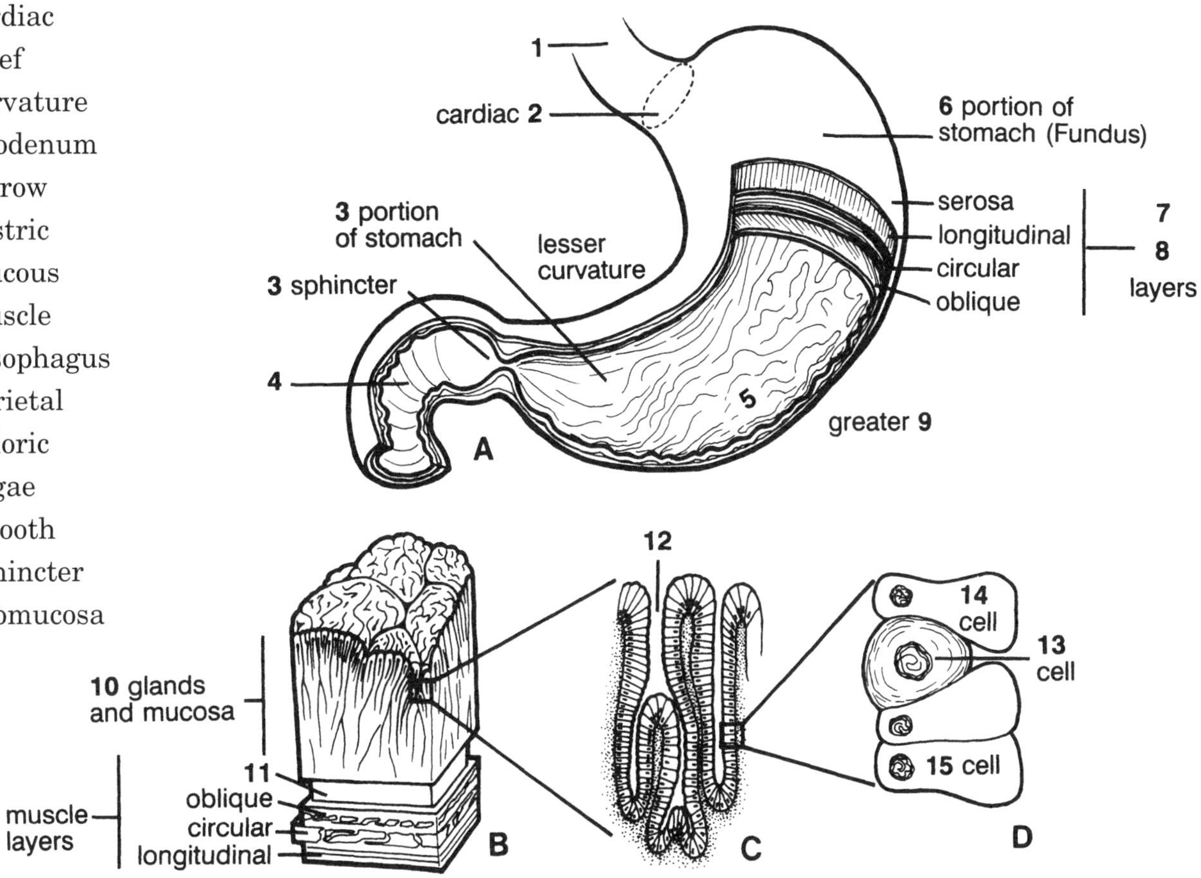

Figure 17.2 Stomach. **A.** External and internal anatomy of the stomach, showing the layers of muscle, the rugae, and the pyloric valve. **B.** Schematic representation of the gastric mucosa, showing all the layers of the stomach. **C.** Gastric glands from the greater curvature of the stomach. **D.** Detail of the gastric glands.

1. __________
2. __________
3. __________
4. __________
5. __________
6. __________
7. __________
8. __________
9. __________
10. __________
11. __________
12. __________
13. __________
14. __________
15. __________

Exercise 17.3

Labelling. Write the name of the structure on the space provided. Colour each organ differently.

Key:

ampulla	duodenum	pancreas
bile	gallbladder	pancreatic
cells	hepatic	sinusoids
cystic	Kupffer	
duct	liver	

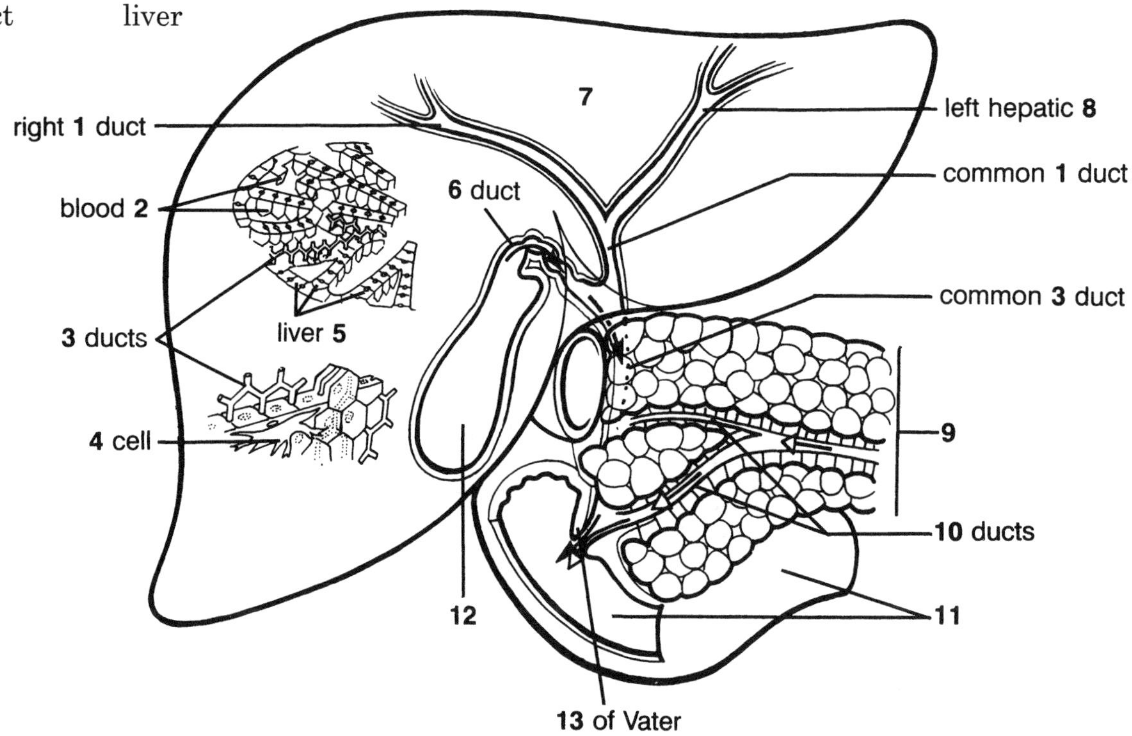

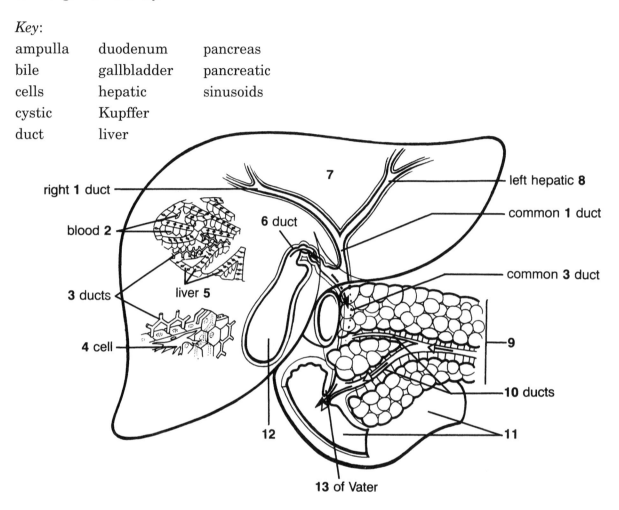

Figure 17.3 Liver and its interrelationship with the gallbladder, pancreas, and duodenum. A section has been removed from the liver and the area enlarged to show the arrangement of liver cells, bile ducts, Kupffer cells, and blood sinusoids. Arrows indicate the direction of flow of bile from the gallbladder and liver and of digestive juices from the pancreas into the duodenum.

1. ______________________
2. ______________________
3. ______________________
4. ______________________
5. ______________________
6. ______________________
7. ______________________
8. ______________________
9. ______________________
10. ______________________
11. ______________________
12. ______________________
13. ______________________

Exercise 17.4

Labelling. Write the name of the hormone or organ on the space provided. Colour the organs in reference to Figures 17.2 and 17.3.

Key:

cholecystokinin	gastrin	secretin
enterogastrone	liver	stomach
enterokinin	pancreas	villikinin
gallbladder	pancreozymin	

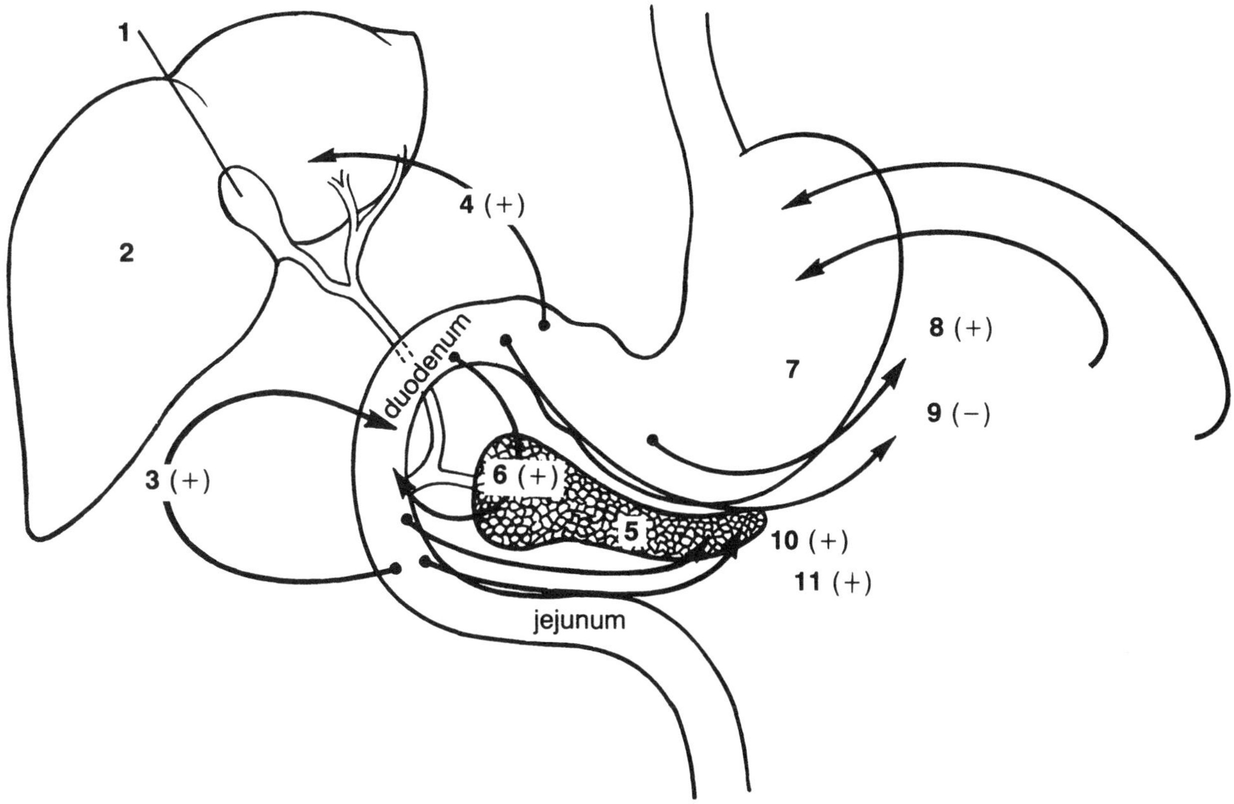

Figure 17.4 Hormonal control of digestion. The + sign indicates stimulation; the − sign indicates inhibition.

1. ____________________
2. ____________________
3. ____________________
4. ____________________
5. ____________________
6. ____________________
7. ____________________
8. ____________________
9. ____________________
10. ____________________
11. ____________________

V. TEST ITEMS

A. *Multiple Choice.* There is only one answer that is either correct or most appropriate. Circle the best answer for each question.

1. An inflammation of the abdominopelvic cavity lining is called
a. gastritis
b. diverticulitis
c. peritonitis
d. peristalsis

2. The exit of the stomach is guarded by a strong ring of muscle called the
a. cardiac sphincter (lower oesophageal sphincter)
b. rugae
c. pyloric sphincter
d. duodenum

3. The first 22 cm of the small intestine is called the
a. jejunum
b. colon
c. ilium
d. duodenum

4. An average adult requires a daily intake of about 2.4 litres of
a. minerals
b. water
c. carbohydrates
d. vitamins

5. Amino acids are the main building blocks of
a. proteins
b. fats
c. minerals
d. vitamins

6. Oxygen-rich blood is brought to the liver by the
a. common bile duct
b. hepatic arteries
c. oesophagus
d. hepatic portal vein

7. The amount of energy used by the body per unit of time is called
a. calories
b. watts
c. metabolic rate
d. nutrition

8. The gallbladder
a. produces bile
b. is attached to the pancreas
c. stores and concentrates bile
d. produces secretin

9. The enzyme that is present in saliva and pancreatic juice that digests starch into the disaccharide sugar maltose is
a. sucrase
b. amylase
c. pepsin
d. trypsin

10. If you have just digested fat molecules, you would expect to find increased amounts of
a. glucose
b. amino acids
c. fatty acids and glycerol
d. nucleic acids

11. Between meals, the glucose level of the blood is maintained by
    a. insulin
    b. glycogenolysis
    c. lipogenesis
    d. glycogenesis

12. Starvation, low carbohydrate diets, and metabolic abnormalities are all factors that contribute to
    a. ketosis
    b. alkalosis
    c. oxygen debt
    d. increased carbonic acid in the blood

13. The synthesis of glycogen molecules for storage in the liver and skeletal muscles is referred to as
    a. glycogenolysis
    b. ketosis
    c. beta oxidation
    d. glycogenesis

14. An inability of the body to synthesise cholecystokinin would hamper or inhibit
    a. swallowing of food
    b. the production of saliva
    c. the emulsification of fats
    d. mass peristalsis of the colon

15. The replacement of hepatic cells by fibrous connective tissue and frequently adipose tissue is called
    a. jaundice
    b. hepatitis
    c. peritonitis
    d. cirrhosis

16. In which organ is the chemical digestion of carbohydrates initiated?
    a. stomach
    b. small intestine
    c. mouth
    d. large intestine

17. Inflammation of the periodontal membrane and adjacent gingivae is referred to as
    a. peritonitis
    b. pyorrhea
    c. mumps
    d. pancreatitis

18. Trypsinogen is produced by which of the following?
    a. liver
    b. stomach
    c. pancreas
    d. duodenum

19. Insulin is secreted by the
    a. exocrine portion of the pancreas
    b. beta cells of the pancreas
    c. ampulla of Vater
    d. liver

20. An X-ray examination of the gallbladder is called a
    a. barium enema
    b. GI series
    c. cholecystogram
    d. gastric analysis

B. *Matching.* Each of the definitions in Column B refers to a term in Column A. Insert the letter of the definition from Column B that best describes each term in Column A. Some words or phrases may be used more than once or not at all.

Column A

1. ___ calculus
2. ___ mumps
3. ___ cholecystitis
4. ___ diarrhoea
5. ___ diverticulosis
6. ___ flatus
7. ___ heartburn
8. ___ constipation
9. ___ hepatitis
10. ___ hernia
11. ___ vomiting
12. ___ pancreatitis
13. ___ colitis
14. ___ colostomy

Column B

a. expulsion of the stomach contents through the mouth by reverse peristalsis

b. excessive amount of gas in the stomach or intestine

c. inflammation of the gallbladder

d. infrequent or difficult defaecation

e. a stone in an organ

f. inflammation of the colon and rectum

g. burning sensation in the region of the oesophagus and stomach

h. painful inflammation and enlargement of the salivary glands

i. frequent defaecation of liquid faeces

j. protrusion of an organ or part of an organ through a membrane or wall of a cavity

k. inflammation of the liver

l. inflammation of the pancreas

m. abnormal sacs or outpockets of the intestinal wall

n. cutting the colon in half and bringing the upper, lower, or both halves through the abdominal wall to the exterior

C. *True or False.* Place a *T* or an *F* in the space provided to indicate true or false.

___ **1.** Contractions of the stomach macerate food, mix it, and eventually reduce it to a thin liquid called a bolus.

___ **2.** Cells within gastric glands that secrete hydrochloric acid are called zymogenic cells.

___ **3.** Distention of the stomach is permitted by folds of the mucosa called rugae.

___ **4.** Failure of the muscle fibres of the pyloric valve to relax normally is called pyloric stenosis.

___ **5.** The portion of the stomach closest to the oesophagus is the cardiac sphincter.

___ **6.** Proteins are formed by linking together different types of amino acids in a number of different sequential patterns.

___ **7.** Fatty acids which do not have double bonds in their structures are known as polyunsaturated fatty acids.

___ **8.** The salivary glands whose secretions are discharged on either side of the frenulum are the parotids.

___ **9.** Projections of the lamina propria of the tongue that are covered with epithelium are called papillae.

___ **10.** All enzymes are proteins.

___ **11.** Glycogen, a polysaccharide composed of many molecules of glucose, is an example of an important carbohydrate.

___ **12.** Increased peristaltic activity of the small intestine will lead to diarrhoea because of a decreased time for absorption of material.

___ **13.** Two types of contractions, peristalsis and segmenting, occur in the small intestine.

___ **14.** Secretion of digestive enzymes by the stomach is brought about exclusively by hormonal stimulation.

___ **15.** Following their absorption, simple sugars, fats, and amino acids are transported to the liver via the hepatic portal vein.

Answer Sheet—Chapter 17

Exercise 17.1

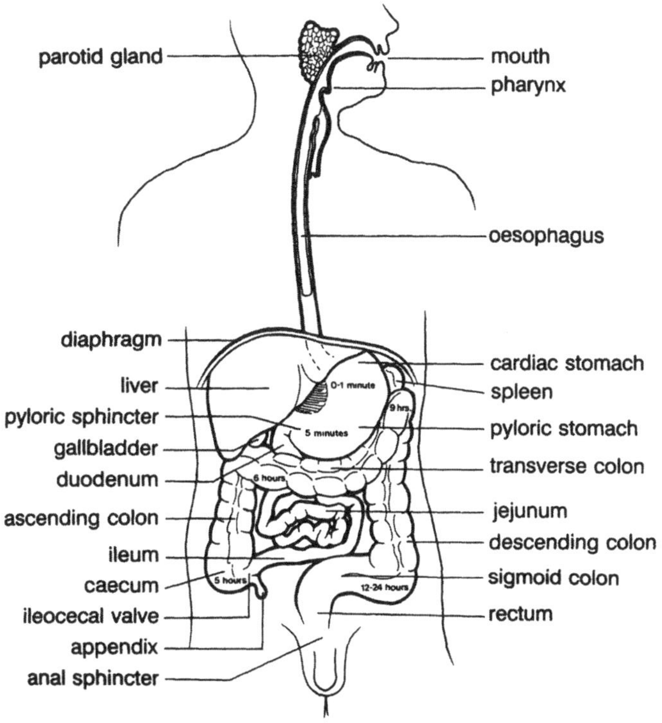

Figure 17.1 Human digestive tract. Times indicated along the tract represent how long it takes food to pass through each area during the process of digestion.

Exercise 17.2

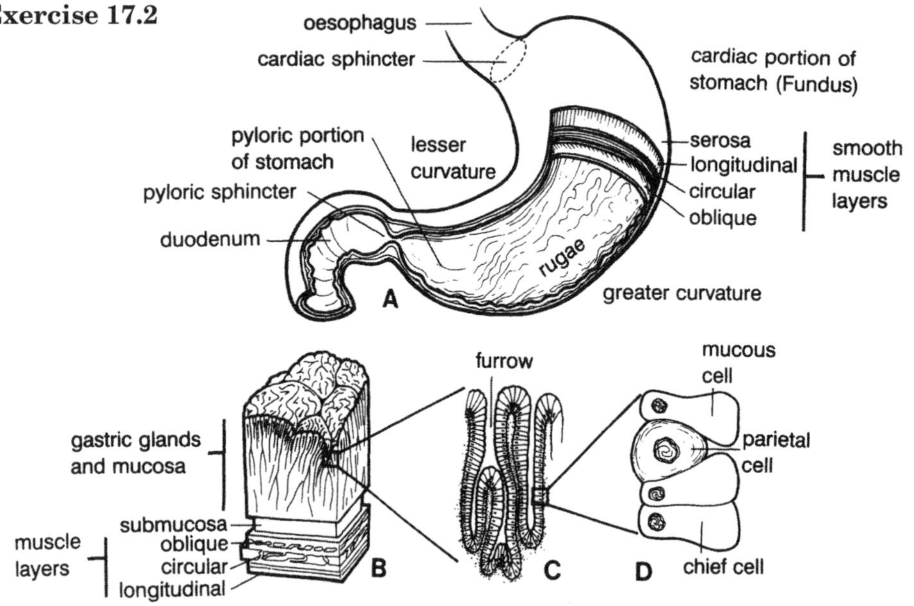

Figure 17.2 Stomach. **A.** External and internal anatomy of the stomach, showing the layers of muscle, the rugae, and the pyloric valve. **B.** Schematic representation of the gastric mucosa, showing all the layers of the stomach. **C.** Gastric glands from the greater curvature of the stomach. **D.** Detail of the gastric glands.

Exercise 17.3

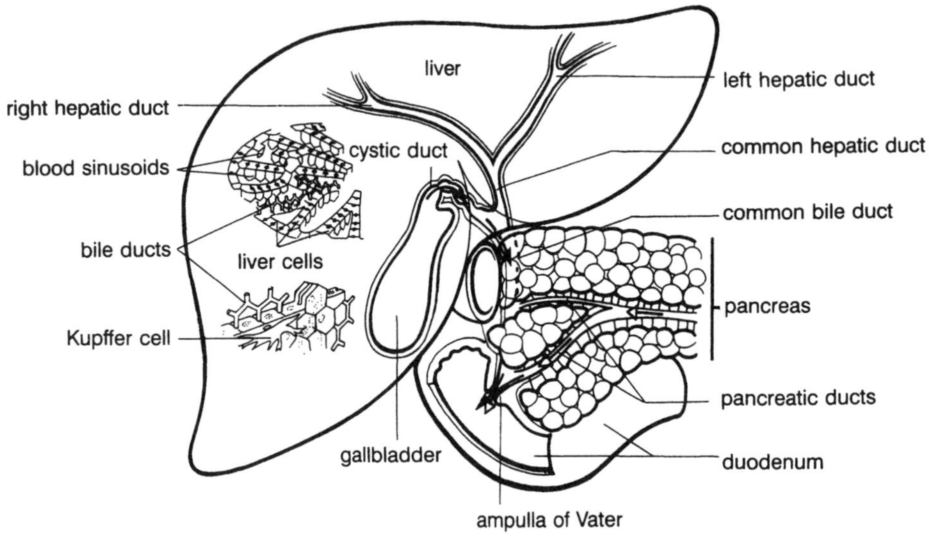

Figure 17.3 Liver and its interrelationship with the gallbladder, pancreas, and duodenum. A section has been removed from the liver and the area enlarged to show the arrangement of liver cells, bile ducts, Kupffer cells, and blood sinusoids. Arrows indicate the direction of flow of bile from the gallbladder and liver and of digestive juices from the pancreas into the duodenum.

Exercise 17.4

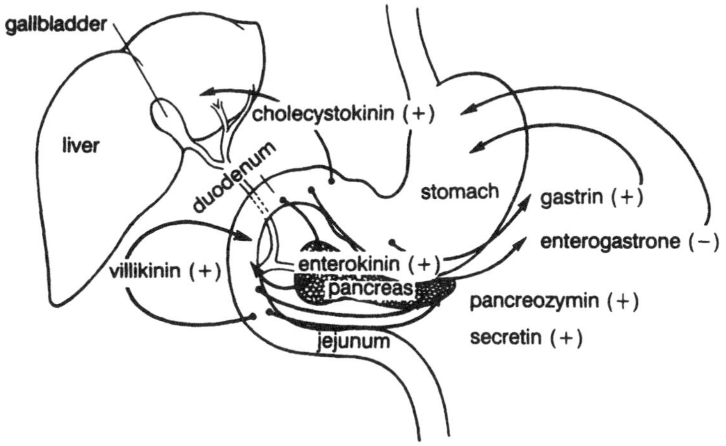

Figure 17.4 Hormonal control of digestion. The + sign indicates stimulation; the − sign indicates inhibition.

Test Items

A. 1. c, 2. c, 3. d, 4. b, 5. a, 6. b, 7. c, 8. c, 9. b, 10. c, 11. b, 12. a, 13. d, 14. c, 15. d, 16. c, 17. b, 18. c, 19. b, 20. c.

B. 1. e, 2. h, 3. c, 4. i, 5. m, 6. b, 7. g, 8. d, 9. k, 10. j, 11. a, 12. l, 13. f, 14. n.

C. 1. F, 2. F, 3. T, 4. F, 5. T, 6. T, 7. F, 8. F, 9. T, 10. T, 11. T, 12. T, 13. T, 14. F, 15. F.

18

Excretion

I. CHAPTER SYNOPSIS

As seen in Chapter 16, the lungs excrete the major metabolic waste product of the body—carbon dioxide. Other waste products, especially urea, the end product of nitrogen metabolism, are excreted by the kidneys into the urine. However, the excretion of waste products is of secondary importance in relation to the role of the kidneys in the regulation of the salt and water content of the internal environment. The salt and water content of the body depends upon the balance between intake and excretion. The major control point is the regulation of excretion by the kidneys.

The amounts of water and salt excreted by the kidneys depend upon the magnitude of the glomerular filtration, tubular reabsorption, and secretion. These basic operations of the kidney are influenced by several hormones whose release is determined by the amounts of salt and water in the blood. Thus, this chapter examines the structure of the kidney and urinary system, basic principles of renal physiology, micturition, and kidney disease.

II. OBJECTIVES

After reading the chapter, the student should be able to:

- Label the anatomy of the urinary system.
- Identify all urinary structures and relate their separate functions.

- Define micturition and identify the factors involved in glomerular filtration rates.
- Define diuresis and explain how it works.
- Explain the role of antidiuretic hormone (vasopressin) and aldosterone in renal tubular absorption.
- Identify the active and passive processes occurring during tubular reabsorption.
- Explain how renal failure disturbs the body's homeostasis.
- Define nephritis, glomerulonephritis, pyelonephritis, cystitis, and urethritis.
- Explain dialysis and identify the two major methods.

III. IMPORTANT TERMS

Using your textbook, define the following terms:

adrenal (a-dree′nul) ______________________________

____

antidiuretic (ant-ee-dye′yoo-ret-ik) ______________________________

____

calculi (kal′kew-lye) ______________________________

____

calyx (kay′liks) ______________________________

____

cystoscope (sis′tah-skope) ______________________________

____

dehydration (dee-high-dray′shun) ______________________________

____

diuresis (dye-yoo-ree′sis) ______________________________

____

dysuria (dis-yoo′ree-uh) ______________________________

____

excretion (ek-skree′shun) ______________________________

____

glomerulus (glom-err′yoo-lus) ______________________________

____

haemodialysis (hee-mo-dye-al′i-sis) ______________________________

____

hilus (high′lus) ______________________________

____

incontinence (in-kon′ti-nunce) ______________________________

____

micturition (mik-tew-rish′un) ______________________________

____

nephron (nef′ron) ______________________________

____

pyramid (pirr′uh-mid) ______________________________

____

renal (ree′nul) ______________________________

____

retroperitoneal (re-tro-per-ri-to-nee′ul) ______________________________

____

transitional (tran-zish′un-ul) ______________________________

____

tubule (tew′bew-lur) ______________________________

____

urea (yoo-ree′uh) ______________________________

____

uraemia (yoo-ree′mee-uh) ______________________________

____

urination (yoo-ri-nay′shun) ______________________________

____

IV. EXERCISES

Complete the following exercises in the order given. A precise set of terms and diagrams has been chosen to describe excretion.

Exercise 18.1

Labelling. Write the name of the structure on the space provided. Colour the vessels and organs separately.

Key:
adrenal
aorta
artery
external
iliac
kidney
prostate
renal
ureter
urethra
urinary
vena cava

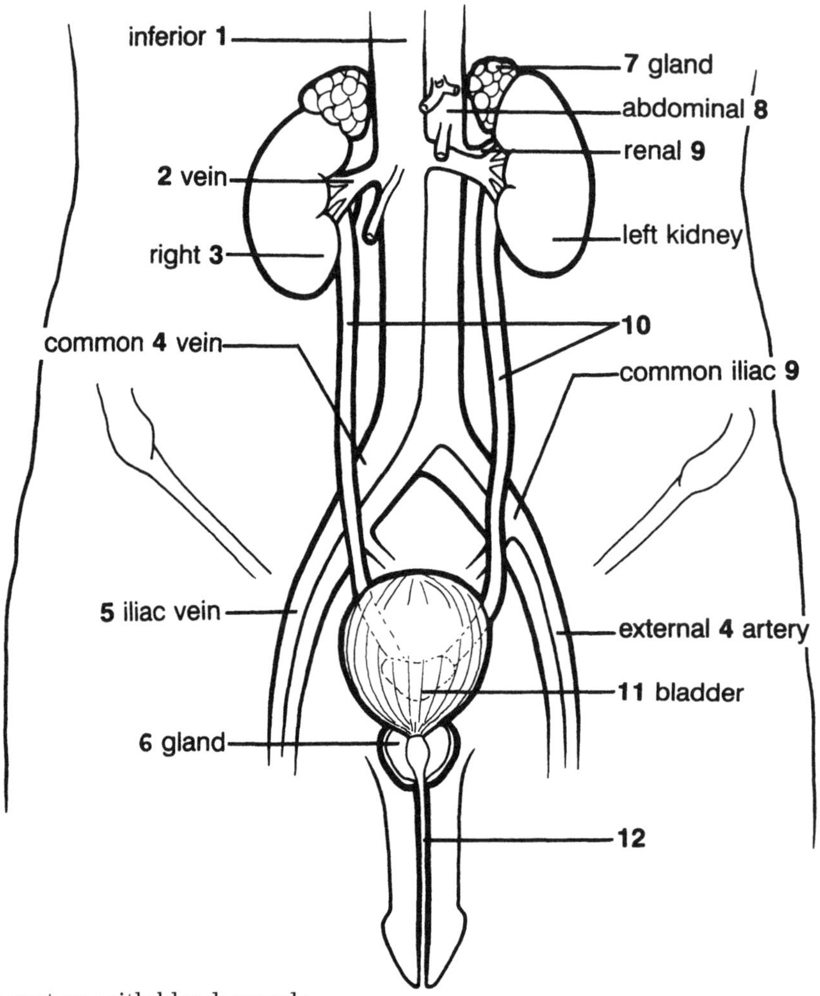

Figure 18.1 Urinary system with blood vessels.

1. ______________________
2. ______________________
3. ______________________
4. ______________________
5. ______________________
6. ______________________
7. ______________________
8. ______________________
9. ______________________
10. ______________________
11. ______________________
12. ______________________

Exercise 18.2

Labelling. Write the name of the structure on the space provided. Colour the three areas of the kidney differently.

Key:

calyx	minor
capsule	opening
cortex	pelvis
fibrous	pyramids
hilus	renal
medulla	ureter

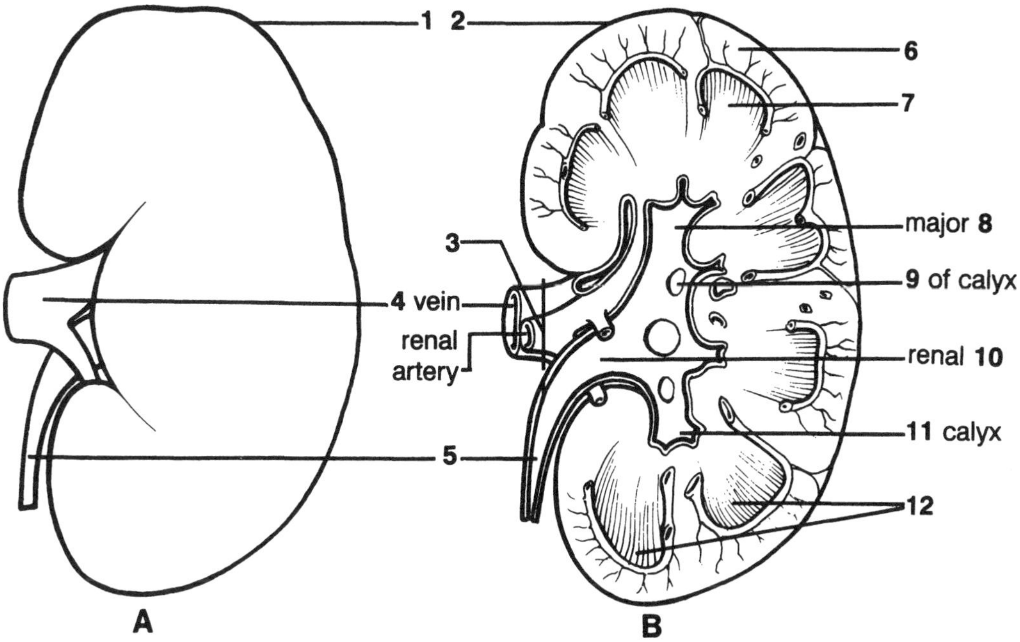

Figure 18.2 The left kidney. **A.** External anatomy. **B.** Internal anatomy.

1. ______________________
2. ______________________
3. ______________________
4. ______________________
5. ______________________
6. ______________________
7. ______________________
8. ______________________
9. ______________________
10. ______________________
11. ______________________
12. ______________________

Exercise 18.3

Labelling. Write the name of the structure on the space provided. Colour the vessels different from the tubules.

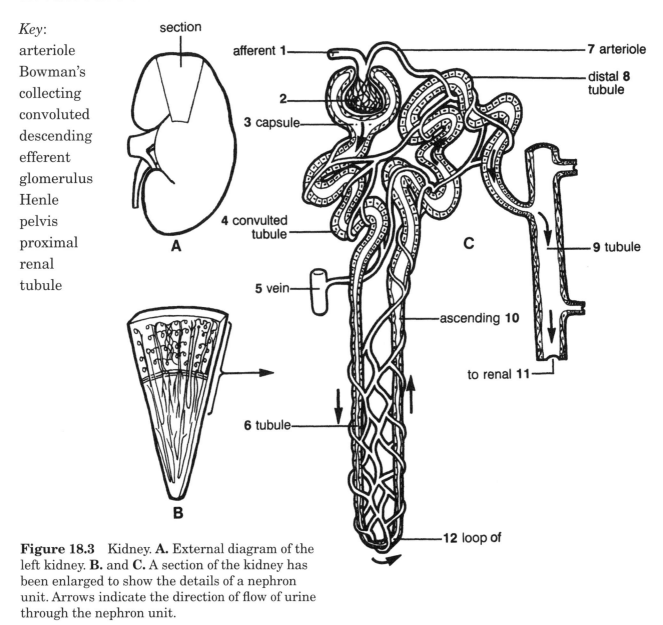

Key:
arteriole
Bowman's
collecting
convoluted
descending
efferent
glomerulus
Henle
pelvis
proximal
renal
tubule

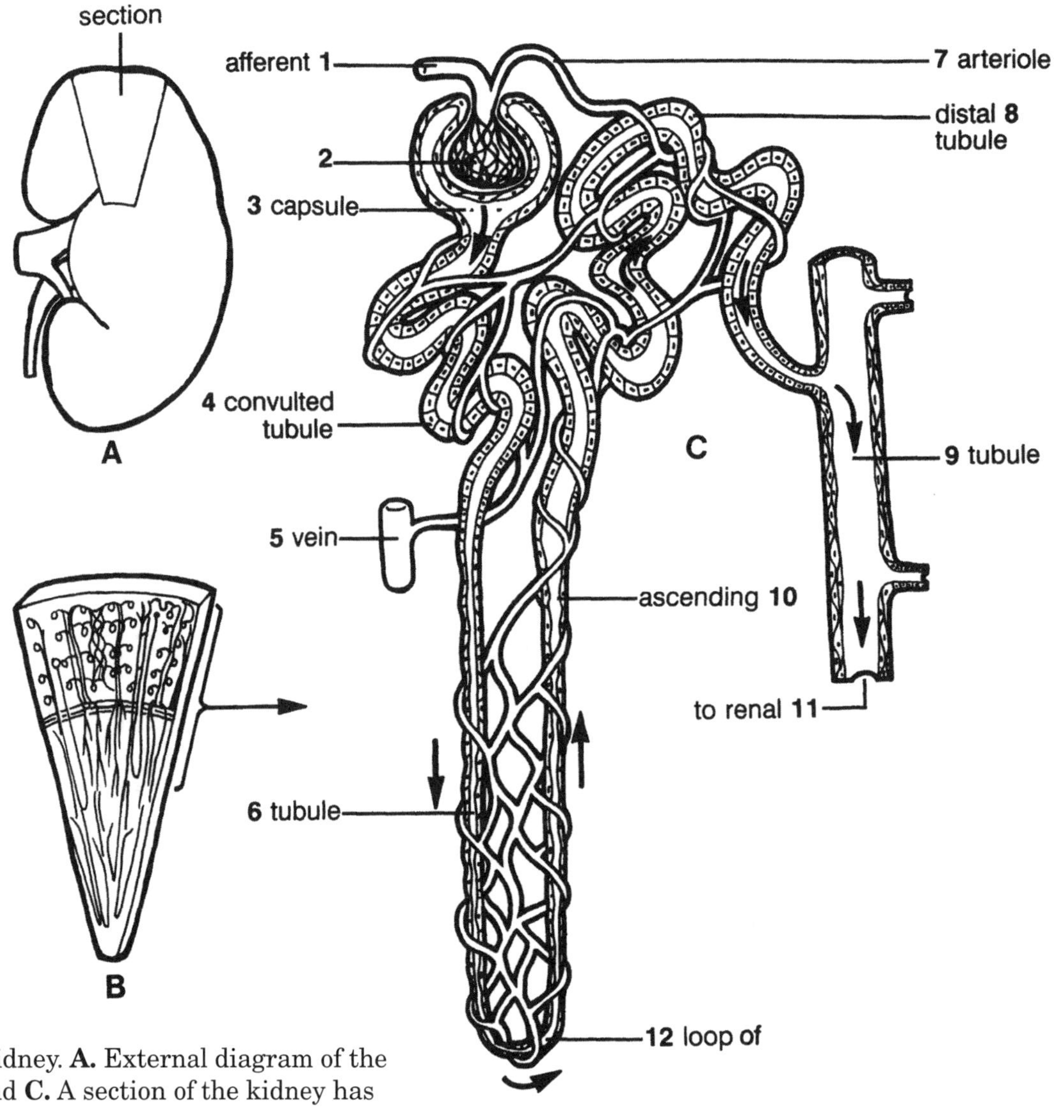

Figure 18.3 Kidney. **A.** External diagram of the left kidney. **B.** and **C.** A section of the kidney has been enlarged to show the details of a nephron unit. Arrows indicate the direction of flow of urine through the nephron unit.

1. ______________________
2. ______________________
3. ______________________
4. ______________________
5. ______________________
6. ______________________
7. ______________________
8. ______________________
9. ______________________
10. ______________________
11. ______________________
12. ______________________

Exercise 18.4

Labelling. Write the name of the structure on the space provided. Colour the organs and tubes differently.

Key:
bulbourethral (Cowper's)
connective
fibrous
internal
muscle
prostate
smooth
sphincter
transitional
ureter
ureters
urethra

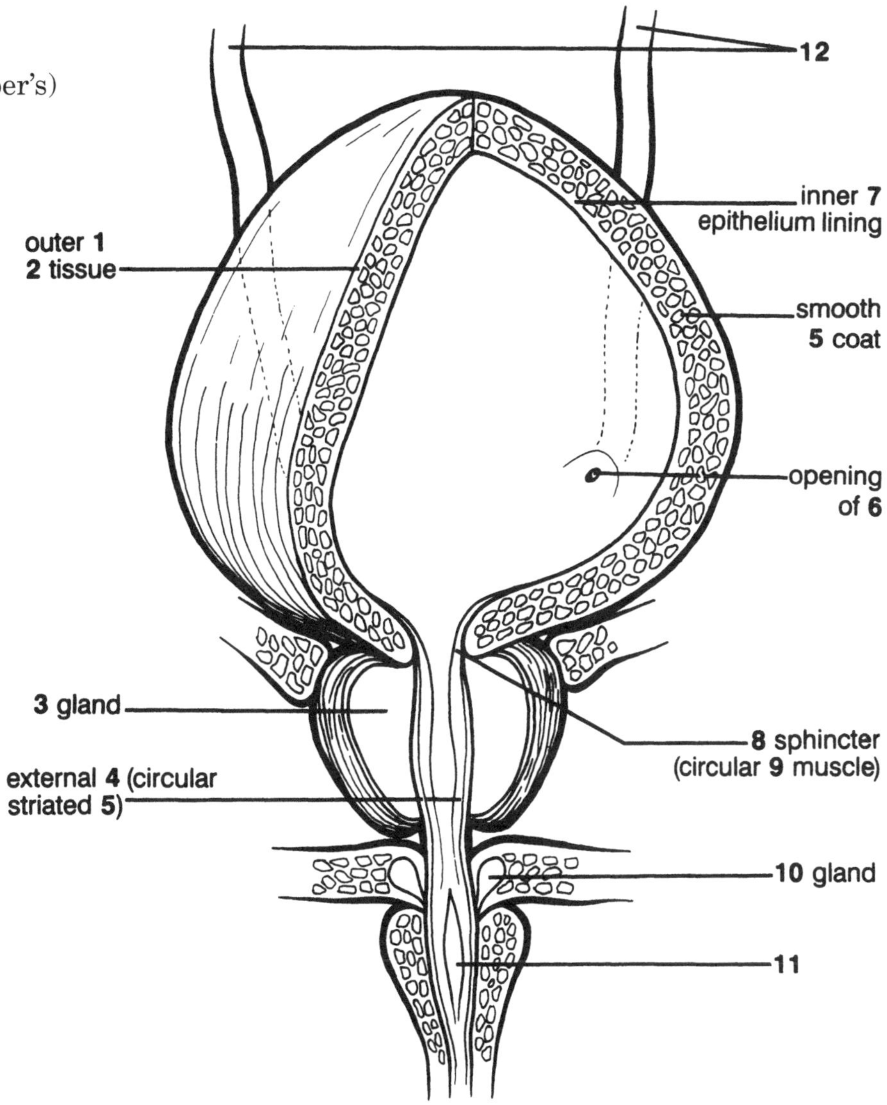

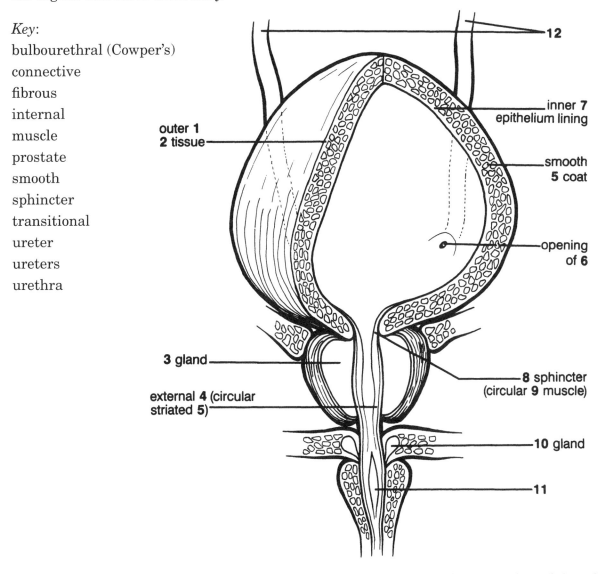

Figure 18.4 Urinary bladder, ureters, and urethra of an adult male.

1. ______________________
2. ______________________
3. ______________________
4. ______________________
5. ______________________
6. ______________________
7. ______________________
8. ______________________
9. ______________________
10. ______________________
11. ______________________
12. ______________________

V. TEST ITEMS

A. *Multiple Choice.* There is only one answer that is either correct or most appropriate. Circle the best answer for each question.

1. Which system helps to regulate the volume and composition of body fluid?
a. reproductive
b. digestive
c. respiratory
d. urinary

2. The blood capillary network found inside Bowman's capsule is called the
a. pyramid
b. calyx
c. glomerulus
d. nephron

3. Micturition is another word for
a. malnutrition
b. reabsorption
c. chewing
d. urination

4. Which of the following is a hormone that regulates the levels of sodium and potassium in the blood?
a. ADH
b. aldosterone
c. adenosine triphosphate (ATP)
d. angiotensin

5. In which of the following areas of a nephron is glucose usually reabsorbed back into the blood
a. Bowman's capsule
b. proximal convoluted tubule
c. loop of Henle
d. distal convoluted tubule

6. The ability to store urine would be affected by which of the following conditions?
a. pyelitis
b. nephrosis
c. cystitis
d. renal suppression

7. An obstruction in the glomerulus would affect the flow of blood into the
a. renal artery
b. efferent arteriole
c. afferent arteriole
d. intralobular artery

8. The most abundant cation in extracellular fluid is
a. Na^+
b. K^+
c. Cl^-
d. HPO_4^-

9. Urine that leaves the distal convoluted tubule passes through the following structures in which sequence?
a. collecting duct, hilum, calyx, ureter
b. collecting duct, calyx, pelvis, ureter
c. calyx, collecting duct, pelvis, ureter
d. calyx, hilum, pelvis, ureter

10. Which of the following hormones would promote the production of a more dilute urine?
a. ADH (vasopressin)
b. cortisol
c. atrial natriuretic peptide (ANP)
d. calcitonin

11. A high level of uric acid in the blood that may crystallise in the kidneys and joints results in a disorder called
a. pyuria
b. gout
c. pyelonephritis
d. anuria

12. As the amount of ADH (vasopressin) in the blood increases,
a. urine is made more acidic
b. more urine is formed
c. tubular reabsorption of water increases
d. diuresis is accelerated

13. Under normal circumstances, filtrate passing from the glomerulus into the Bowman's capsule is free of
a. water
b. glucose
c. proteins
d. chloride

14. Hypertension and inflammation are two conditions that may lead to
a. dehydration
b. oedema
c. excessive water loss
d. alkalosis

15. Conditions such as diabetes mellitus, starvation, and low carbohydrate diets are closely linked to
a. ketosis
b. pyuria
c. haematuria
d. calculi

16. Incontinence is distinguished from retention in that the former is
a. a failure to void urine
b. an inability of the kidneys to make urine
c. a lack of voluntary control over micturition
d. voluntarily controlled by the cerebral cortex

17. The primary function of ADH (vasopressin) is to
a. cause active re-absorption of potassium
b. decrease the permeability of the collecting duct
c. cause active re-absorption of calcium
d. increase the permeability of the distal convoluted tubule

18. Osmoreceptors in the hypothalamus control
a. release of ADH (vasopressin)
b. release of aldosterone
c. electrolyte reabsorption
d. glucose reabsorption

19. The kidney contributes to the maintenance of acid-base balance primarily by
a. secreting urea
b. excreting H^+ in exchange for Na^+
c. excreting Na^+ in exchange for H^+
d. excreting HCO_3^-

20. Another means by which the kidney controls the pH of the blood is by
a. excreting CO_2
b. excreting the buffers that transport acid substances in the blood
c. excreting Na^+
d. secreting ammonia

B. *Matching Questions.* Each of the phrases in Column B refers to a word or phrase in Column A. Insert the letter of the word or phrase from Column B that best describes each word or phrase in Column A. Some of the words or phrases may be used more than once or not at all.

Column A	Column B
1. ___ glomerulus	**a.** the deep fissure on the kidney
2. ___ renal pyramids	**b.** cone-shaped masses in the medulla
3. ___ micturition	**c.** epithelial cells within Bowman's capsule
4. ___ aldosterone	**d.** a hormone that regulates blood glucose
5. ___ hypocalcemic tetany	**e.** urination
6. ___ ureter	**f.** antidiuretic hormone (ADH)
7. ___ HCl	**g.** stimulates sodium reabsorption
8. ___ lactic	**h.** drains urine from the kidneys
9. ___ haemoglobin	**i.** drains urine from the bladder
10. ___ urethra	**j.** a disease caused by low calcium
11. ___ insulin	**k.** plays a role in calcium metabolism
12. ___ hilum	**l.** a strong acid
13. ___ vasopressin	**m.** the vascular component of the nephron
14. ___ vitamin D	**n.** a weak acid
15. ___ podocytes	**o.** a buffer

Column A	Column B
1. ___ respiratory alkalosis	**a.** abnormal decrease in pH due to a decrease in the rate of respiration
2. ___ buffer system	**b.** a chemical substance that dissociates into ions
3. ___ oedema	**c.** a weak acid and salt of that acid that prevents drastic changes in pH
4. ___ metabolic acidosis	**d.** abnormal decrease in pH due to the buildup of metabolic acids in the blood and/or loss of bicarbonate
5. ___ electrolyte	**e.** abnormal increase in pH due to an increase in the minute volume of respiration
6. ___ extracellular fluid	**f.** a larger than normal volume of interstitial fluid produce swelling of the tissue
7. ___ respiratory acidosis	**g.** body fluid found inside cells
8. ___ intracellular fluid	**h.** abnormal increase in pH due to a loss of acid by the body or excessive intake of alkaline substances
9. ___ metabolic alkalosis	**i.** fluid outside of body cells such as plasma and interstitial fluid

C. *True or False.* Place a *T* or an *F* in the space provided.

___ **1.** In the normal adult, the glomerular filtration rate is about 500 mL/minute.

___ **2.** The term renal suppression applies to a condition in which glomerular blood hydrostatic pressure falls to about 50 mm Hg.

___ **3.** Because the afferent arteriole is smaller in diameter than the efferent arteriole, it offers more resistance to the outflow of blood from the glomerulus.

___ **4.** The three steps involved in urine formation are filtration, reabsorption, and secretion.

___ **5.** A renal corpuscle is a Bowman's capsule together with its glomerulus.

___ **6.** The part of a nephron that passes the filtrate into the collecting duct is the proximal convoluted tube.

___ **7.** The triangular-shaped structures inside the medulla of a kidney are called the calyces.

___ **8.** Inflammation of the kidney pelvis and its calyces is referred to as pyelitis.

___ **9.** Urine always has an acid reaction.

___ **10.** Angiotensin II stimulates aldosterone secretion and causes vasoconstriction and elevation of blood pressure.

___ **11.** Glomeruli are small arteries present in the kidney.

___ **12.** The volume of urine secreted is regulated mainly by mechanisms that control the glomerular filtration rate.

___ **13.** A decrease in glomerular blood pressure tends to decrease glomerular filtration rate.

___ **14.** An increase in the hydrostatic pressure in Bowman's capsule tends to increase the glomerular filtration rate.

___ **15.** A decrease in blood protein concentration tends to decrease the glomerular filtration rate.

___ **16.** Osmoreceptors lie in the anterior portion of the hypothalamus.

___ **17.** The functioning renal unit of the kidney is called the nephron.

___ **18.** Glomerular capillary pressure is higher than blood capillaries in other body tissues.

___ **19.** The kidneys lie behind the peritoneum, i.e., retroperitoneally.

___ **20.** The bases of the pyramids rest on the renal medulla.

Answer Sheet—Chapter 18

Exercise 18.1

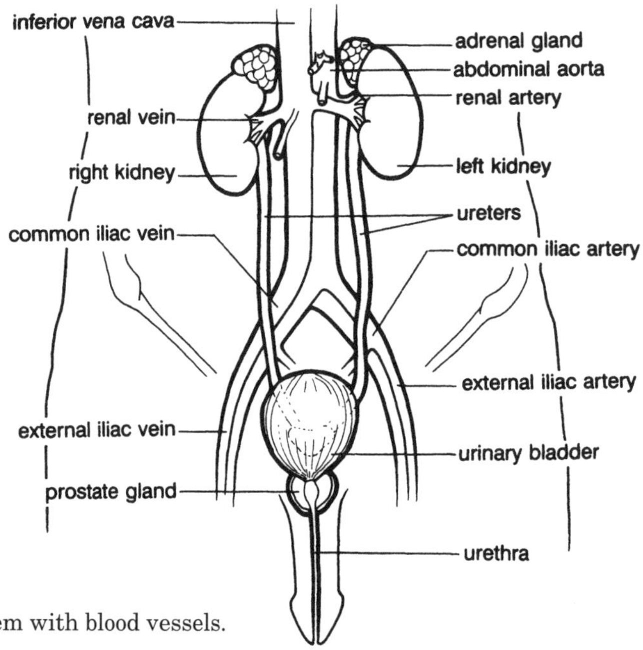

Figure 18.1 Urinary system with blood vessels.

Exercise 18.2

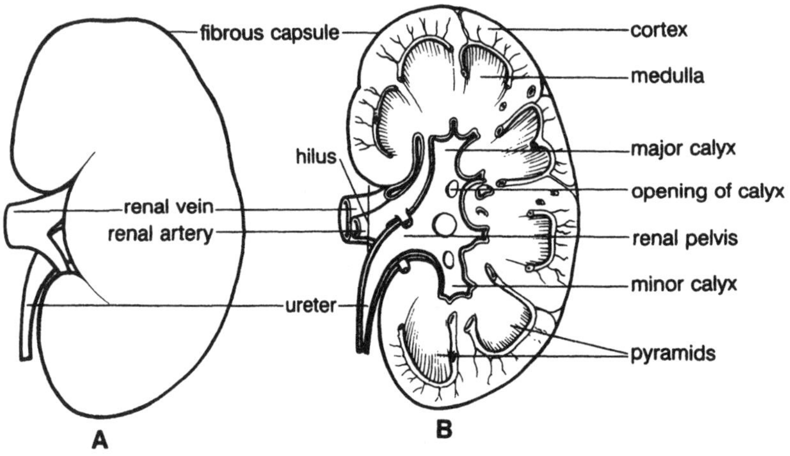

Figure 18.2 The left kidney. **A.** External anatomy. **B.** Internal anatomy.

Exercise 18.3

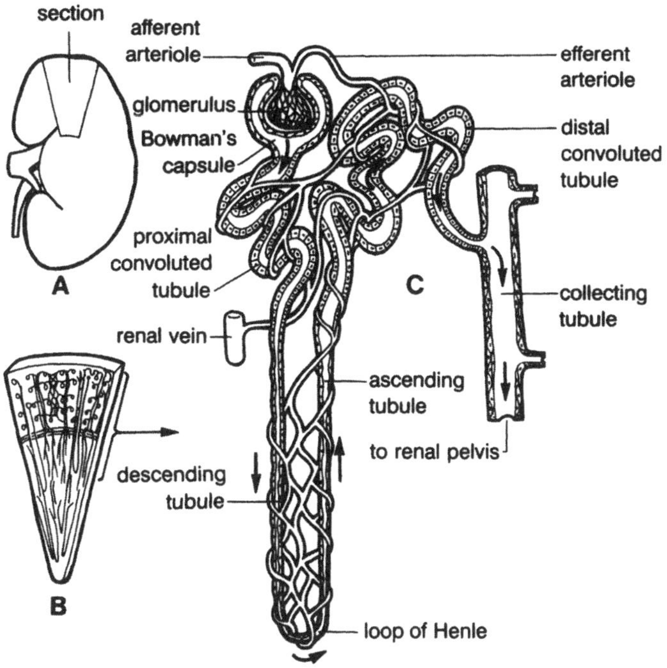

Figure 18.3 Kidney. **A.** External diagram of the left kidney. **B.** and **C.** A section of the kidney has been enlarged to show the details of a nephron unit. Arrows indicate the direction of flow of urine through the nephron unit.

Exercise 18.4

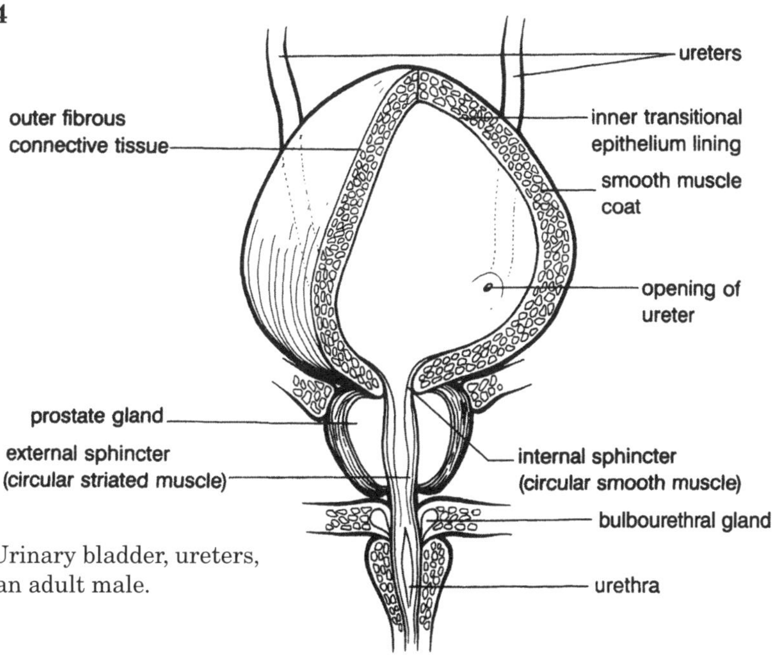

Figure 18.4 Urinary bladder, ureters, and urethra of an adult male.

Test Items

A. 1. d, 2. c, 3. d, 4. b, 5. b, 6. c, 7. b, 8. a, 9. b, 10. c, 11. b, 12. c, 13. c, 14. b, 15. a, 16. c, 17. d, 18. a, 19. b, 20. d.

B. 1. m, 2. b, 3. e, 4. g, 5. j, 6. h, 7. l, 8. n, 9. o, 10. i, 11. d, 12. a, 13. f, 14. k, 15. c.
1. e, 2. c, 3. f, 4. d, 5. b, 6. i, 7. a, 8. g, 9. h.

C. 1. F, 2. T, 3. F, 4. T, 5. T, 6. F, 7. F, 8. T, 9. F, 10. T, 11. F, 12. F, 13. T, 14. F, 15. F, 16. T, 17. T, 18. T, 19. T, 20. F.

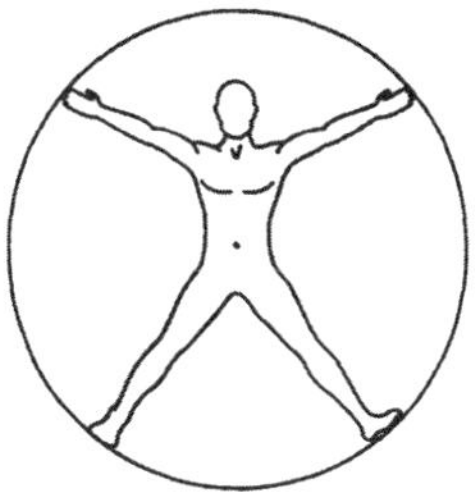

19

Reproduction

I. CHAPTER SYNOPSIS

In addition to allowing the production of offspring and the passing of genes down the generations, the reproductive organs produce several key hormones that influence body composition. The student is introduced to the anatomy and physiology of the organs of reproduction. Emphasis is placed on the endocrine relations of the male and female systems, particularly those of the menstrual dysfunctions, ovarian cysts, leucorrhoea, tumours of the breasts, and cervical cancer.

II. OBJECTIVES

After reading the chapter, the student should be able to:

- Contrast mitosis and meiosis in terms of tissue, location, and number of chromosomes.
- Define spermatogenesis and explain the role of the pituitary gland.
- Identify the structures of the male and female reproductive systems.
- Contrast spermatogenesis and oogenesis.
- List the constituents of semen.
- Name the ovarian and pituitary hormones that regulate the menstrual cycle.
- Define myometrium, perimetrium, endometrium, and endometriosis.

- Describe the changes that occur in the uterus during menstrual cycle.
- Define puberty, menopause, and menarche in relation to hormonal production and cessation.
- Describe the glandular structure of the breast and the hormonal influences of lactation.
- Describe the physiology of breast feeding.

III. IMPORTANT TERMS

Using your textbook, define the following terms:

abortion (uh-bor′shun) ______________________________

alveolus (al-vee′o-lus) ______________________________

amenorrhoea (a men-o-ree′-uh) ______________________________

ampulla (am-pul′uh) ______________________________

autosome (aw′to-sohm) ______________________________

chromosome (kro′muh-sohm) ______________________________

copulation (kop-yoo-lay′shun) ______________________________

corpus (kor′pus) ______________________________

cryptorchidism (krip-tor′kid-izm) ______________________________

dysmenorrhea (dis-men-o-ree′-uh) ______________________________

ectopic (ek-top′ik) ______________________________

ejaculation (e-jak′yoo-lay′shun) ______________________________

endometriosis (en-do-mee-tree-o′sis) ______________________________

endometrium (end-o-mee′tree-um) ______________________________ fertilisation (fur-ti-ly-zay'shun) ______

foetus (fee'tus) ______

gamete (gam'eet) ______

lactation (lak-tay'shun) ______

meiosis (my-o'sis) ______

menopause (men'o-pawz) ______

menstruation (men-stroo-ay'shun) ______

mitosis (my-to'sis) ______

myometrium (my-o-mee'tree-um) ______

ovulation (ov-yoo-lay'shun) ______

ovum (o'vum) ______

perimetrium (per-ee-mee'tree-um) ______

proliferation (pro-lif-ur-ay'shun) ______

semen (see'men) ______

somatic (so-mat'ik) ______

sperm (spurm) ______

vasectomy (vas-ek'tuh-mee) ______

zygote (zy'gote) ______

IV. EXERCISES

Complete the following exercises in the order given. A precise set of terms and diagrams has been chosen to describe the reproductive system.

Exercise 19.1

Labelling. Write the term on the space provided. Colour the various stages a different colour.

Key:
fertilisation
growth
maturation
meiosis
oocyte
oogenesis
ovum
polar body
proliferation
second
sperm
spermatocyte
spermatogenesis
spermatids
zygote

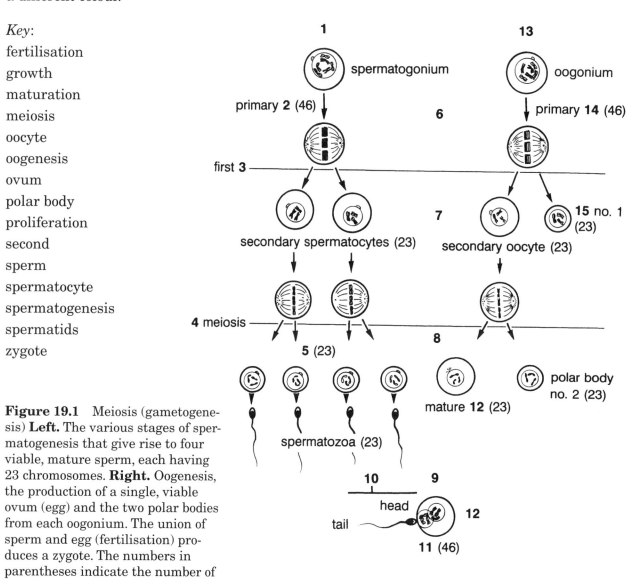

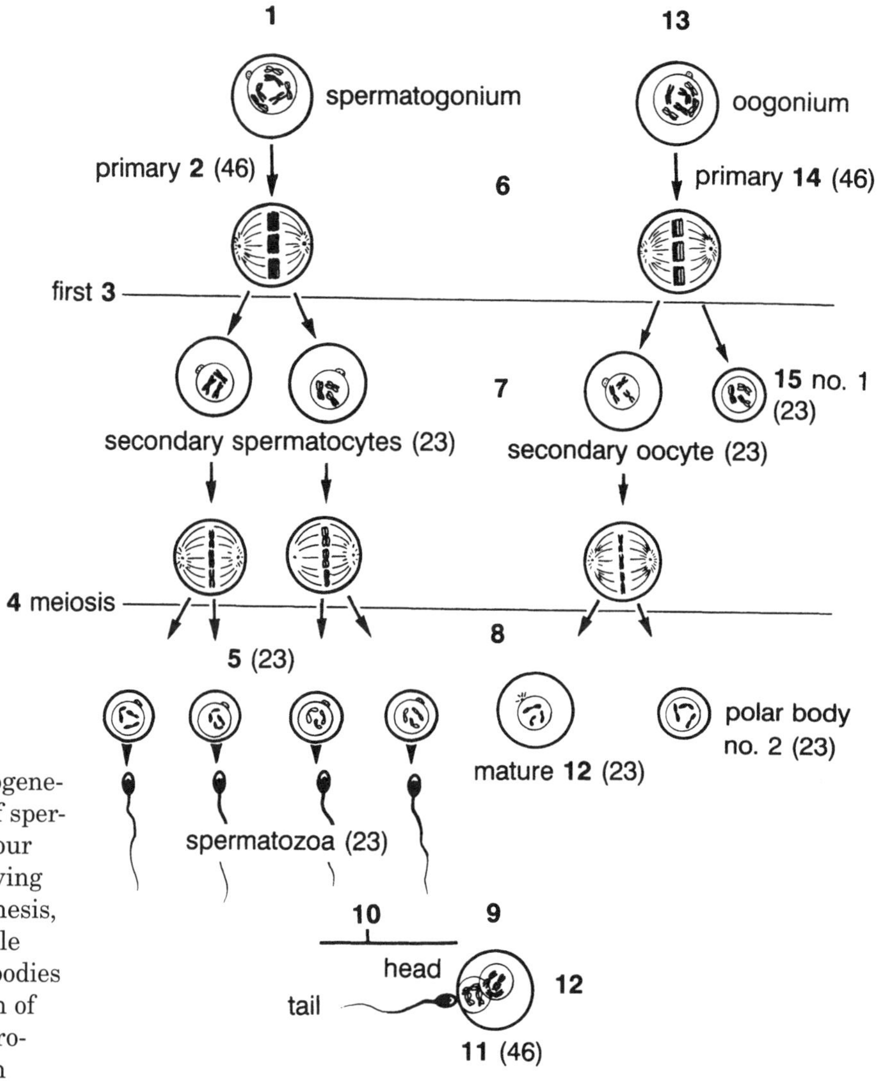

Figure 19.1 Meiosis (gametogenesis) **Left.** The various stages of spermatogenesis that give rise to four viable, mature sperm, each having 23 chromosomes. **Right.** Oogenesis, the production of a single, viable ovum (egg) and the two polar bodies from each oogonium. The union of sperm and egg (fertilisation) produces a zygote. The numbers in parentheses indicate the number of chromosomes.

1. ______________
2. ______________
3. ______________
4. ______________
5. ______________
6. ______________
7. ______________
8. ______________
9. ______________
10. ______________
11. ______________
12. ______________
13. ______________
14. ______________
15. ______________

Exercise 19.2

Labelling. Write the name of the structure on the space provided. Colour the reproductive tract different from the surrounding tissue.

Key:

anus	corpus	prepuce	scrotum	testis	urethral
bladder	epididymis	prostate	seminal	ureter	vas
bulbourethral	penis	rectum	sigmoid	urethra	

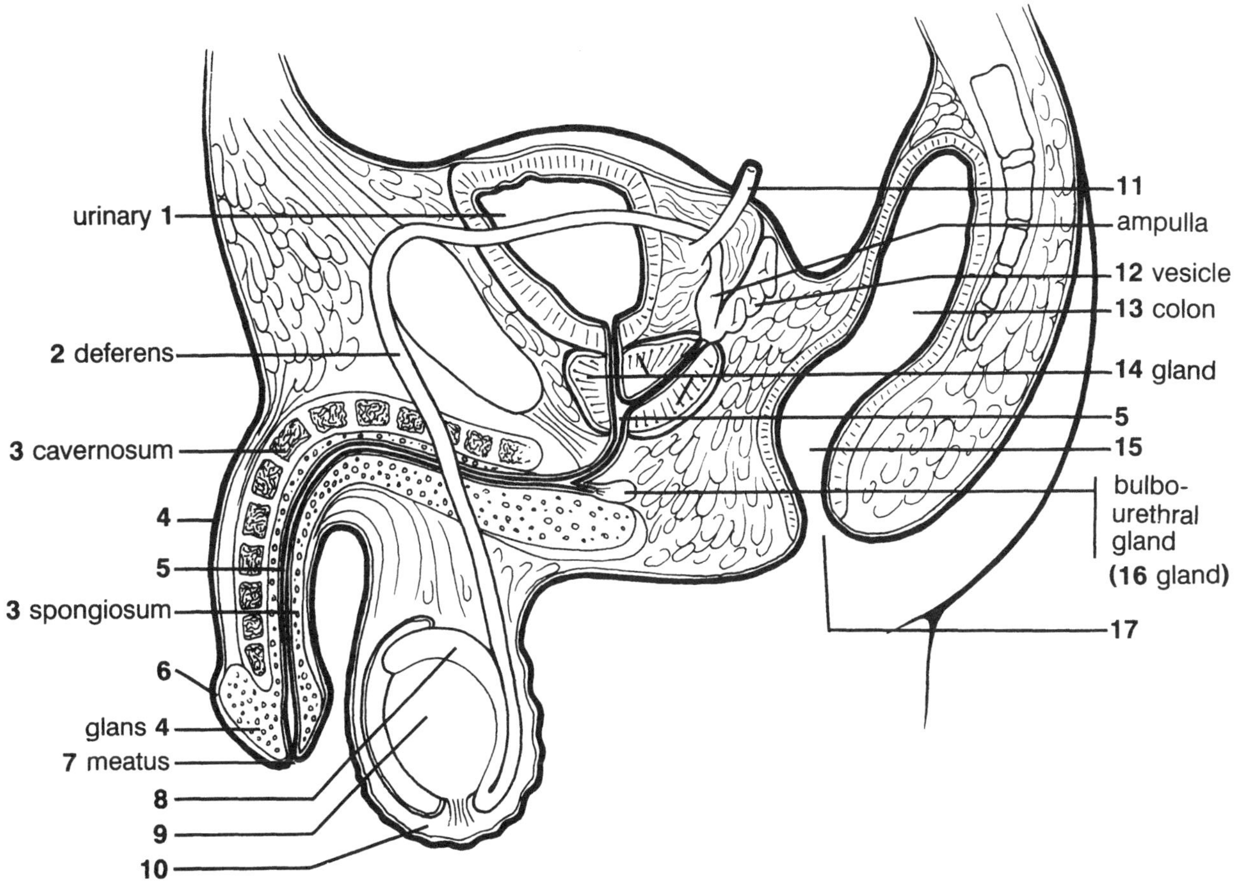

Figure 19.2 Midsagittal section of the male reproductive system.

1. ______________________
2. ______________________
3. ______________________
4. ______________________
5. ______________________
6. ______________________
7. ______________________
8. ______________________
9. ______________________
10. ______________________
11. ______________________
12. ______________________
13. ______________________
14. ______________________
15. ______________________
16. ______________________
17. ______________________

Exercise 19.3

Labelling. Write the name of the structure on the space provided. Colour the systems differently.

Key:
anus
bladder
broad
cervix
clitoris
endometrium
fallopian
hymen
ligament
majora
myometrium
ovary
oviduct
posterior
pubis
rectum
sigmoid
urethra
vagina

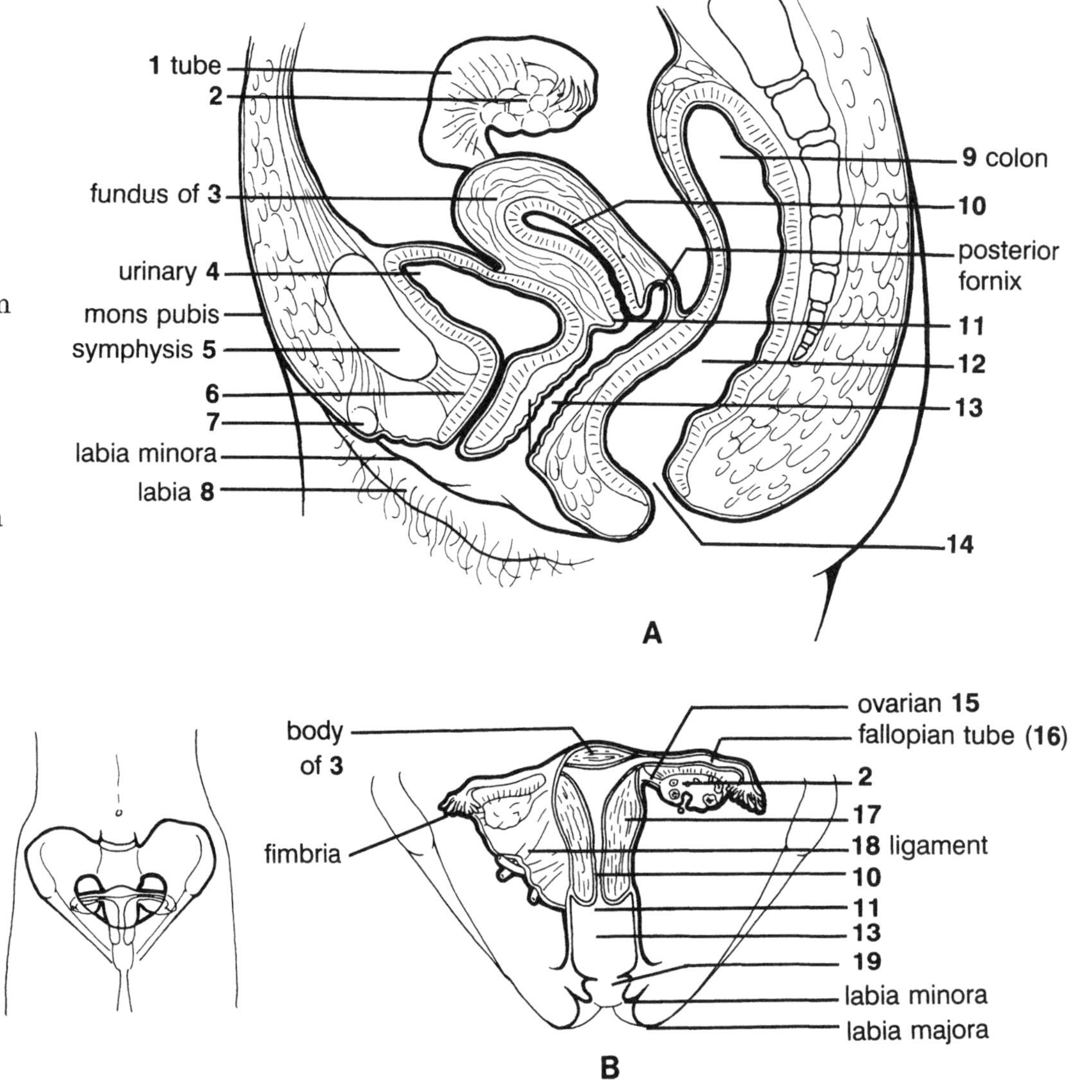

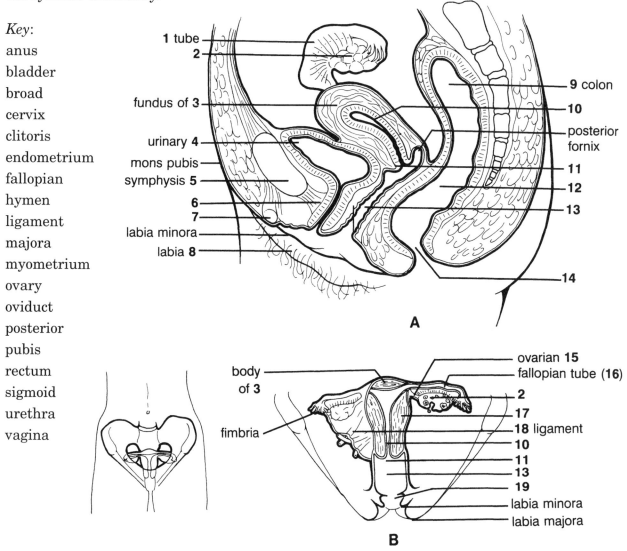

Figure 19.3 Female reproductive system. **A.** Midsagittal section of the reproductive organs of the human female. **B.** Anterior aspect of the female reproductive organs, with the left tube, ovary, and entire ureters cut away to show their internal anatomy. At the left is the position of the female reproductive organs in relation to the pelvis.

1. ______________
2. ______________
3. ______________
4. ______________
5. ______________
6. ______________
7. ______________
8. ______________
9. ______________
10. ______________
11. ______________
12. ______________
13. ______________
14. ______________
15. ______________
16. ______________
17. ______________
18. ______________
19. ______________

Exercise 19.4

Labelling. Write the name of the structure on the space provided. Colour the tissues differently.

Key:
afferent
alveolus
ampulla
areola
clavicle
fat
hypothalamus
lactiferous
lobe
muscles
nerves
nipple
pituitary
posterior
ribs

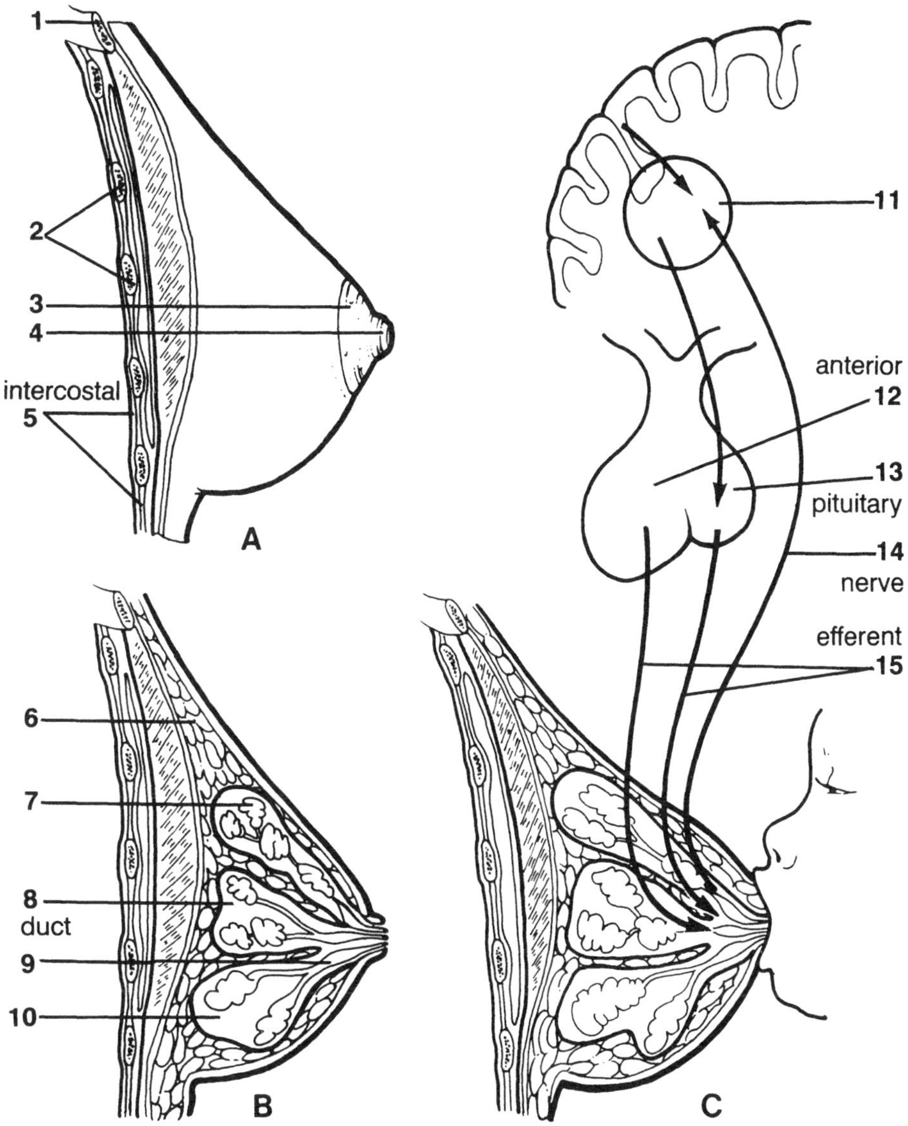

Figure 19.4 Mammary glands. **A.** and **B.** Lateral aspect and sagittal section of the mammary glands, showing the external and internal anatomy of the milk (lactiferous) glands and duct system. **C.** Lactation—The child's suckling gives rise to afferent nerve impulses, which, in turn, stimulate the mammary glands to secrete milk.

1. ____________________
2. ____________________
3. ____________________
4. ____________________
5. ____________________
6. ____________________
7. ____________________
8. ____________________
9. ____________________
10. ____________________
11. ____________________
12. ____________________
13. ____________________
14. ____________________
15. ____________________

V. TEST ITEMS

A. *Multiple Choice.* There is only one answer that is either correct or most appropriate. Circle the best answer for each question.

1. Reproduction involves several processes including those conducted by specialised sex cells called
   a. gonads
   b. gametes
   c. ovaries
   d. testicles

2. A very short duct passing through the prostate gland and then opening into the urethra is called the
   a. vas deferens
   b. spermatic cord
   c. ejaculatory duct
   d. testis

3. Circumcision is the removal of the loose-fitting skin of the penis called the
   a. urethra
   b. glans
   c. prepuce (foreskin).
   d. scrotum

4. Normally, fertilisation takes place in the upper third of the
   a. cervix
   b. ovaries
   c. uterine tubes (fallopian tubes)
   d. vagina

5. Production of an ovum each month and preparation of the uterus for pregnancy is called
   a. orgasm
   b. menstrual cycle
   c. menopause
   d. ejaculation

6. The male urethra is encircled by which structure?
   a. epididymis
   b. scrotum
   c. prostate gland
   d. seminal vesicle

7. The basic difference between spermatogenesis and oogenesis is that
   a. during spermatogenesis two more polar bodies are produced
   b. the mature ovum contains the haploid chromosome number, whereas the mature sperm contains the diploid number
   c. in oogenesis, one mature ovum is produced, and in spermatogenesis, four mature sperm are produced
   d. spermatogenesis involves mitosis and meiosis, but oogenesis involves meiosis only

8. The union of a sperm nucleus and an ovum nucleus resulting in the formation of a zygote is referred to as
   a. implantation
   b. fertilisation
   c. gestation
   d. parturition

9. After ovulation, the corpus luteum (yellow body) forms. If the ovum is not fertilised the corpus luteum degenerates, but if the ovum is fertilised, the corpus luteum persists for several months. Which hormones provide for the maintenance of the corpus luteum during the early months of pregnancy?
   a. follicle-stimulating hormone (FSH)
   b. adrenal corticotrophic hormone (ACTH)
   c. vasopressin
   d. chorionic gonadotropin

10. What is the hormone that suppresses ovulation during pregnancy?
a. luteinising hormone (LH)
b. progesterone
c. oestrogen
d. FSH

11. The male sex hormone is produced where?
a. in the interstitial cells of the testes
b. in the tubules of the testes
c. in the anterior lobe of the pituitary gland
d. in the sustentacular cells of the testes

12. After ovulation, the ruptured follicle
a. disappears, all its cells disintegrating
b. passes as waste material down the oviduct with the egg
c. mends itself and begins the maturation of another egg
d. differentiates into another temporary endocrine gland

13. The cells lying between sperm-forming cells produce a hormone called
a. oesterone
b. testosterone
c. progesterone
d. aldosterone

14. Androgens in men are produced by the
a. prostate
b. seminal vesicles
c. interstitial cells in the testes
d. pituitary

15. In humans, sperm cells are produced in the
a. interstitial tissue
b. urethra
c. seminiferous tubules
d. ductus deferens

16. Which of these is mismatched?
a. ovary–testes
b. oviduct–ductus deferens
c. uterus–epididymis
d. vagina–penis

17. Semen
a. contains many sperm in a fluid medium
b. is ejaculated during copulation
c. is used for artificial insemination
d. all of these

18. The major portion of the volume of semen is contributed by the
a. bulbourethral glands
b. testes
c. prostate gland
d. seminal vesicles

19. The chief ligament supporting the position of the uterus and keeping it from dropping into the vagina is the
a. cardinal ligament
b. round ligament
c. broad ligament
d. ovarian ligament

20. The sex chromosomes of a normal male are designated as
a. YY
b. XY
c. XX
d. none of these

B. *Matching.* Each of the phrases in Column B refers to a term in Column A. Insert the letter of the phrase from Column B that best describes each term in Column A. Some words may be used more than once or not at all.

Column A		*Column B*	
1. ___	mutation	**a.**	removal of the uterine mucous lining
2. ___	abortion	**b.**	a gene that results in embryonic death or death shortly after birth
3. ___	lethal gene	**c.**	a permanent heritable change in a gene that causes the gene to express a different trait
4. ___	autosome	**d.**	any chromosome that is not a sex chromosome
5. ___	endometrectomy	**e.**	removal of a foetus and placenta through an abdominal incision in the uterine wall
6. ___	cesarean section	**f.**	premature expulsion from the uterus of the products of contraception—embryo or nonviable foetus

Column A		*Column B*	
1. ___	Leydig cells	**a.**	suspended in the scrotum
2. ___	seminal vesicles	**b.**	contains one or more seminiferous tubules
3. ___	spermatids	**c.**	interstitial cells
4. ___	interstitial cells	**d.**	undifferentiated germ cells
5. ___	impotence	**e.**	transformed into mature spermatozoa
6. ___	testes	**f.**	the tip of the sperm
7. ___	ovum	**g.**	a supporting cell type in the testes
8. ___	acrosome	**h.**	drain into the vas deferens
9. ___	antrum	**i.**	corpora cavernosa
10. ___	castration	**j.**	frequently due to psychological problems
11. ___	Sertoli cell	**k.**	cells that secrete testosterone
12. ___	lobule	**l.**	removal of the testes
13. ___	corpus luteum	**m.**	the female germ cell
14. ___	erectile tissue	**n.**	a fluid-filled space
15. ___	spermatogonia	**o.**	follicular cells become the __________

C. *True or False.* Place a *T* or an *F* in the space provided to indicate true or false.

___ **1.** In older males, enlargement of the prostate gland may obstruct the flow of urine.

___ **2.** The inability of a male to attain or hold an erection is known as infertility.

___ **3.** Low levels of progesterone may cause painful menstruation, a condition known as amenorrhea.

___ **4.** Each duct of a seminal vesicle joins a ductus deferens to form the ejaculatory ducts that open into the prostatic portion of the urethra.

___ **5.** In males, FSH stimulates spermatogenesis and interstitial cell stimulating hormone (ISCH) stimulates the production and secretion of testosterone.

___ **6.** The greater vestibular (Bartholin's) glands lie on either side of the female urethral orifice.

___ **7.** Oestrogens are responsible for the preovulatory changes in the uterus following menstruation, and progesterone is responsible for the postovulatory (secretory) phase.

___ **8.** Ovulation is initiated by a sharp rise in LH secretion.

___ **9.** Oestrogens are secreted by the ovarian follicle, oestrogens and progesterone by the corpus luteum.

___ **10.** Spermatogenesis takes place in the epididymis.

___ **11.** Progesterone and oestrogens are secreted by the placenta after several weeks of pregnancy.

___ **12.** Oestrogens promote the growth of the alveoli of the mammary gland, and progesterone promotes the growth of the ducts.

___ **13.** The disintegration of the corpus luteum (about 10 days after ovulation) is prevented by chorionic gonadotropin.

___ **14.** Oestrogens decrease the motility of the uterus and its sensitivity to oxytocin, while progesterone has the opposite effect.

___ **15.** Destruction of the hypothalamus prevents ovulation.

___ **16.** The hypothalamus produces a hormone that travels in the blood to the anterior pituitary, causing the release of luteinising hormone.

___ **17.** During the process of meiosis, the 46 human chromosomes are separated into 23 male chromosomes and 23 female chromosomes.

___ **18.** Removal of the gonadal tissue of a male embryo prior to the sixth week of development results in the embryo developing female sexual characteristics.

___ **19.** The undifferentiated sex cells, e.g., spermatogonia, increase in number by mitosis during childhood and throughout life.

___ **20.** Mature sex cells are called gametes.

Answer Sheet—Chapter 19

Exercise 19.1

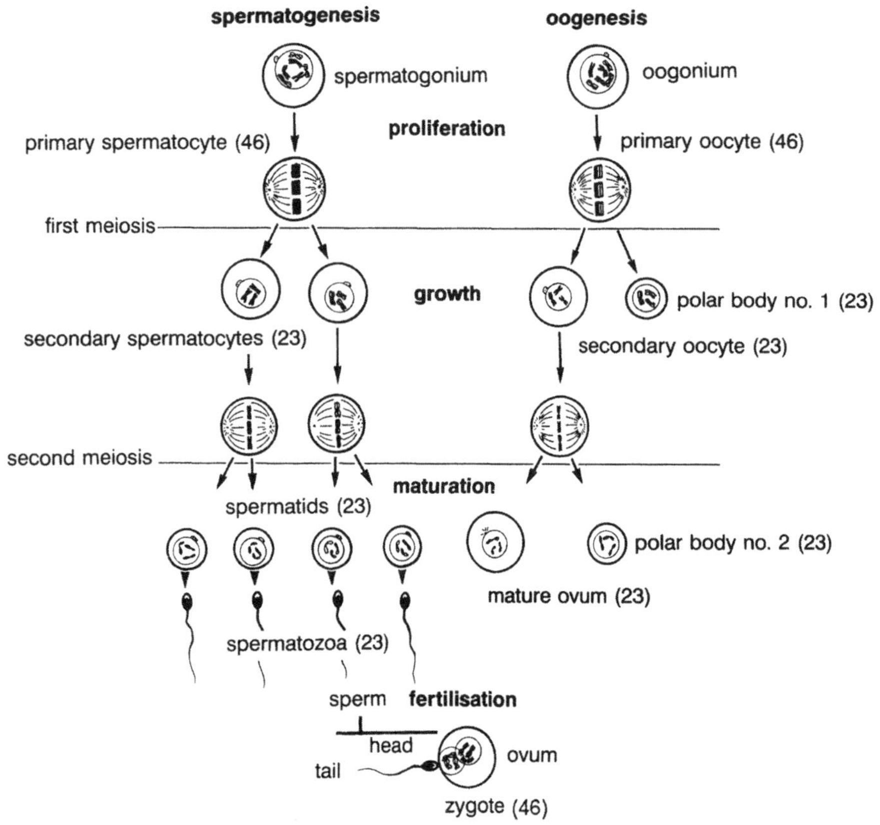

Figure 19.1 Meiosis (gametogenesis). **Left.** The various stages of spermatogenesis that give rise to four viable, mature sperm, each having 23 chromosomes. **Right.** Oogenesis, the production of a single, viable ovum (egg) and the two polar bodies from each oogenium. The union of sperm and egg (fertilisation) produces a zygote. The numbers in parentheses indicate the number of chromosomes.

Exercise 19.2

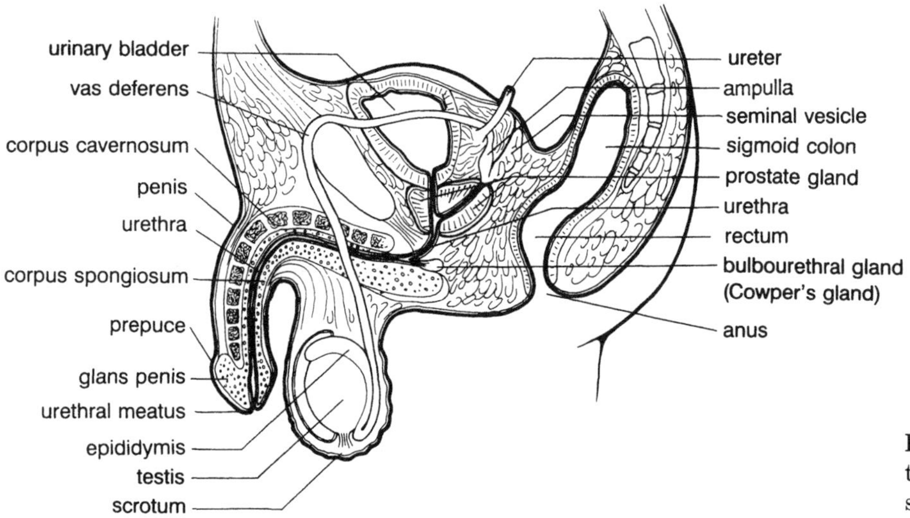

Figure 19.2 Midsagittal section of the male reproductive system.

Exercise 19.3

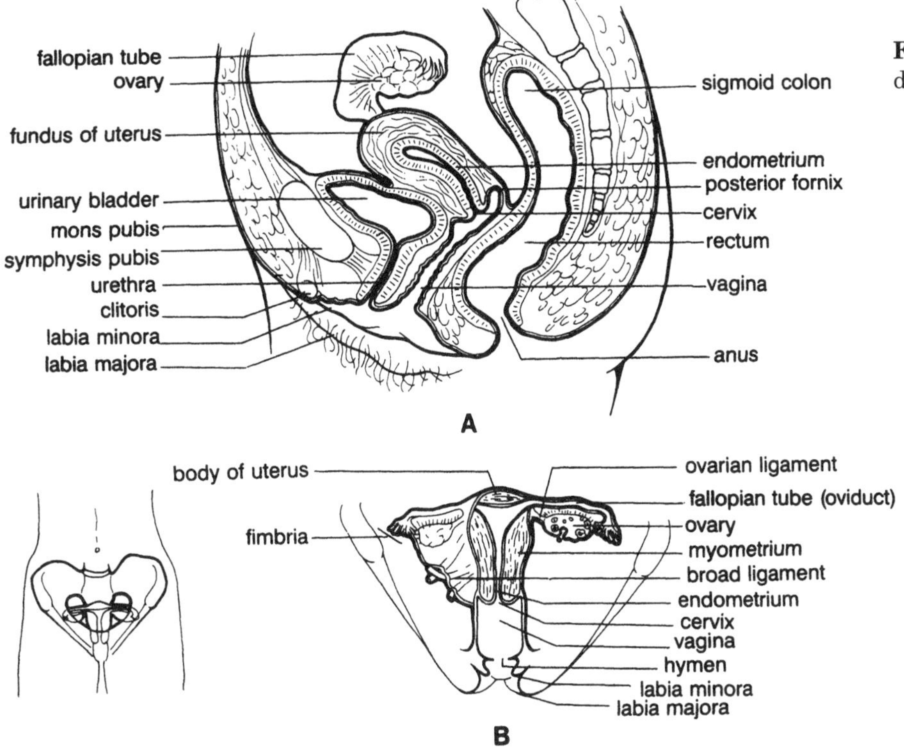

Figure 19.3 Female reproductive system.

Exercise 19.4

Figure 19.4 Mammary glands. **A.** and **B.** Lateral aspect and sagittal section of the mammary glands, showing the external and internal anatomy of the milk (lactiferous) glands and duct system. **C.** Lactation—The child's suckling gives rise to afferent nerve impulses, which, in turn, stimulate the mammary glands to secrete milk.

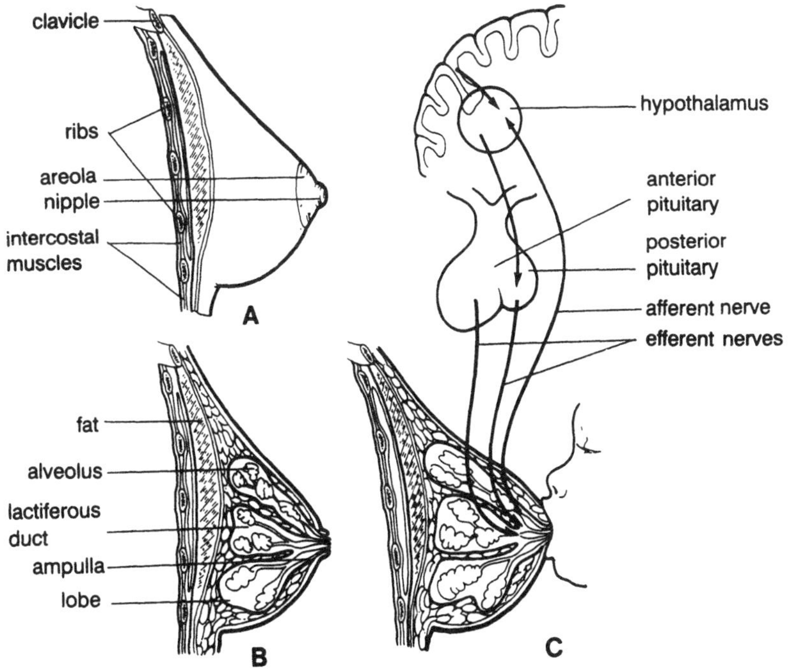

Test Items

A. 1. b, 2. c, 3. c, 4. c, 5. b, 6. c, 7. c, 8. b, 9. d, 10. b, 11. a, 12. d, 13. b, 14. c, 15. c, 16. c, 17. d, 18. d, 19. c, 20. b.

B. 1. c, 2. f, 3. b, 4. d, 5. a, 6. e.
1. c, 2. h, 3. e, 4. k, 5. j, 6. a, 7. m, 8. f, 9. n, 10. l, 11. g, 12. b, 13. o, 14. i, 15. d.

C. 1. T, 2. F, 3. F, 4. T, 5. T, 6. F, 7. T, 8. T, 9. T, 10. F, 11. T, 12. F, 13. T, 14. F, 15. T, 16. T, 17. F, 18. T, 19. T, 20. T.

Glossary

abdominal superior portion of the abdominopelvic cavity
abduction movement away from the body midline
abortion termination of a pregnancy before birth
absorbed dose amount of ionising radiation absorbed per unit of mass of irradiated material as it passes through matter
accommodation ability of the eye to focus on objects at different distances
acetylcholine neurotransmitter substance
acid any substance containing hydrogen that tends to increase the concentration of hydrogen positive ions in a water solution
acidosis disorder of body chemistry in which the hydrogen ion concentration of the blood is increased, decreasing the pH
acromegaly disease of the pituitary marked by progressive enlargement of face, hands, and feet—overproduction of somatotropin (growth hormone) by the anterior pituitary after normal growth has ceased
actin muscle protein found on the I band
active transport movement of a substance across a membrane against the concentration gradient by the expenditure of energy
adaptation adjustment to changes in the environment
adduction movement to or toward the body midline
adenohypophysis anterior pituitary gland
adenoma benign glandular tumour
adenosine triphosphate (ATP) compound of one molecule each of adenine and D-ribose with three molecules of phosphoric acid that is concerned with energy transformations in metabolism
adrenal at or on the kidney
adrenal glands glands that produce hormones, located above the kidneys
adrenergic nerve fibres that release a chemical that stimulates the sympathetic nervous system
adrenocorticotropic hormone (ACTH) a hormone produced by the anterior pituitary, which stimulates the adrenal cortex to function
aerobic reacting chemically or growing only in the presence of oxygen
afferent toward an organ or area
agglutination clumping of cells
agglutinin molecule that causes agglutination
agglutinogen antigen that causes the formation of an antibody
ageing measurement of the degree of physical maturity of a cell or individual
agranulocyte cell with a clear cytoplasm—no granules
aldosterone a hormone produced by the adrenal cortex that regulates sodium and potassium concentrations in the blood
alkaline (base) a pH over 7.0
alkalosis disorder of body chemistry in which the hydroxyl ion concentration of the blood is increased, elevating the pH
allergen substance that induces an allergic response
allergy hypersensitivity to normally harmless substances
alveolar a hollow cavity
alveolus air sacs in the lungs where exchange of gasses occurs
amphiarthroses semimovable or partially moving joints
ampulla saccular dilation of canal
anabolism constructive phase of metabolism, during which protoplasm and other complex compounds such as hormones are synthesised from simpler substances, within the cell
anaerobic chemical reaction or growth without benefit of oxygen
anaphase third stage of mitosis; chromosomes separate
androgen hormone that stimulates development of male sex characteristics
anaemia lack of blood or lack of sufficient red blood cells

anaesthetic drug that produces loss of feeling or sensation

aneurysm saclike enlargement of a blood vessel caused by a weakening of the vessel wall

angiography X-ray of vessels after injection with an opaque dye

ankylosis fixation of a joint

anorexia loss of appetite commonly associated with significant weight loss

antagonist muscle that balances the effects of another muscle

antibody specific substance formed in response to antigen that provides protection against the antigen

anticoagulant substance that prevents clotting of the blood

antidiuretic hormone (ADH) also known as vasopressin; a hormone secreted by the posterior pituitary gland that regulates water re-absorption in the kidneys

antigen substance that stimulates the production of antibodies or reacts with them

anus ring of muscle (sphincter) at the terminal portion of the large intestine

aorta the main trunk of the arterial system, emerging from the left ventricle

apex pointed portion of a conical structure, as in the apex of the lung or heart

apnoea temporary cessation of respiration

aponeuroses sheets of connective or membranous tissue, connecting muscle and the part it moves

apoplexy sudden loss of consciousness, followed by paralysis due to cerebral haemorrhage

appendicular skeleton that part of the skeleton that forms the arms and the legs (appendages) that are suspended from the central supporting frame of the axial skeleton

appendix wormlike projection opening into the cecum

arteriography X-ray of an artery after injection of a radiopaque dye

arteriole small artery

arteriosclerosis thickening, hardening, and loss of elasticity of arteries

artery vessel that carries blood away from the heart

arthritis inflammation of a joint

arthrology the science of joints

articulate to join together so as to permit motion between parts

articulation the point of union of any two bones

asphyxiation loss of consciousness due to inadequate oxygen supply; suffocation

aspiration removal of fluids or gases by suction; also, the accidental inhalation of an object into the trachea

assimilation absorption of food; constructive metabolism

association nerve fibres that link one area of the brain to another area

astigmatism faulty vision due to irregular curvature of cornea or lens

ataxia loss of the power of muscular coordination

atherosclerosis accumulation of fatty plaque in artery walls which reduces blood flow

atlas first cervical vertebra; supports the head and, with the second cervical vertebra, forms the axis of rotation of the skull

atom smallest bit of matter that can be identified

atrium receiving chamber of the heart

atrophy wasting or decrease in the size of a part of the body

audiometer instrument used to measure range of hearing

auditory pertaining to sound

auricle also known as the pinna, forms the external part of the ear

autoimmune disease antibodies act against the body's own tissue

autolysis process by which lysosomes break open within the cell, resulting in the self-digestion of the cell

autonomic nervous system independent, self-controlling

autosome first 22 pairs of human chromosomes, not involved in determining gender

axial skeleton bones of the vertebral column, thorax, and skull

axis second cervical vertebra; with the first cervical vertebra, forms the axis of rotation

axon extension from the cell body of a neuron that conducts a nerve impulse (action potential)

azotaemia excess of urea in the blood

B cells lymphocytes that produce antibodies and that are derived from bone marrow

base any substance containing a hydroxyl group that acts to increase the concentration of hydroxyl ions in a water solution

benign not a threat to life; nonmalignant

bicuspid also known as the mitral valve; a heart valve with two cusps

bilateral found on both sides of the body or a body part

bile bitter, alkaline, yellow-green fluid secreted by the liver

bilirubin orange pigment derived from haemoglobin
binocular having two eyes
biopsy examination of living tissue removed from an organism
blastula hollow ball of cells found in the early stages of prenatal human development
bolus rounded mass of soft consistency
bond force holding two atoms or ions together in a molecule
bradycardia abnormally slow heart rate usually defined as a resting heart rate below 60 bpm
brachial pertaining to the upper arm
bronchiole small tubes branching off from the bronchi
bronchus a main branch of the trachea leading to the bronchioles
buffer any substance in a fluid that tends to resist the change in pH when acid or alkali is added
bunion swollen, inflamed bursa of the large toe
bursa fluid-filled sac or space located in areas where friction may develop between moving parts, such as near joints, under muscles, and over bony projections.
bursitis inflammation or irritation of a bursa sac

calcification process of hardening caused by deposits of calcium compound
calcitonin hormone produced by the thyroid gland that is involved in calcium homeostasis
calculi stones formed within a body part
callus hard substance formed between fragments of broken bone or a hardened area of skin that forms when the skin is subjected to increased friction
calorie unit of heat; calorie (cal.) is the standard unit and is the amount of heat required to raise 1 g of water from 15°C to 16°C
calyx small cavity in the kidney
canal narrow tubular passage or channel
cancellous sponge-like material
cancer malignant neoplasm
capillary small vessels connecting arterioles and venules
carbohydrate organic compound containing carbon, hydrogen, and oxygen that is used as the major energy source of the body
carcinoma malignant tumour of epithelial or glandular tissue
cardiac pertaining to the heart
cardiac muscle branching involuntary muscle tissue found in the myocardium of the heart
caries tooth decay
catabolism the breaking-down process of metabolism, during which complex substances are converted into simpler compounds within the cells
cataract loss of transparency of the crystalline lens of the eye or of its capsule
catecholamine amine compounds such as epinephrine (adrenaline) and norepinephrine (nor-adrenaline) act to stimulate the sympathetic nervous system
celiac relating to the abdominal cavity
centriole organelle involved with moving chromosomes during cell division
centromere constricted part of the chromosome to which the spindle fibres attach during mitosis and meiosis
cerebrovascular blood supply to the brain
cerebrovascular accident (CVA) medical term for stroke caused by either a blockage in or rupturing of a cerebral blood vessel
cerumen earwax
cervical refers to the neck or the ring of muscle at the neck of the uterus (womb)
chemoreceptor receptors sensitive to chemical stimuli
chemotherapy treatment of disease by means of various chemicals
cholecyst gallbladder
cholinergic nerve fibres or receptors that release or interact with the neurotransmitter acetylcholine
cholinesterase an enzyme that causes the breakdown of acetylcholine
choroid middle layer of the eye that helps prevent internal reflection of light
chromatin nucleic acid and protein substance that make up a chromosome
chromosome gene-containing filamentous structure in a cell nucleus
chyle milky fluid taken up by the lacteals from the food in the intestine after digestion; it consists of lymph and emulsified fat
chyme semifluid mass of partly digested food passed from the stomach into the duodenum
circumduction circular movement of a part
circumflex posterior portion of the left coronary artery
cirrhosis pathological change that usually involves the deposition of fibrous scar tissue in an organ e.g. the liver
cisterna enclosed space

cleavage splitting of a molecule or fertilised egg during cell division
clonus spasm in which a muscle contracts and relaxes alternately
coagulation clotting
coarctation abnormal narrowing of the aorta
cochlear snail-like portion of the inner ear concerned with hearing
codon three adjacent nucleotides coding a specific amino acid
coenzyme nonprotein substance that activates an enzyme
coitus sexual intercourse
collagen chief structural protein of skin and connective tissue
collateral side branches of an axon
colostrum first fluid secreted from the mother's breast following childbirth rich in antibodies that are important for immunity in early infancy
colposcopy vaginal examination
coma state of profound unconsciousness from which one cannot be roused
comedo blackhead
commissure groups of nerve fibres connecting opposite corresponding portions of the central nervous system
communicans connecting neurons in the cerebrum
compact hard and dense portion of bone
compound substance in which the molecules are composed of two or more different elements
computerised fluoroscopy computerised analysis of direct examination of the body using a fluoroscope
computerised tomography (CT) cross-sectional X-ray utilising a computer for analysis
concave curved inward
concentration gradient difference in concentration between two areas
concha bones of the nasal septum
conductance transmittance of an impulse from one point to another
conduction transmission of energy from one point to another
condyle rounded projection
cones photoreceptors in the eyes responsible for detailed vision and colour
conjunctivitis inflammation of the conjunctivia
connective tissue supporting tissue of the body
constipation decreased bowel action that results in progressive collection of faecal material in the colon
contractility ability of a muscle to become short and thick
contraction shortening of a structure
convex curved outward
convulsion involuntary contraction or series of contractions of voluntary muscles
copulation sexual intercourse
cornea anterior transparent portion of the eye
corneum outer layer of the epidermis
coronary pertaining to the blood vessels that supply blood to the heart muscle (myocardium)
corpus pertaining to a body or structure
cortex outer portion of an organ
Corti inner canal of the cochlea concerned with hearing
cortisone long term steroid stress hormone produced by the adrenal cortex
covalent bond sharing of electrons by two atoms in a chemical compound
cranial pertaining to the head
creatine phosphate (CP) an intermediate source of energy in muscle contraction
crenation shriveling of a cell due to the passage of its fluid into the surrounding medium
crest ridge surrounding a bone or its border
cross-bridges extensions of the A-bands in muscle
cryptorchidism failure of the testes to descend into the scrotum
curie unit of radioactivity
cutaneous skin
cyanosis dark, bluish appearance of the skin, lips, and nails due to inadequate oxygenation of the blood
cystoscope instrument used to examine the inside of the bladder
cytoplasm region of a cell between the nuclear envelope and plasma membrane where most organelles are located

deafness impairment or defect in ability to hear sounds
deamination removal of an amino group from a substance
defaecation expulsion of faecal matter from the bowel
defibrillator device to correct ventricular fibrillation
deglutition swallowing
dehydration inadequate water content in the body tissues
dementia deterioration of intellectual function
dendrite extension of a nerve body that conducts an impulse toward the nerve body

deoxyribonucleic acid (DNA) nucleic acid that stores the genetic blueprint; found in the nucleus and in small amounts in the mitochondria of cells
dermatitis inflammation of the skin
dermatosis general term for any skin disorder
dermis connective tissue layer under the epidermis; the location of structural components of the skin such as hair follicles, sweat glands and blood vessels
dextroposition out of position
dialysis separation of crystalloids from colloids in solution by using a selectively permeable membrane
diapedesis passage of blood cells, especially white cells (leukocytes), through the intact blood vessel walls
diaphysis shaft of a long bone
diarrhoea abnormally liquid discharges from the bowels
diarthroses joint that permits free movement
diastole rhythmic period of relaxation and dilation of the heart
dichromatic having two-colour vision instead of three-colour vision
diffusion passage of a liquid or gas from a region of greater concentration of its molecules to a region of lesser concentration of its molecules
diplopia double vision
dislocation displacement of a limb or organ from its original position
distal farthest away from a point
diureses increased urine output
diverticulum outpouching from a main tubular structure or organ cavity
dominant trait that will always be expressed
dorsal pertaining to the back; posterior
dose rate radiation dose delivered per unit of time, usually roentgens per minute
dosimeter device that measures radiation exposure (e.g., film badge, ionisation chamber, Geiger counter)
duct a bypass tube connecting two structures
dysfunction impaired function
dysmenorrhoea painful menstruation
dysphagia difficulty in swallowing
dyspnoea difficult or labored breathing
dystrophy degenerative disease of the body tissues
dysuria painful urination

ectopic out of the normal place
efferent away from an organ
ejaculation ejection of semen
elasticity ability to be stretched and return to normal shape
electrocardiogram (ECG) graphic record of the electrical activity of the heart muscle
electrolyte solution containing free ions and, therefore, having the ability to conduct an electrical current
electromagnetic ionising radiations that have energy only
electron particle in motion outside the nucleus of an atom that carries a negative charge
elements substances that cannot be decomposed or transformed by chemical means
elephantiasis poor lymphatic drainage commonly caused by parasitic worm infestation that blocks lymphatic vessels leading to severe swelling and enlargement of limbs and organs
embolism solid mobile debris in the blood, commonly a clot, fatty plaque or a bone fragment that can cause a blockage and obstruct blood flow
eminence prominence or projection
emphysema dilation of the pulmonary air vesicles, usually through atrophy of the septa between the alveoli
emulsification process by which bile lowers the surface tensions of fat inducing the breakup of large fat globules into tiny fat droplets
endocardium inner layer of the heart
endochondral within cartilage
endocrine a ductless gland that produces hormones
endocrine glands ductless glands that release their secretions (hormones) directly into the blood
endometriosis proliferation of endometrial tissue outside of the uterus
endoplasmic reticulum interconnected flattened membranes within the cytoplasm of a cell
endorphin peptide involved in pain inhibition
endoscope instrument used to look inside hollow organs
endoskeleton internal supporting bony framework
endothelial innermost tissue layer of a blood vessel
endothermic characterised by the storage of energy
energy power exercised with vigor
enkephalin peptide found in the brain and involved in pain inhibition

enteric pertaining to the intestines
enzyme organic catalyst; made in a cell
epicardium outer layer of the heart
epicondyle projection above a condyle
epidermis outer layer of the skin
epigastric area of the abdomen above the umbilicus
epiglottis one of the cartilaginous portions of the larynx that functions as a "trap door" and closes over the airway during swallowing
epimysium sheath of connective tissue surrounding individual muscles
epinephrine (adrenaline) hormone that stimulates the sympathetic nervous system
epineurium connective tissue covering of a bundle of nerve bundles
epiphysis ends of long bones
epistaxis nosebleed
epithelium nonvascular cellular layer that covers the internal and external surfaces of the body
equilibrium state of balance, resulting in a stable system
erythema redness of the skin
erythrocyte a red blood cell
erythropoiesis manufacture of red blood cells
eupnoea normal, easy respiration
eustachian hollow tube connecting the middle ear with the nasopharynx
eversion turning a body part outward away from the body midline
excitability ability to respond to a stimulus
excretia discharged natural waste
excretion separation and removal of substances by the cell
exocrine epithelial gland secreting material to the outside using ducts
exocrine glands glands that release their secretions into ducts
exoskeleton external supporting bony framework
exothermic characterised by the release of energy
expiration movement of air out of the lungs
extensibility ability of a muscle to be stretched
extension straightening a limb or body part
exteroceptors nerve endings that detect environmental changes that directly affect the skin
extracellular area outside a cell
extracorporeal outside the body
extrasystole premature contraction of heart muscle
extrinsic originating from the outside

facet small flat surface
familial affecting several members of the same family
fascia sheet of connective tissue
fasciculus small bundle of nerve fibres or muscle cells
fat group of organic molecules also termed lipids which includes triglycerides, phospholipids and steroids
fatigue inability to respond to a stimulus
feedback a regulatory system detecting changes in homeostasis
fertilisation union of the ovum and sperm
fetus name given to a developing human organism after the second month of pregnancy
fibrillation uncoordinated contractions of individual muscle fibres
fibrositis inflammation of connective tissue
filtrate liquid that has passed through a membrane or filter
filtration passage of a liquid through a filter or membrane by a force that is exerted on the mixture
fissure relatively deep cleft or groove
flaccid flabby, soft
flare diffuse redness of the skin, surrounding an injured or pressured point
flexion bending a limb or body part
flutter fast, irregular motion
follicle-stimulating hormone (FSH) pituitary hormone that stimulates the enlargement of ovarian follicles (sacs containing ova) in females and the maturation of sperm cells in males
fontanel unossified area between cranial bones
foramen natural opening or passage
fossa trench or channel, which denotes a hollow or depressed area
fovea a depression in the retina of the eye
fracture broken bone
frontal a plane dividing the body into anterior and posterior sections

gamete sexual haploid cell produced by meiosis
gamma ray electromagnetic radiation that originates from a radioactive nucleus and causes ionisation in matter
ganglion aggregation of nerve cells within the brain, along the course of a sensory nerve
gastrulation formation of the third embryonic germ layer
gene unit of heredity located in the chromosome and made mostly of DNA
glands secreting organs or tissues

glaucoma disease characterised by abnormally high pressure within the eye, resulting in blindness
glomerulus small coil of blood capillaries that sits inside Bowman's capsule
glottis opening of the trachea
glucagon hormone that stimulates the breakdown of glycogen in the liver to increase blood glucose
glucocorticoids steroid hormones such as cortisol that stimulate production of glucose from noncarbohydrate sources
gluconeogenesis formation of glucose from noncarbohydrate sources
glycocalyx carbohydrate-rich outer covering on the surface of cells
glycogenesis formation of glycogen from simple sugars
glycogenolysis breakdown of glycogen into simple sugars
glycoprotein carbohydrate–protein compound; a conjugated protein
glycosuria presence of glucose in urine
goiter enlargement of the thyroid
Golgi apparatus cellular organelle responsible for refining proteins and preparing material for export out of cells
granulocyte cell with granules in the cytoplasm
grey ramus nonmyelinated nerve fibres of the autonomic nervous system
growth hormone (GH) interior pituitary hormone that stimulates skeletal and soft tissue growth before maturity also known as somatostatin
gustation sense of taste
gyrus smooth surface of an organ

half-life time (specific for each radioactive substance) required for radioactive material to decay to half its initial activity
helical spiral
haematocrit formed element content of the blood
haematopoietic producing blood cells
haemodialysis removal of wastes from blood through a semipermeable membrane
haemodynamics forces connected with circulation of blood
haemoglobin an iron-protein compound that carries gases in the blood
haemolysis disintegration of red blood cells that results in the appearance of haemoglobin in the surrounding fluid
haemopoietic blood producing
haemophilia sex-linked, hereditary disease characterised by prolonged coagulation time and abnormal bleeding
haemorrhage bleeding through vessel walls
haemostasis checking flow of blood through any part of the body
heparin an anticoagulant produced by the liver and by mast cells and basophils
hepatic pertaining to the liver
hermaphroditism condition of having both male and female sex organs
hernia weakened opening in the abdominal wall
hilus an opening of an organ
histamine inflammatory mediator produced predominantly by mast cells and basophils which triggers vasodilation (vasodilatation)
histocompatibility tolerance of host tissue to donor or foreign tissue, such as occurs in transplants
Hodgkin's a form of lymphatic cancer
homeostasis consistency and uniformity of the internal body environment, which maintains normal body functions
hormone chemical substance produced in one organ, which, when carried to another organ by the circulation, stimulates the latter organ to functional activity
hyaline glossy membrane found in the newborn lung
hydrocortisone steroid hormone with anti-inflammatory effects
hydronephrosis accumulation of urine in the kidney due to an obstruction
hydrophilic affinity for water
hydrophobic tending to repel water
hydrostatic pressure pressure created by fluid content
hyperactive marked by increased activity or overactiveness
hypercapnia high carbon dioxide content of the air or blood
hyperaemia swelling due to increased blood supply
hyperglycaemia excess of sugar in the blood
hyperkalaemia elevated potassium concentration in the blood
hypermenorrhea prolonged menstruation
hyperopia farsightedness
hyperplasia increased size of an organ or tissue
hyperpnoea increased breathing rate and depth of breathing
hypertension elevated blood pressure

hypertonic property of higher osmotic pressure than some other solutions
hypertrophy increase in size of a tissue or organ
hypoactive marked by diminished activity or underactivity
hypochondriac upper outer regions of the abdomen
hypogastric positioned below the stomach region
hypoglycaemia deficiency of sugar in the blood
hypophysis pituitary gland
hypothalamic pertaining to the hypothalamus
hypothalamus part of the brain located under the thalamus
hypotonic property of lower osmotic pressure than some other solutions
hypoxia insufficient oxygen in the body tissues

iliac pertaining to the upper thigh region
immunity properties of the host that protect it from foreign agents
immunodeficiency disease disease due to failure of some immune function
immunoglobulin antibody against a particular antigen; humoral immunity
immunosuppression use of drugs to weaken immune response
incontinence inability to control the passage of urine or faeces
incus middle ear bone
infarction death of tissue due to loss of blood supply
infectious capable of producing disease in a susceptible host
inferior toward the foot
inflammation a series of normal physiological reactions in the body caused by injury, microorganisms or irritants and marked by redness and swelling of the affected area
inguinal lower outer region of the abdomen
inhibit to stop
insertion attachment of a muscle to the more movable bone
inspiration active mechanism by which air is taken into the lungs
insulin hormone produced by the beta cells of the pancreas which stimulates glucose uptake by cells and reduces blood glucose
integument covering, especially the skin
intercellular inside a cell
intercostals between the ribs
interferon protein produced by virally infected cells
internuncial microscopic horizontal neurons of the spinal cord
interoceptors receptors within organs concerned with maintenance of the internal environment
interphase longest period of the cell cycle; the period between active cell division
interstitial between cells
interstitial cell-stimulating hormone (ICSH) pituitary hormone that stimulates androgen production in the testes also known as luteinising hormone (LH)
intoxication pathological state produced by a drug, serum, alcohol, or any toxic substance
intrapulmonary space within the alveolar sacs
intrathoracic space in the thoracic cavity between the pleura
intrinsic pertaining to an internal activation process
intussusception infolding of one segment of the intestine within another segment
inversion turning a body part toward the body midline
involuntary performed without free will
ion charged particle
ionisation production of ions from neutral atoms or compounds
iris coloured portion of the eye
ischaemia lack of blood in an area of the body
isometric contraction of a muscle without shortening its length
isotonic condition of equal osmotic pressure between two different solutions
isotope element that has the same atomic number as another but a different atomic weight

jaundice yellowness of skin and eyes
joint point of connection between two or more bones

keratin tough fibrous protein produced by keratinocytes
kinesthetic referring to the ability to sense movement
kyphosis increased curvature of the thoracic spine, giving a hunchback appearance

lactation secretion of milk by the mammary glands
lacteal one-celled vessel of the lymphatic system
lactogenic hormone (prolactin) pituitary hormone that stimulates milk production
lacuna small hollow, depression or pit
lamina thin, flat layer in a portion of tissue, consisting of layers of cells; also a flat plate; e.g., the laminae of vertebrae

larynx medical/anatomical term for the voice-box
lateral toward the side of the body
leukaemia disease of the blood-forming tissues marked by increase in the number of leukocytes (leukocytosis)
leukocyte (leucocyte) white blood cell
leukocytosis increase in the number of leukocytes caused by the host body's response to an injury or infection
leukopaenia decrease in the number of leukocytes
leucorrhoea vaginal discharge other than blood
ligament band of fibrous tissue, connecting bones and strengthening joints
lingual referring to the tongue
lipid fat, oil, or their derivatives
loop a curved tube
lordosis forward curvature of the lumbar spine
lumbar refers to the lower back
luteinising hormone (LH) pituitary hormone that stimulates formation of the corpus luteum in the ovary and production of testosterone in the testes of men
lymph fluid that circulates within the lymphatic system
lymph nodes oval structures located along a lymphatic vessel that filter foreign matter
lymphangiogram injection of an opaque dye into a vein for X-ray purposes
lymphatic pertaining to lymph nodes
lymphokines soluble substances produced by lymphocytes that can affect other cells
lymphoma proliferation of lymphatic tissue
lysis rupture of a cell
lysosome an organelle containing digestive enzymes

macrocyte large cell
macrophage large phagocytic cell derived from blood cells termed monocytes responsible for trapping foreign material
malignant referring to disorders that tend to worsen and cause death
malleolus hammer-shaped protuberance
malleus outermost bone of the middle ear
mastectomy removal of breast tissue
mastication act of chewing food
matrix intercellular substance of a tissue
medial toward the middle of the body
mediastinum central cavity within the thorax between the right and left lung
medulla inner core of a structure; brain stem
medullary centrally located soft tissue
meiosis special method of cell division, occurring during the development of sex cells (ova and sperm) in which the number of chromosomes is halved from the diploid number of 46 to the haploid number of 23
melanin dark pigment found in skin, hair, and retina
melanocyte pigment cell of the skin that produces melanin
melanocyte-stimulating hormone (MSH) a pituitary hormone that regulates melanin production in the skin
menarche first episode of menstrual bleeding occurring in early puberty in females
meninges three membranes that envelop the brain and the spinal cord
menopause period of life when menstruation normally ceases; change of life
menorrhagia excessive menstrual flow
menorrhalgia painful menstruation
menstruation monthly event characterised by a bloody discharge from the uterus
mesenchyme embryonic connective tissue
messenger transmits information between structures
metabolism physical and chemical processes by which living organisms produce the necessary energy to maintain life
metaphase third phase of mitosis; chromosomes line up in pairs
metric relating to the meter as a basis of measurement
metrorrhagia irregular bleeding from the uterus
microcyte small cell
microfilament a slender rod-like structure in a cell
microtubule a slender hollow structure in a cell
micturition urination
midsagittal a middle plane dividing the body into right and left segments
mineralocorticoids steroidal hormones produced by the adrenal cortex that help regulate electrolytes such as sodium and potassium
mitochondria organelles responsible for cellular respiration and the formation of the energy storage molecule adenosine triphosphate (ATP)
mitosis normal cell division where the diploid number of 46 chromosomes is maintained
mixture two or more substances that are not chemically combined
molecule smallest unit of a particular substance formed from two or more atoms
monochromatic having only one-colour vision

monosomy when one of a pair of homologous chromosomes is missing
mosaic inlaid network of pattern of small pieces
motor action
motor end plate axonic terminals of motor neurons also known as a neuromuscular junction
motor unit that which produces movement
mucin substance secreted by mucous membranes that contains mucopolysaccharides
mucoprotein compound composed of proteins and mucopolysaccharides
murmur abnormal sound indicating a pathological condition of the heart valve
muscle contractile electrochemical tissue that exists in three forms: skeletal (striated), cardiac and smooth
myalgia muscle pain or aching
myelin fatty protective sheath around a nerve that speeds up conduction of nerve impulses (action potentials)
myelocytic produced in the bone marrow
myeloma tumour found in the bone marrow
myocardium middle layer of the heart that is composed of cardiac muscle
myofibril contractile fibres within a muscle fibre
myopathy any disease of the muscles
myometrium the middle layer of the uterus (womb) composed of smooth muscle
myopia nearsightedness
myosin muscle protein found on the A-bands
myositis inflammation of a muscle

nasopharynx part of the pharynx above the soft palate
necrosis tissue death, usually in a localised area
neoplasm new growth; a tumour
nephron functional unit of the kidney
nerve fibre extension of the nerve body
neuralgia severe pain along the course of a nerve
neuritis inflammation along a nerve
neurofibril microscopic part of a nerve
neuroglia supporting cells to the nervous system
neurohypophysis posterior portion of the pituitary gland
neurilemma outer protective membrane of a neuron
neuron basic functional unit of the nervous system
neurosecretory secretion of hormones by neurons
neurotransmitter chemical substance able to transmit an impulse between two structures
neutron particle found in the nucleus of an atom that does not carry a charge; neutral
nodes of Ranvier a gap in the myelin covering of an axon
norepinephrine (noradrenaline) hormone that stimulates the sympathetic nervous system
nucleic acid one of a class of molecules composed of joined nucleotide complexes; the principal types are deoxyribonucleic acid (DNA) and ribonucleic acid (RNA)
nucleolus an organelle in the nucleus that synthesises ribosomal RNA (rRNA) which is used to synthesise ribosomes
nucleoplasm living substance in the nucleus
nutrition utilisation of food for growth
nystagmus involuntary side-to-side movements of the eyes

obesity excess fat
occlusion closing of an opening or passage
oedema swelling caused by accumulation of excess fluid
oestrogens hormones that stimulate development of female sex characteristics
oncology study and treatment of tumours
oncotic pertaining to water pressure
oncotic pressure osmotic pressure exerted by colloids
oocyte ovum or egg cell
oogenesis process of formation of ova or egg cells
ophthalmoscope instrument used to visualise the retina
opsonisation combination of antibody and antigen that makes them susceptible to phagocytosis
optic pertaining to the eye; vision
organelle tiny specific region of living material present in most cells and serving a specific function in the cell
orgasm culmination or climax of sexual intercourse
origin attachment of a muscle to the less movable bone
oropharynx part of the pharynx in the back of the mouth
osmosis passage of molecules of a pure solvent, such as water, from a region of lesser solute concentration to a region of greater solute concentration across a selectively (semi) permeable membrane
osseous bony or bonelike
ossification process of forming bone or the conversion of fibrous tissue, or cartilage, into bone

osteoblast young bone-forming cell
osteoclast cell that absorbs bone tissue
osteocyte mature bone cell
osteogenic derived from bone
otoliths calcium carbonate masses of the inner ear
ovaries female reproductive organ that produces ova and hormones
ovulation explosive release of an ovum from an ovarian follicle midway through the menstrual cycle
ovum female sex gamete
oxygenated to infuse with oxygen
oxytocin hormone produced by the posterior pituitary gland that stimulates smooth muscle contraction of the uterus initiating childbirth (parturition) and promotes bonding behaviour

palsy loss or impairment of nerve or muscle function
pancreas abdominal gland that secretes enzymes for digestion and hormones that regulate carbohydrate metabolism and appetite
papilla any small projection or elevation
paralysis loss of muscle function; inability to move
parasympathetic conservative branch of the autonomic nervous system most active when the body is relaxed
parathyroid glands a set of small glands behind the thyroid that produce a hormone to regulate calcium levels in the blood
parietal pertaining to the outer wall of a cavity
particles small portions of matter
particulate radiation pertaining to having small particles that emit energy
parturition birth
pathogenic capable of producing disease
peduncle a stalk-like attachment
pelvic bowl-like area in the lower abdominal cavity
pepsin enzyme produced in the stomach responsible for chemical breakdown of proteins
perfusion passage of fluid through the vessels of an organ
pericardium protective combination membrane surrounding the heart consisting of an outer fibrous layer and a serous inner layer that produces pericardial fluid which surrounds and lubricates the beating heart
perichondrium fibrous membrane, covering cartilage
periosteum fibrous membrane covering bone tissue
peripheral towards the outer regions of the body
peristalsis rhythmical waves of smooth muscle contractions
peritoneum large serous membrane that lines the abdominal cavity and is reflected over the organs within the abdominal cavity
permeability the extent to which molecules of various kinds can pass through cellular membranes
permeable membrane that allows passage of all particles
phagocytosis process by which a cell engulfs and digests a particle or substance
phosphocreatine source of energy found in muscle
photon unit of energy of a light wave
photoreceptor receptor sensitive to visible light
phrenic nerve controlling the diaphragm
pigmentation coloration by deposition of pigments
pineal gland cone-shaped gland in the middle of the brain that produces melatonin, which inhibits secretions of male sex hormones and is important in regulating the sleep/wake cycle
pinocytosis process by which a cell engulfs and digests a droplet of liquid
pituitary gland almond-shaped gland at the base of the brain that produces hormones that regulate many body functions
placebo chemical substance given in place of medication
placenta organ within the uterus through which the fetus derives its nourishment
plasmalemma flexible cell membrane
platelet also known as thrombocytes, platelets are fragments of much larger cells termed megakaryocytes and play a key role in blood clotting
pleura membrane covering the lungs
pleurisy inflammation of the pleura
plexus network or tangle of interweaving nerves, veins, or lymphatic vessels
pneumonia inflammation of the lungs
pneumotaxic breathing control centre of the pons
pneumothorax air in the thoracic cavity
polycythaemia abnormally large number of red blood cells (erythrocytes)
polymerise process of joining small compounds to form a compound of high molecular weight
polyuria abnormally large quantity of urine
pore an opening in a membrane

portal an opening or entrance
postganglionic distal to or after a ganglion
precipitation conversion of a soluble substance to an insoluble substance
preganglionic the first neuron fibre in the autonomic nervous system structure prior to (before) a ganglion
presbyopia difficulty focusing on close objects such as text in a book, caused by age-related thickening and loss of flexibility in the lens, typically corrected by reading spectacles
pressoreceptors receptors sensitive to mechanical stimuli
process prominence or projection
progestin hormone of the ovary that stimulates uterine (endometrial) development
prolactin hormone of the pituitary that stimulates milk secretion
proliferation production of new cells
pronation moving the arm so that the palm of the hand is facing backward
prophase second phase of mitosis; nuclear membrane dissolves
proprioceptors receptors that provide the body with information about its position in space
prostaglandin family of lipid derived local hormones (autocoids) that have multiple functions
protein complex nitrogenous compound of high molecular weight
proton particle found in the nucleus of an atom, carrying a positive charge
protoplasm living part of a cell, including the nucleus, cytoplasm,and organelles
protraction movement of the jaw forward
proximal closest to the trunk of the body
pruritus itching
pseudostratified a false layered effect
pulmonary pertaining to the lungs
pulse rhythmic pressure waves that can be felt in the major arteries and which correspond to the ventricular contraction (systole) of the heart and the ejection of blood
pupil opening of the iris
Purkinje microscopic nerve fibres in the heart
pustule small, pus-containing elevation on the skin
pyloric distal opening of the stomach
pyogenic producing pus
pyramid microscopic collection of nephrons in the kidney

radiation emission and projection of energy
radiation therapy medical specialty of treatment with ionising radiations
radical atom or molecule that is usually highly reactive
radioactive pertaining to atoms of elements that undergo spontaneous transformation, resulting in emission of radiation
radiography photographic film produced by X-ray
radioisotope radioactive isotope of an element
radioresistance resistance of cells to radiation
radiosensitivity responsiveness of cells to radiation
ramus branch
receptor sensory nerve ending that responds to stimuli
recessive trait that is masked by dominant genes and only expressed if dominant genes are not present
reflex an involuntary response to a stimulus
refraction bending of light rays
releasing factors hormonelike chemicals that stimulate a gland to release its hormone into the bloodstream
renal pertaining to the kidney
respiration a physical and chemical process in which an organism takes in oxygen, uses it to produce energy, and releases a waste product—carbon dioxide
response reaction to a stimulus
resuscitation restoration to consciousness after respiration has ceased
reticulum a fine network of material
retina innermost layer of the eye where photoreceptor cells termed rods and cones are present
retraction moving of the jaw backward
retroperitoneal located behind the peritoneum
rhodopsin photoreceptor chemical of the rods in the eye
ribonucleic acid (RNA) single stranded nucleic acid chain
ribosome cellular organelle that produces proteins
rods photoreceptors in the eyes involved in detection of faint light
rotation movement around a vertical axis
rugae folds of the empty stomach

saphenous superficial vessels of the leg
sarcolemma cell membrane of a muscle cell
sarcoma malignant tumour of connective tissue
sarcomere structural and functional unit of a myofibril
sarcoplasm specialised endoplasmic reticulum of muscle cells and fibres
sclera outer protective layer of the eye

scoliosis lateral curvature of the spine
sebum oily secretion of sebaceous gland that acts as a natural conditioner to the skin and hair follicles
seizure attack of convulsions
semen ejaculatory fluid, consisting of sperm cells and secretions of the prostrate and bulbourethral glands and seminal vesicles
semipermeable permitting the passage of some particles (molecules) and not others
sense organ any organ of special sense
sensory transmission of impulses to the brain and nervous system
septum partition
sesamoid seedlike bone
sex chromosomes the final 23rd pair of human chromosomes that determine physical gender, typically XX for female or XY for male
shock acute peripheral failure of blood circulation
sinoatrial node (SAN) the heart's natural pacemaker
sinus cavity or hollow space
sinusoid deep depression for veins
skeletal muscle a striated, voluntary muscle that is usually attached to bones
smooth muscle unstriated, involuntary muscle found in organs and blood vessels
solute substance that can be dissolved in a solvent to form a solution
solvent vehicle capable of dissolving a solute to form a solution
somatic pertaining to body cells
somesthetic bodily awareness
spasm involuntary, convulsive muscular contraction
sperm male sex gametes
spermatogenesis process of formation and development of the spermatozoa
sphincter circular muscle at an opening of an organ
sphygmomanometer instrument for measuring arterial blood pressure
spinal pertaining to nerves in the vertebral column
spine thornlike process or projection
splenomegaly enlarged spleen
sprain joint injury, resulting from wrenching or twisting
squamous scalelike (thin and flat)
stapes innermost bone of the middle ear
stenosis narrowing of an opening, duct, or canal
steroid lipid molecules synthesised from cholesterol
sterol unsaturated alcohol
stethoscope device used to measure or detect sounds
stimulus irritant or excitant
strabismus squinting
stratified having layers of tissue
stratum layer
stretch receptors sensory receptors that recognise mechanical distention
stroke blockage in or haemorrhage from a cerebral blood vessel that deprives the affected region of the brain of oxygen and usually results in brain damage
subcutaneous located beneath the skin
substrate any substance acted upon by an enzyme
sulcus depression or separation
supination moving the arm so that the palm of the hand is facing forward
suppuration formation of pus
suture junction line between two immovable bones
sympathetic part of the autonomic nervous system that prepares the body for action
symphysis partially movable joint between two bones
synapse region where parts of two neurons are anatomically related so that impulses are transmitted from one neuron to another
synarthroses immovable joints between two bones
syncytium mass of cytoplasm with several nuclei
synergist two or more structures or chemicals that work together
synovial of or pertaining to synovia
synovial fluid the lubricating liquid found in the cavities of articular (movable) joints
systole contraction of the heart muscle

T cells lymphocytes that mature in the thymus gland before being released into the general circulation
tachycardia excessively fast heart rate usually defined as a resting heart rate above 100 bpm
target a tissue with specific receptors
taste buds receptors for taste on the tongue
teleceptors nerve endings that detect environmental changes occurring some distance from the body
telophase final phase of mitosis
tendon connective tissue that connects muscle to bone

tenosynovitis inflammation of the sheath around a tendon
testes male reproductive organs that produce sperm and hormones
testosterone steroid male sex hormone derived from cholesterol
tetany intermittent tonic muscular contractions of the extremities
thermodynamics concerned with heat and its conversion to other forms of energy
thoracic refers to the thorax
thorax the chest
thrombocyte a blood clotting platelet
thrombocytopenia lack of platelets, causing haemorrhages
thrombophlebitis condition in which inflammation of the vein wall has preceded the formation of a thrombus or intravascular clot
thrombus blood clot
thymus gland major lymphoid organ located on the superior (top) portion of the heart that plays a key role in programming the immune system to recognise "self" in infancy, gradually atrophies (shrinks) with age
thyroid gland gland found in the neck that produces hormones that regulate metabolism and calcium homeostasis
thyroid-stimulating hormone (TSH) hormone from the anterior pituitary gland that controls the release of thyroid hormones
thyrotropin hormone from the pituitary that stimulates the growth and function of the thyroid
thyroxine iodine-containing hormone from the thyroid that regulates the body metabolism
tinnitus ringing or singing sound in the ears
tissues groups of cells similar in origin, structure, and function
tonsil lymphatic nodules located in the oropharynx
tonus partial, continual contraction of a muscle
toxins poisonous substances that come from a variety of sources including pathogens, plants, animals and environmental pollutants
trabeculae supporting network of tissue fibres
transamination addition of an amino group to a substance
transcription copying of genetic information from DNA to messenger RNA (mRNA) for use in protein synthesis
transitional epithelium tissue that forms the lining of the bladder with cells that change shape depending on the amount of urine present
translation process of directing the production of proteins using mRNA at the ribosome and transfer RNA (tRNA) which delivers the correct amino acids for insertion into the protein
transverse across
trauma an injury or wound that may be produced by external force or shock
trichromatic having normal three-colour vision
tricuspid valve found between the right atrium and right ventricle characterised by the presence of three cusps
triiodothyronine (T_3) iodine containing thyroid hormone that aids in maintaining body metabolism
tropomyosin muscle protein that inhibits contraction
troponin muscle protein that inhibits contraction
tubule a small hollow structure
tubercle nodule or small, rough, rounded eminence
tuberosity elevation or protuberance
tumour new growth or neoplasm that may be benign or malignant
tympanic medical/anatomical term for the eardrum

ulcer lesion of a mucous membrane
ultrafiltration the process by which renal filtrate is formed in the renal corpuscles of the kidney
umbilical technical term for the central region of the abdomen
uraemia presence of toxic substances in the blood
urea the major nitrogenous waste product of protein metabolism
urination act of voiding urine also referred to as micturition

vagus cranial nerve X
valence combining power of an atom
valve structure that regulates the movement of material between two locations
varices abnormally swollen veins
varicose veins vein that has become overdistended and swollen, most frequently affecting the saphenous veins of the legs
vascular pertaining to or consisting of vessels
vasectomy common form of male sterilisation/contraception involving surgical cutting or sealing of the vas deferens (sperm ducts)
vasoconstriction narrowing of blood vessels by a nerve or a chemical substance

vasodilation also known as vasodilatation; a dilation and widening of blood vessels via either nervous or chemical stimulation to increase blood flow
vasomotor regulating the contraction and dilation of the blood vessels
vasopressin also known as antidiuretic hormone (ADH); released from the posterior pituitary to increase water re-absorption in the kidney and reduce urine output.
vein vessel that carries blood to the heart
ventilation process of bringing air into and out of the lungs
ventral the front portion of the trunk
ventricle thick muscular pumping chamber of the heart
venule small veins
vertebra one of 33 bones that form the spinal column
vertebral bones and supporting structures of the back
vertigo dizziness
vesicle small sac or blister filled with fluid
vessel hollow tubule
vestibular a chamber of the inner ear
vital capacity total of inspiratory capacity and expiratory reserve
vitamin organic substance necessary for normal metabolism

wart small, horny outgrowth of the skin
wheal ridgelike swelling of the skin commonly associated with the inflammatory response
white matter region of myelinated axons
white ramus a series of connecting nerve bodies in the autonomic nervous system

zygote the result of the union between a haploid spermatozoon and a haploid ovum following fertilisation